Comprehensive Atlas of High-Resolution Endoscopy and Narrowband Imaging

This book is dedicated to JJC and EJC for their lifelong inspiration. AEL-CFI-S!

JC

Comprehensive Atlas of High-Resolution Endoscopy and Narrowband Imaging

EDITED BY

Jonathan Cohen, MD, FASGE, FACG

Clinical Professor of Medicine
NYU Langone School of Medicine
New York, NY, USA

SECOND EDITION

WILEY Blackwell

This edition first published 2017 © 2017 by John Wiley & Sons, Ltd
First edition © 2007 by Blackwell Publishing Ltd

Registered office: John Wiley & Sons, Ltd, The Atrium, Southern Gate, Chichester,
West Sussex, PO19 8SQ, UK

Editorial offices: 9600 Garsington Road, Oxford, OX4 2DQ, UK
1606 Golden Aspen Drive, Suites 103 and 104, Ames, Iowa 50010, USA

For details of our global editorial offices, for customer services and for information about how to apply
for permission to reuse the copyright material in this book please see our website at
www.wiley.com/wiley-blackwell

Library of Congress Cataloging-in-Publication Data

Names: Cohen, Jonathan, 1964- editor.
Title: Comprehensive atlas of high resolution endoscopy and narrowband imaging/edited by
   Jonathan Cohen.
Description: Second edition. | New York, NY : John Wiley & Sons, Inc., 2017. | Includes bibliographical
   references and index.
Identifiers: LCCN 2016023805 (print) | LCCN 2016024982 (ebook) | ISBN 9781118705933 (cloth) |
   ISBN 9781118706015 (pdf) | ISBN 9781118706039 (epub)
Subjects: | MESH: Endoscopy, Gastrointestinal—methods | Gastrointestinal Neoplasms—diagnosis | Atlases
Classification: LCC RC804.E6 (print) | LCC RC804.E6 (ebook) | NLM WI 17 | DDC 616.3/307545—dc23
LC record available at https://lccn.loc.gov/2016023805

A catalogue record for this book is available from the British Library.

Wiley also publishes its books in a variety of electronic formats. Some content that appears in print may not
be available in electronic books.

Cover images courtesy of J. Cohen and Y. Sano

Set in 8.5/11pt MeridienLtStd by Aptara Inc., New Delhi, India
Printed and bound in Singapore by Markono Print Media Pte Ltd

1 2017

Contents

Preface

Since the introduction of the flexible endoscope, physicians have been able to explore the images of the gastrointestinal tract in health and in disease and use this information to make diagnoses and direct therapies. As technology has advanced, endoscopists have steadily been able to reach more locations and visualize the mucosa with increasing clarity.

Over the past decade, the growing use and capabilities of competing noninvasive imaging technologies have cast some doubt as to the future utility of performing endoscopy for purely diagnostic purposes. To survive as more than a purely therapeutic modality, endoscopy had to evolve not only to provide better-quality images than available by other new technologies, but also to reveal more useful diagnostic information than previously possible with standard optical imaging. By providing immediate intelligence about the lesions detected and their extent at the same time as interventions are carried out, advanced imaging technology might also confer greater efficiency and effectiveness to minimally invasive endoscopic therapy.

Numerous advances have been introduced during the past decade that allow the gastrointestinal endoscopist to see more and to better define abnormalities of the gastrointestinal mucosal lining. Specifically, the development of high-resolution endoscopy (HRE) and optical contrast technology such as narrowband imaging (NBI) has breathed critically needed new attention into the endoscopic examination of the gastrointestinal tract. To paraphrase Mark Twain, reports of the demise of diagnostic endoscopy have been greatly exaggerated.

In 2007, the first edition of this atlas introduced academic and practicing endoscopists around the world to the new look of high-resolution imaging and NBI. For many of the potential applications, data supporting its value was limited. The general purpose of the book was to allow readers to understand the technology, to recognize the defining features of key pathologies, and to interpret the images they encountered in their clinical practices.

The limitations to the initial adoption of the technology were access to the new equipment, knowledge about how to properly use it, and motivation that using it made a significant difference. Over the past 10 years, much has transpired to eliminate these barriers. Since the release of the first edition of the atlas, investigators have generated a much clearer understanding of what applications of HRE and NBI lead to specific patient benefits. In the key areas of Barrett's esophagus and colon polyps, wider acceptance of the value of targeted biopsy and the potential benefits of optical polyp diagnosis has resulted. As more and more practicing endoscopists have access to high-resolution scopes, and as motivation grows to take advantage of the technology, the need for guidance is perhaps even greater than it was in 2007 to provide the resources needed to use it to maximum advantage. In this context, the current atlas has been produced to support the efforts of clinicians to learn to use and adopt this technology in their practices.

The chapters of this volume explore in detail the critical literature in HRE and NBI since 2007 and will allow readers to apply this evidence to guide when to use advanced imaging in their practice. For readers from North American and European countries using the EXERA system scopes, the improvements in lighting and magnification conferred by the H190 EXERA III instruments and processors have resulted in much sharper and brighter images in which the signature features of important pathologic findings are easier to discern and to illustrate.

The desire to provide a thorough guide to accelerate the learning curve for individuals wishing to adopt this new imaging capability remains the primary motivating force behind this book. Emphasis is naturally placed on those conditions for which NBI is considered particularly useful, such as detecting dysplasia in Barrett's esophagus and squamous mucosa, and distinguishing between adenomatous and hyperplastic colon polyps. However, since HRE and NBI generate such dramatic new images throughout the gastrointestinal tract, we aim to provide a comprehensive look at the bowel using this lens. It is intended that the images selected will generate the excitement that resulted at each of the earlier major steps forward in endoscopic imaging technology.

This book begins with a series of introductory chapters to review the theoretical framework for HRE and NBI, the historical development of this technology, the way it actually works, and the essential practical information needed to start using these endoscopes. The subsequent sections include chapters examining the clinical applications of HRE and NBI along with supportive data, organized by organ system. Finally, the atlas contains color plates of images in high-resolution white and narrowband light, in low and high magnification, along with some pathology confirmation, to illustrate normal and abnormal pathology throughout the gastrointestinal tract.

In this second edition, all chapters have been reviewed and revised wherever new evidence was available to assess applications and benefits. In addition, three new chapters have been included on the topics of colon polyp optical diagnosis for resect and discard strategies, the use of HRE and NBI in the bile duct and pancreatic duct, and the use of NBI to enhance therapeutic endoscopy in real time. Over 500 new images have been added to the atlas section, primarily new H190 EXERA III images. One feature is the inclusion of many more examples of some of the key pathologic findings than appeared in the first edition, in order to provide readers with the best resources to learn the characteristic findings.

Instead of the CD-ROM provided in 2007, this book comes with access to a special accompanying website that will contain searchable access to all atlas images, and over 80 video clips, to provide a more complete sense of how HRE NBI works and looks in real time. This is fitting as this imaging modality is geared to enhance endoscopic decision-making during the procedure, to facilitate therapeutic maneuvers, and to make tissue sampling more precise and of higher diagnostic yield.

The reader will note that this atlas contains many images from both Japan, using the LUCERA system, and from throughout Europe and North America, using the EXERA system. The reader should note that all images appearing in the atlas section of this volume from Japanese contributors are taken from LUCERA series endoscopes; all other images taken using EXERA series instruments will be designated in the captions as coming from the EXERA III H190 or the older H180 series instruments. Contributing centers are credited for all photos, and differences between the two systems are explained in the introductory chapters.

Many of the contributing authors to this volume are pioneers in developing this technology and in discovering the clinical implications of the patterns that are revealed. I am indebted to their efforts to collaborate on this project and help generate this atlas to rapidly disseminate their expertise and demonstrate the way endoscopy will look in the years to come.

Jonathan Cohen MD, FASGE, FACG
Clinical Professor of Medicine
NYU Langone School of Medicine

Acknowledgments

I wish to thank the many colleagues throughout the world who have submitted text, images, and video clips to this volume. Their enthusiasm and excitement for this field are reflected in their commitment to teaching and in the high quality of their contributions.

The detailed explanations and images of NBI in the laryngopharynx (Dr. M. Muto), esophagus (Dr. H. Inoue), stomach (Dr. K. Yao and Dr. M. Kaise), and colon (Dr. Y. Sano and Dr. T. Matsumoto) are abstracted from a book published in Japan, entitled *Atlas of New Endoscopic Imaging Technologies – Unique Diagnostic Imaging Using NBI, AFI and IRI*, Nihon Medical Center, Inc. 2006 (edited by Hisao Tajiri). I am indebted to this publisher for the use of this material.

Special thanks are due to Dr. Brian West for his assistance in reviewing the pathology images and captions included in this volume.

Finally I want to thank Cori, Juliette, and Ben for their tremendous love, understanding, and support.

Contributors

Pathology editor

A. Brian West
Director of Gastrointestinal Pathology Services,
AmeriPath New York Gastrointestinal Diagnostics,
Shelton, CT; and Adjunct Professor of Pathology,
NYU School of Medicine, New York, NY, USA

Contributing authors

Ajay Bansal
University of Kansas School of Medicine, Kansas City,
MO, USA

Michael J. Bartel
Gastroentrology and Hepatology, Mayo Clinic School of
Medicine Jacksonville, FL, USA

Robert Bechara
Digestive Diseases Center, Showa University,
Koto-Toyosu Hospital, Koto-ku, Tokyo, Japan

Jacques J. Bergman
Department of Gastrointestinal Endoscopy,
University of Amsterdam, Amsterdam,
The Netherlands

Michael Bourke
Professor of Medicine, University of Sydney and Director
Gastrointestinal Endoscopy, Westmead Hospital,
Sydney, NSW, Australia

Jonathan Cohen
NYU Langone School of Medicine, New York, NY, USA

Guido Costamagna
Digestive Endoscopy Unit, Catholic University of the
Sacred Heart and A. Gemelli University Hospital,
Rome, Italy

Wouter L. Curvers
Department of Gastroenterology and Hepatology,
Academic Medical Center, University of Amsterdam,
Amsterdam, The Netherlands

Evelyn Dekker
Faculty of Medicine, University of Amsterdam,
Amsterdam, The Netherlands

Jacques Deviere
Erasmus University Hospital, Brussels, Belgium

James DiSario
University of Utah Health Sciences Center, Salt Lake
City, UT, USA

James East
Wolfson Unit for Endoscopy, St Mark's Hospital,
Harrow, Middlesex, UK

Fabian Emura
Advanced GI Endoscopy, EmuraCenter LatinoAmerica,
Bogotá, D.C.; and Medical School, Universidad de La
Sabana, Chía, Colombia

Kazuhiro Gono
Research Department, Olympus Medical Systems Corp.,
Tokyo, Japan

Neil Gupta
Department of Gastroenterology, Loyola University
Health System, Maywood, IL, USA

Gregory Haber
Lenox Hill Hospital, New York, NY, USA

Rob Hawes
Medical University of South Carolina, Charleston,
SC, USA

Fumihito Hirai
Department of Gastroenterology, Fukuoka University;
Chikushi Hospital, Fukuoka, Japan

Haruhiro Inoue
Digestive Disease Center, Showa University,
Northern Yokohama Hospital, Yokohama, Japan

Takao Itoi
Associate Professor, Department of Gastroenterology and Hepatology, Tokyo Medical University, Shinjuku, Tokyo, Japan

Akinori Iwashita
Department of Pathology, Fukuoka University, Chikushi Hospital, Fukuoka, Japan

Dennis M. Jensen
Professor of Medicine in Digestive Diseases at David Geffen School of Medicine at UCLA, Staff Gastroenterologist at the Ronald Reagan UCLA and West Los Angeles VA Medical Centers, Key Investigator and Associate Director of the CURE Digestive Diseases Research Center, Los Angeles, CA, USA

Lijia Jiang
Gastroentrology and Hepatology, Mayo Clinic, Jacksonville, FL, USA

Mitsuru Kaise
Department of Gastroenterology, Toranomon Hospital, Tokyo, Japan

Tonya Kaltenbach
Veterans Affairs Palo Alto Health Care System; Stanford University School of Medicine, Stanford, CA, USA

Philip Kaye
Department of Pathology, University Hospital, Queen's Medical Centre, Nottingham, UK

Tetsuji Kudo
Department of Medicine and Clinical Science, Graduate School of Medical Sciences, Kyushu University, Fukuoka, Japan

James Lau
Department of Surgery, Faculty of Medicine, The Chinese University of Hong Kong, Hong Kong

Mitsuo Lida
Department of Medicine and Clinical Science, Graduate School of Medical Sciences, Kyushu University, Fukuoka, Japan

Guilherme Macedo
Servico de Gastrenterologia, Hospital Sao Marcos, Braga, Portugal

Toshiyuki Matsui
Department of Gastroenterology, Fukuoka University, Chikushi Hospital, Fukuoka, Japan

Takayuki Matsumoto
Department of Medicine and Clinical Science, Graduate School of Medical Sciences, Kyushu University, Fukuoka, Japan

Manabu Muto
Department of Therapeutic Oncology, Kyoto University Graduate School of Medicine, Kyoto University Hospital Cancer Center, Kyoto, Japan

Takashi Nagahama
Department of Gastroenterology, Fukuoka University, Chikushi Hospital, Fukuoka, Japan

Takashi Nakayoshi
Department of Endoscopy, Jikei University School of Medicine, Tokyo, Japan

Atsushi Ochiai
Pathology Division, National Cancer Center Research Institute East, Chiba, Japan

Thierry Ponchon
Edouard Herriot Hospital, Lyon, France

Krish Ragunath
Wolfson Digestive Disease Centre, University Hospital, Queen's Medical Centre, Nottingham, UK

Gottumukkala S. Raju
Department of Gastroenterology, Hepatology and Nutrition, UT MD Anderson Cancer Center, Houston, TX, USA

Douglas K. Rex
Indiana University School of Medicine, Indianapolis, IN, USA

Jean-François Rey
Institute Arnault Tzanck, St Laurent du Var, France

Richard Rothstein
Dartmouth Hitchcock Medical Center, Lebanon, NH, USA

Yasushi Sano
Gastrointestinal Center, Sano Hospital, Kobe, Japan

Stefan Seewald
Internal Medicine, Gastro Hirslanden, Zurich, Switzerland

Prateek Sharma
University of Kansas Medical Center, Kansas City, MO, USA

Rajvinder Singh
University of Adelaide; and Lyell McEwin Hospital, Adelaide, South Australia, Australia

Roy Soetikno
Stanford University, Stanford, CA, USA

Suketo Sou
Department of Gastroenterology, Fukuoka University, Chikushi Hospital, Fukuoka, Japan

Stavros N. Stavropoulos
Temple University, New York, NY, USA

Anne-Fré Swager
Department of Gastroenterology and Hepatology, Academic Medical Center, University of Amsterdam, Amsterdam, The Netherlands

Hisao Tajiri
Division of Gastroenterology and Hepatology, Department of Internal Medicine, Jikei University, School of Medicine, Tokyo, Japan

Hiroshi Tanabe
Department of Pathology, Fukuoka University, Chikushi Hospital, Fukuoka, Japan

David Tate
Westmead Hospital, Sydney, NSW, Australia

Michael B. Wallace
Gastroentrology and Hepatology, Mayo Clinic School of Medicine, Jacksonville, FL, USA

Jerome Waye
Gastrointestinal Endoscopy Unit, Mount Sinai School of Medicine, New York, NY, USA

Nobuaki Yagi
Kyoto Prefectural University of Medicine, Kyoto, Japan

Kenshi Yao
Department of Gastroenterology, Fukuoka University, Chikushi Hospital, Fukuoka, Japan

Naohisa Yoshida
Department of Molecular Gastroenterology and Hepatology, Kyoto Prefectural University of Medicine, Graduate School of Medical Science, Kyoto, Japan

Shigeaki Yoshida
National Cancer Center Hospital East, Chiba, Japan

About the Companion Website

Don't forget to visit the companion website for this book:

www.wiley.com/go/cohen/NBI

There you will find valuable material designed to enhance the book, including:

- Videos illustrating key procedures
- Images from the print book available in digital format

Scan this QR code to visit the companion website:

List of videos illustrating key procedures

Video 1 NBI examination of the oropharynx (see Chapters 4 and 12)

Video 2 Benign lesion, hyperplasia (see Chapters 4 and 12)

Video 3 Neoplastic lesion, low-grade intraepithelial neoplasia (see Chapters 4 and 12)

Video 4 Diagnosis of superficial squamous cell carcinoma (see Chapters 4 and 12)

Video 5 Pharyngeal squamous cell carcinoma, type V IPCL pattern (see Chapter 4)

Video 6 Hyperplastic changes following radiation and chemotherapy (see Chapter 4)

Video 7 Inflammatory change (see Chapter 4)

Video 8 Residual carcinoma, coexisting with hyperplastic change post radiation and chemotherapy (see Chapter 4)

Esophagus

Video 9 Superficial squamous cell cancer, IIc+IIa (see Chapter 5)

Video 10 Detection and cap EMR of minute focus of early squamous cancer (HGD) (see Chapter 5)

Video 11 NBI patterns in a patient with nondysplastic Barrett's esophagus (see Chapter 3)

Video 12 Measuring hiatal hernia and Barrett's landmarks (see Chapter 6)

Video 13 NBI detection of focal dysplasia in Barrett's esophagus using cap examination (see Chapters 3 and 6)

Video 14 Band EMR of focal high-grade dysplasia in Barrett's (see Chapters 6 and 13)

Video 15 Radiofrequency ablation of Barrett's tongues (see Chapters 6 and 13)

Video 16 Barrett's cap EMR of high-grade dysplasia (see Chapters 6 and 13)

Video 17 Barrett's HGD cap EMR: bleeding management (see Chapter 13)

Video 18 Advanced obstructing esophageal adenocarcinoma (see Chapter 13)

Video 19 NBI examination of esophageal varices

Video 20 Diagnosis of Boorhaave's syndrome with management of leak using Polyflex self-expanding plastic stent

Stomach

Video 21 Normal squamous esophageal mucosa (see Chapter 5)

Video 22 Esopahgeal squamous high-grade intraepithelial neoplasia (see Chapter 5)

Video 23 Barrett's high-grade intraepithelial neoplasia (see Chapter 6)

Video 24 Barrett's carcinoma of the gastroesophageal junction (see Chapter 6)

Video 25 Long-segment Barrett's esophagus with low-grade dysplasia (see Chapter 6)

Video 26 NBI in a patient with C9M9 Barrett's esophagus (see Chapter 6)

Video 27 Normal stomach (see Chapter 7)

Video 28 Systematic white light EGD examination (see Chapter 7)

Video 29 Systematic NBI H190 EGD examination (see Chapter 7)

Video 30 Gastric body: gastritis (see Chapter 7)

Video 31 Gastric body: early gastric cancer, type IIb, differentiated type (see Chapter 7)

Video 32 Gastric angle: early gastric cancer, type IIb, differentiated to undifferentiated type (see Chapter 7)

Video 33 Gastric body: early gastric cancer, type IIc, differentiated type (see Chapter 7)

Video 34 Gastric cardia: early cancer, type IIc, undifferentiated type (see Chapter 7)

Video 35 Low-grade gastric dysplasia (see Chapters 7 and 8)

Video 36 NBI detection of poorly differentiated superficial gastric cancer not seen on white light (see Chapters 7, 8 and 13)

Video 37 Endoscopic submucosal dissection of superficial gastric cancer (see Chapters 7, 8 and 13)

Video 38 Submucosal GIST tumor

Video 39 GAVE with APC treatment

Duodenum

Video 40 Normal duodenum (see Chapter 7)

Video 41 Duodenal AVMs (see Chapter 7)

Video 42 Saline injection polypectomy of sessile duodenal adenoma (see Chapter 7)

Video 43 Large duodenal adenoma in patient with familial adenomatous polyposis (see Chapter 7)

Video 44 Bleeding vessels in nodular cholangiocarcinoma (see Chapter 12)

Video 45 Nodular cholangiocarcinoma with abnormal tumor vessels (see Chapter 12)

Video 46 Benign bile duct stricture (see Chapter 12)

PART 1
The Basics of NBI

1 Narrowband imaging: historical background and basis for its development

Shigeaki Yoshida

In Japan, where the incidence of gastric cancer is very much higher than in the rest of the world, greater attention has been paid to early diagnosis since the beginning of the 1950s when the "gastrocamera" was first introduced. In those days, the finding of early gastric cancer (EGC) was not frequent and most of these lesions were identified from the differential diagnosis of deeply ulcerated (type III) or polypoid (type I) lesions, which can be easily detected. In the 1970s, early diagnosis progressed and it became possible to detect those cancers showing the appearance of ulcer scar (type IIc) and plateau-like elevation (type IIa). Furthermore, at the beginning of the 1980s, early diagnosis of gastritis-like malignancy (type IIb-like) became more readily possible following the results of retrospective studies of rapidly growing advanced cancer [1]. With this increased appreciation of the appearance of early superficial lesions, the widespread use of biopsy and with careful scrutiny of the mucosa using dye-spraying techniques, EGCs appearing as just faint mucosal irregularities or discoloration came to be the most frequent EGC being diagnosed by the late 1980s [2].

Such results were also applied to esophageal and colorectal malignancies, and there has been a general acceptance in Japan that early malignancies in the alimentary tract may not appear polypoid or ulcerative. The desire to better recognize such malignancies, which may be difficult to distinguish from nonspecific inflammation or trauma, had prompted us to envision new endoscopic technology capable of revealing cancer-specific images of the surface structure of the mucosa. It is within this context that the field of narrowband imaging (NBI) was developed as a promising way to facilitate the endoscopic diagnosis of early neoplastic and pre-cancerous lesions in the alimentary tract.

NBI is an optical image enhancement technology that visualizes vessels on the surface of the mucosa and patterns on the surface of mucosa by employing the characteristics of the visible light spectrum. The development of NBI goes back to the study of spectroscopy more than 20 years ago. The Japanese government implemented the Second Term Comprehensive 10-Year Strategy for Cancer Control in 1994. Together with Professor N. Oyama of the Tokyo Institute of Technology and Olympus Medical Systems Corp., we received funding from the project and started the study in which we intended to digitalize the color and structure of mucosa in order to establish a more objective/quantitative pathologic diagnosis and hence better diagnostic yield. At that time, multiple facilities and industries had conducted studies to achieve optical biopsy using the characteristics of the visible light spectrum. We aimed to achieve differentiation of normal and abnormal mucosa using a custom-made spectrophotometer developed by Olympus Medical Systems Corp.

Using the method described in Figure 1.1, we obtained and analyzed more than 2000 samples from esophagus, stomach, and colon. However, we faced multiple challenges to establish a stable diagnostic standard. The spectrum showed different patterns in normal and abnormal tissues but the spectral pattern differed from patient to patient, so that it was quite difficult to achieve stable classification between normal and abnormal. Furthermore, spectral data were not stable under the measuring conditions employed.

However, throughout the study we noticed a specific spectral pattern when selecting certain narrowband wavelengths (Figure 1.2). To highlight the specific pattern, we shifted our study from qualitative analysis using spectroscopy to qualitative imaging that enhanced details of the mucosal surface. As a result, when employing a

Comprehensive Atlas of High-Resolution Endoscopy and Narrowband Imaging, Second Edition. Edited by Jonathan Cohen.
© 2017 John Wiley & Sons, Ltd. Published 2017 by John Wiley & Sons, Ltd.
Companion website: www.wiley.com/go/cohen/NBI

narrowband filter, we found excellent light enhancement deep in the mucosa at red light wavelengths, shallow mucosal surface features at blue light wavelengths, and levels in between at green light wavelengths [3]. Based on the findings, we continued the study with the research and development group at Olympus and finally found that narrowband blue light wavelengths matched the light absorption characteristics of blood hemoglobin and enhanced details of the mucosal surface.

In December 1999, we obtained the world's first clinical images using NBI in our facility (Figures 1.3–1.6). The original technology only generated black and white monochrome images with limited information for diagnosis, making it impractical for clinical applications. The challenge was shortly solved by the introduction of newer improved filters and the development of a prototype incorporating a circuit board exclusively for NBI color display.

Since these first clinical NBI pictures were achieved, we have actively expanded the study in cooperation with multiple research facilities. As a result of this collaborative investigation, the application of NBI diagnosis has expanded rapidly [4,5]. Starting with the diagnosis of colonic tumor and squamous cell carcinoma of esophagus, the applications of NBI were established in other fields such as superficial carcinoma in pharynx, Barrett's esophagus and adenocarcinoma, stomach cancer, and inflammatory bowel disease. Multiple studies have been published in these areas; the results have been published in academic society proceedings, research committee reports and clinical papers in peer-reviewed journals. Much of this data is discussed in detail in subsequent chapters of this book.

In December 2005, the NBI system became commercially available from Olympus, and the technology and diagnosis expanded further, not only in Japan but also worldwide.

In summary, endoscopic diagnosis has been rapidly progressing. Beyond technical advances such as chromoendoscopy and improvements in image quality, endoscopic diagnosis has now advanced to the area of pathology. This is possible because the imaging technology now allows assessment of the three-dimensional architecture of tissue by fine examination of the mucosal surface with magnifying endoscopy. In the coming years,

special light observation such as NBI may be able to provide even more information about a targeted lesion, in order to clarify the indication of new cancer therapies.

Such endoscopic diagnosis through special light observation holds great promise. None of these advances could have been achieved without the great contribution of Professor H. Niwa, Board Chairman of the Japan Gastroenterological Endoscopic Society, and his colleagues who have devoted themselves to the development of multiple modalities of optical diagnosis, such as ultraviolet gastrocamera, infrared and autoflorescence imaging, since the project was first initiated while working together at Tokyo University. We must recognize the history of endoscopic diagnosis and the contribution and diligence of these individuals in bringing the field to where it is today. I hope that special light diagnosis through NBI will become an increasingly reliable tool with more clinical evidence to support its applications. As this occurs, the technology should make important contributions to improve and facilitate diagnosis in clinical practice.

 Video clips to accompany this book can be found in the online material at www.wiley.com/go/cohen/NBI

References

1 Yoshida S, Yoshimori M, Hirashima T *et al.* Nonulcerative lesion detected by endoscopy as an early expression of gastric malignancy. *Jpn J Clin Oncol* 1981;11:495–506.

2 Yoshida S, Yamaguchi H, Tajiri H *et al.* Diagnosis of early gastric cancer seen as less malignant endoscopically. *Jpn J Clin Oncol* 1984;14:225–41.

3 Gono K, Obi T, Yamaguchi M *et al.* Appearance of enhanced tissue features in narrowband endoscopic imaging. *J Biomed Opt* 2004;9:568–77.

4 Sano Y, Kobayashi M, Hamamoto Y *et al.* New diagnostic method based on color imaging using narrowband imaging (NBI) endoscopy system for gastrointestinal tract. *Gastrointest Endosc* 2001;53:AB125.

5 Kara MA, Fockens P, Peters F *et al.* Narrowband imaging (NBI) in Barrett's esophagus: what features are relevant for detection of high-grade dysplasia (HGD) and early cancer (EC)? *Gastroenterology* 2004;126:A50.

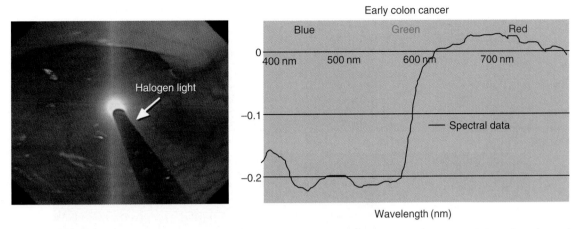

Figure 1.1 Spectral reflectance analysis. Spectral data were sampled at intervals of 2 nm ranging from 400 to 800 nm. In each examination, we measured spectral reflectance in both normal and neoplastic areas. (Copyright S. Yoshida.)

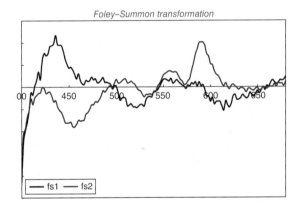

Figure 1.2 Spectral sensitivity functions for discrimination of cancerous regions. (Copyright S. Yoshida.)

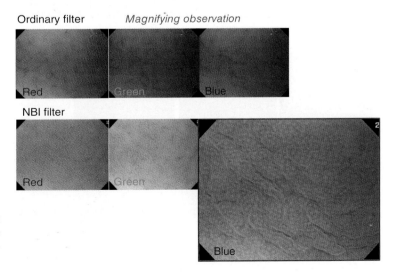

Figure 1.3 Normal gastric mucosa: mucosal crypt pattern of the stomach can be observed without dye spraying by blue-filtering of NBI. (Copyright S. Yoshida.)

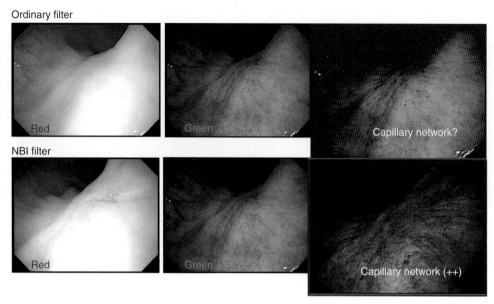

Figure 1.4 Gastric ulcer scar: capillary network can be observed without dye spraying by blue-filtering of NBI. (Copyright S. Yoshida.)

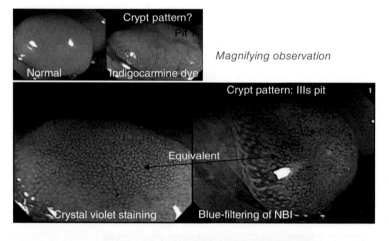

Figure 1.5 Flat adenoma of sigmoid colon: crypt pattern of the depressed area can be observed without dye spraying by blue-filtering of NBI. (Copyright S. Yoshida.)

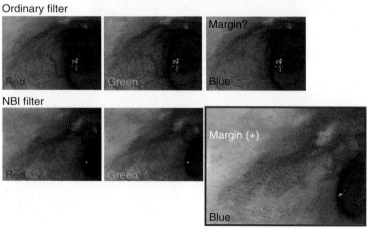

Figure 1.6 Esophageal cancer (type 0–IIc): the margin of the lesion is clearly detected by blue-filtering of NBI. (Copyright S. Yoshida.)

2 An introduction to high-resolution endoscopy and narrowband imaging

Kazuhiro Gono

Introduction

The development of narrowband imaging (NBI) started in May 1999. To confirm the idea of NBI, a study using a multi-spectrum camera capable of producing spectroscopic images and high-power light source was conducted, with this author volunteering as a test subject. The study revealed that the use of 415-nm narrowband light can improve the contrast of capillary images, which are difficult to observe under conventional white light. The first image of living tissue ever produced on NBI is shown in Figure 2.1. The development of an NBI endoscopy system proceeded in cooperation with Dr Sano of the National Cancer Center Hospital East. On December 14, 1999, based on a study using the NBI prototype, we confirmed that the technology was promising for endoscopies of colon, stomach, and esophagus. Since that time, we have developed products in cooperation with not only Japanese endoscopists, but also endoscopists from around the world in an effort to expand the capacity of the prototype. EXERA II, the next generation system equipped with both high-definition TV (HDTV) and NBI, was introduced in December 2005.

At present, Olympus has two types of video endoscopy systems in use worldwide. The difference between these two systems is based on how a color image is produced. One is based on a color charge-coupled device (CCD) chip which has several tiny color filters in each pixel. This system is the 100 series and is branded as EVIS EXERA II. The second system is based on a black and white CCD, in which color separation is achieved through the use of an RGB color filter wheel within the light source unit. This system is the 200 series and is branded as EVIS LUCERA SPECTRUM. Both systems possess NBI technology. Research and development for NBI was first attempted with the EVIS LUCERA SPECTRUM system, the system predominant in Japan, the UK, and Asian countries. Once success was achieved

with that system, research and development was focused on the use of NBI with the color CCD system or EVIS EXERA II. Both systems possess the same optical filter in the light source, which enables the illumination of two narrowbands within the visible spectrum of light for NBI. As such, both systems are "optically" identical. However, since both technologies are fundamentally different, there are actually some minor differences in image reproduction. For NBI, both systems are the same, as they both provide improved image contrast when viewing microvessel patterns within the superficial mucosa. If images from both systems are compared simultaneously without magnification, some observers may notice slight differences. However, these differences are quite minor and have not been shown to be clinically significant.

Apart from these optical features, the two systems do differ in the method of magnification incorporated into the endoscopes and the resulting ability to magnify the images observed. In the EXERA II system, the endoscope currently has digital zoom at 1.2× and 1.5× magnification. The HDTV format also possesses "physical zoom" properties that allow the scope tip to be advanced up to 2 mm from the mucosal surface without losing resolution. This combined feature results in a capacity for at least a 50-fold magnification. In contrast, the LUCERA system utilizes an optical zoom system, similar to that used in previous non-high-resolution zoom magnification endoscopes, that allows for magnification of the image up to 80 times. However, these numbers for mucosal magnification have somewhat limited reliability, as there are a number of variables that may affect the actual magnification of tissue that is observed, such as the size of the monitor that is used.

HDTV is a video format that provides clear and high-resolution images while NBI offers high-contrast images of blood vessels. In theory, combining these technologies will give the best performance in close observation of

Comprehensive Atlas of High-Resolution Endoscopy and Narrowband Imaging, Second Edition. Edited by Jonathan Cohen.
© 2017 John Wiley & Sons, Ltd. Published 2017 by John Wiley & Sons, Ltd.
Companion website: www.wiley.com/go/cohen/NBI

the mucosa. Knowledge of the design concept underlying the functions of EXERA II, its technical limitations and how to read NBI images should be helpful in learning the practical use of HDTV and NBI.

There are many "high definition" TV formats. At the time of product development, 1080i and 720p were the most popular, as they still are today. Olympus had to consider which format would provide the highest level of resolution for motion and still imaging, as well as maintain its popularity within the market so that current and future peripheral devices such as monitors, printers and digital recorders would remain compatible. As the result, 1080i was selected and has proven to be the most popular high-definition broadcast format to this day.

Unlike conventional image processing, NBI is a technology in which an image is emphasized by light. Designing such light requires an in-depth understanding of the optical characteristics of living tissue. As an introduction, this chapter first discusses the characteristics of light, including wavelength and color, as well as the interaction between living tissue and light, such as absorption and scattering. Next, it describes the value offered by HDTV and NBI in terms of image quality and the method for designing chromatic images on NBI. Finally, the chapter explains how typical endoscopic findings such as fine mucosal pattern and blood vessel images look on NBI and why they look that way, using illustrations.

Light and bio-optics

Light and wavelength
Light is an electromagnetic radiation having the characteristics of both wave and particle. When light is considered as a wave, the distance from peak to peak in each wave is called "wavelength" (Figure 2.2). Visible wavelength ranges from 400 to 700 nm. A different wavelength is perceived as a different color. Although colors look different depending on the psychological state of each individual, 400 nm, on average, is perceived as blue, 550 nm as green, and 600 nm as red. Generally, saturation decreases when light contains more wavelengths. In other words, blue light of narrow bandwidth looks more vivid compared with that of broad bandwidth. Light of broad bandwidth within the range 400–700 nm looks white.

Color, absorption, and reflection
When white light illuminates the surface of an apple, the pigment in apple skin absorbs light at wavelengths of 400–550 nm. The absorbed light is converted to heat. In other words, energy in the blue–green range of the white light is converted to heat. Unabsorbed light at 550–700 nm is reflected. The reflected light reaches our eyes and the apple is perceived to be red. How would an apple look if cyan-colored light, instead of white, illuminated it? Cyan-colored light mainly consists of blue and green light, and because such light is absorbed by pigment and almost no light is reflected, the apple looks black. That is to say, white light is needed to perceive the natural color of an object. Contrarily, the light does not need to be white if it is not intended to reproduce the appearance of an object in natural color. NBI is based on this idea and has been developed for the purpose of highlighting blood vessels, not reproducing natural colors. Therefore, light other than white is used for NBI.

Light scattering
In relation to light propagation in an optically turbid medium such as diluted milk, light scattering needs to be taken into consideration in addition to reflection and transmission. Milk contains a number of fat globules of various sizes (1–100 μm). When light strikes such small particles, it diffuses three- dimensionally. This is called light scattering. When there are a multitude of particles, multiple scattering occurs as scattered light is scattered again by striking another particle. Light propagates diffusively due to this light scattering even when a flux of light such as a laser beam is injected into milk.

Absorption and scattering in tissue
A schematic diagram of the interaction between light and living tissue is shown in Figure 2.3. When light enters biological tissue, some reflects from the surface and some diffuses within the body. Multiple scattering occurs among light and small particles such as cell nuclei, cell organelles and nucleoli in the tissue. As a result, light propagates diffusively through the tissue. The propagation of light is determined by its wavelength. Red light, having a long wavelength, diffuses widely and deeply, while blue light, having a short wavelength, diffuses over a smaller range. This is shown in Figure 2.4.

Part of the scattered light is absorbed by blood. To be accurate, hemoglobin absorbs blue and green light. Hemoglobin is a type of chromophore. Components in the gastrointestinal mucosa apart from hemoglobin, such as cell nuclei and fiber tissue, do not have colors. Therefore, the color of the gastrointestinal mucosa is mainly determined by hemoglobin.

The interaction between light and living tissue is characterized by hemoglobin, which strongly absorbs blue and green light, and multiple scattering in biological tissue.

Resolution and contrast

Resolution and contrast are terminologies to describe image quality. Figure 2.5 shows the relationship between resolution and contrast. A good-quality image cannot be provided when resolution is high but contrast is poor. Image quality is best when the level of both resolution and contrast is high.

Resolution is a term that describes the capacity to present minute patterns. The capacity of an optical device to reveal fineness of detail is defined by using a resolution chart (Figure 2.5). Resolution is determined by the pixel numbers of the CCD, signal processing, and lens characteristics. The resolution of an endoscope capable of producing HDTV standard images is significantly greater than that attained by conventional endoscopes.

Contrast is defined as the ratio of density or brightness between a pattern and its background. The word describes clarity – how vividly the subject stands out against the background or vice versa. As shown in Figure 2.5, a pattern cannot be seen clearly when it is low in contrast though high in resolution. NBI is a technology capable of improving the contrast of blood vessels selectively. Resolution is enhanced by HDTV while NBI improves contrast. As a result, the combination of HDTV and NBI can offer a high-quality image of blood vessels, analogous to the illustration at upper right in Figure 2.5.

Basic principles and system design

Basic principles

Figure 2.6 is a schematic diagram of NBI. Two blood vessels running in living tissue are named BV(A) and BV(B), respectively. Broadband light composed of wavelengths of $\lambda 1$, $\lambda 2$ and $\lambda 3$ is injected into BV(A) and narrowband light composed of wavelength $\lambda 2$ is injected into BV(B). The degree of absorption into blood is $\lambda 2 \gg \lambda 1, \lambda 3$. $\lambda 1$ and $\lambda 3$ diffuse more widely and deeply within the tissue compared with $\lambda 2$. When $\lambda 2$ strikes the blood vessel, most of its energy is absorbed by blood. On the other hand, when $\lambda 1$ and $\lambda 3$ light rays strike the blood vessel, some of the energy transmits to the blood vessel and scatters deeply and widely. As a result, some of the scattered light rays of $\lambda 1$ and $\lambda 3$ re-transmit to the blood vessel or bypass the blood vessel and exit from the mucosal surface. When the vessel is illuminated with light that is rarely absorbed by blood and which scatters widely and deeply like $\lambda 1$ and $\lambda 3$, a blurry image is produced, labeled VI(A) in Figure 2.6. This is analogous to the conventional light source of endoscopes. On the other hand, when $\lambda 2$ strikes the peripheral mucosa, the light is observed at the mucosal surface as scattered light without bypassing the blood vessel. As a result, the contrast of the blood vessel is improved and the vessel shows black due to its strong absorbing capacity

and in brighter colors for other parts, labeled VI(B) in Figure 2.6. Figure 2.7(a) is an image of the blood vessel pattern of the underside of the human tongue mucosa illuminated by conventional broadband blue light. Figure 2.7(b) is an image produced by narrowband blue light. By changing the illumination to narrowband, we can see that the contrast of the capillary patterns of Figure 2.7(a) is improved in Figure 2.7(b). NBI is a technology for observing biological tissue with narrowband light, created by extracting from conventional broadband light wavelengths that are strongly absorbed by blood and which do not diffuse widely and deeply.

System design

Figure 2.8 shows blood vessel images of the underside of the human tongue mucosa produced by narrowband light of 415, 500, 540, and 600 nm. A very fine pattern of blood vessels is reproduced by the 415-nm wavelength, while a thicker pattern is indicated by light of longer wavelength. Blood vessels in the tongue mucosa are believed to become finer at the superficial layer of the mucosa, as shown in the lower part of Figure 2.8. The relationship between the blood vessels and the narrowband images is provided in the figure. It is therefore most appropriate, by the principle of NBI, to select 415 nm for observing capillaries on the surface and 540 nm for thicker vessels. On the other hand, blood vessels in the deeper part are reproduced in the 600-nm image. However, considering the fact that early cancer develops in the superficial layer and changes the blood vessel structure there, using 600-nm images in NBI can only make a small contribution to medical applications. Therefore, the NBI system uses two narrowband illuminations of 415 and 540 nm. Figure 2.9 shows the configuration of the NBI system in the EVIS EXERA II system. A xenon lamp is installed in front of an optical filter for NBI. It is a double-band filter (415 and 540 nm) as described previously. When observing with NBI, the filter is placed in the light path. Under normal observation, the filter is removed from the optical axis. Under NBI observation, the light from the xenon lamp splits into two bands (415 and 540 nm) and the split light illuminates the mucosa.

As shown in Figure 2.9, two narrowband images of 415 and 540 nm are reproduced when the NBI filter is placed. However, in order to create color images, we need three images to be outputted to the R, G and B channels of the monitor. There are variations concerning which bandwidth goes to which channel, but in order to achieve high visibility of blood vessels, first, the capillary patterns on the superficial layer of the mucosa need to be reproduced as a black and white pattern and, second, the relatively thick vessels in the deeper part of the mucosa need to be highlighted with a color different from that of the capillary pattern. Therefore, colors are allocated according to human visual perception.

The human observer finds it easier to perceive very fine patterns when they are brightly lit (Figure 2.10, Pattern A) rather than when they are colored (Figure 2.10, Pattern B). Thicker vessels can be perceived easily with a color pattern (Figure 2.10, Pattern C). Considering such characteristics, 415 nm is allocated to B and G channels so that the blood vessels on the surface are reproduced in a brownish pattern much like the black and white pattern, and 540 nm is allocated to R channel so that the vessels in the deeper parts are indicated in a cyan color pattern (Figure 2.11).

Blood vessels and bleeding

When observing the mucosal surface closely with an HDTV scope, capillaries in the superficial layer of the mucosa are seen as a brownish pattern on NBI (lower part of Figure 2.12a). When a blood vessel is thin and the CCD is unable to produce its image clearly, it is reproduced as a blurry brownish spot. Relatively thick blood vessels located in the deeper part of the mucosa are reproduced in cyan hue.

On the other hand, bleeding is shown in a black tar-like color, because light rays of 415 and 540 nm are absorbed by blood on the mucosal surface and not reflected.

In many tumors, blood vessel density on the superficial layer of the mucosa becomes high. In cases of esophageal squamous cell carcinoma, for example, expansion, growth and meandering of intrapapillary capillary loops are findings characteristic of the disease. These are perceived as brownish areas when observed by NBI from middle to long distance (upper part of Figure 2.12a).

Fine mucosal pattern

Figure 2.12(b) shows a cross-sectional diagram of the colonic mucosa. Microvessels running in the tissue between the crypt foci are reproduced in brownish hue since they are the same as capillaries on the mucosal surface, shown in Figure 2.12(a). On the other hand, no materials around the crypt foci absorb light except cells surrounding the gland. Therefore, a significant amount of light is reflected and the crypt foci present as a white pattern. As a result, the fine mucosal pattern of the large bowel is reproduced as a brown–white pattern. Gastric mucosa and Barrett's mucosa, both having a similar gland structure, are also presented in the same way. NBI is expected to produce an effect similar to chromoendoscopy. NBI can highlight the fine mucosal pattern as long as mucus is transparent, which does not exert influence over observation. On the other hand, when capillaries are not developed in the tissue between the crypt foci, as

seen in hyperplastic polyps, the fine mucosal pattern is not highlighted on NBI.

Squamo-columnar junction

Stratified squamous epithelium of the normal esophageal mucosa has few blood vessels and reflects light strongly when seen optically. Therefore, it presents as a bluish-white image on NBI. On the other hand, because the surface of the gastric mucosa has a number of blood vessels, whole mucosa is observed in brownish hue. Therefore, the esophageal mucosa and gastric mucosa at the squamo-columnar junction are reproduced in a strong contrast of white and brown (Figure 2.12c). The extent of Barrett's mucosa, like the normal squamo-columnar junction, can be detected easily by the contrast with normal esophageal mucosa. Detecting normal esophageal epithelium surrounded by Barrett's mucosa would be especially easy compared with normal observation.

Residue and bile

Residue and bile in the large bowel are reproduced in yellow hue under white light. The yellow pattern is presented in red (as if bleeding) on NBI. Residue and bile strongly absorb the 415-nm light while reflecting 540-nm light strongly. Since NBI produces 540-nm images on R channel and 415-nm images on B and G channels of the output monitor, images on B and G channels become darker while those on R get brighter. Therefore, residue and bile are highlighted in blood red.

Second-generation NBI on EVIS EXERA III

Since the first-generation NBI was introduced onto the market as an advanced imaging technology, branded EVIS EXERA II, Olympus R&D has been committed to improving the performance of NBI. The first-generation NBI has limitations with regard to brightness: in gastric observation, the distal end of the endoscope needs to be carefully advanced towards the mucosa to obtain sufficient brightness in NBI mode. This insufficient brightness adversely affects the operability of the endoscope. To overcome this limitation, we have made various modifications to increase the brightness of NBI. We have developed a high-intensity discharge lamp, intensified the brightness of the lens in the light source, improved the sensitivity of the image sensor, and worked on the image processing in the processor to reduce noise. As a result of these modifications at various parts of the system, from the tip of the endoscope to light source and signal processor, the second-generation NBI has been able to deliver more than one-and-a-half times as much brightness as the first-generation NBI and to achieve twice the viewable distance in the lumen. The difference in brightness of test models between first-generation and second-generation NBI is shown in Figure 2.13.

In addition, the dual focus function has been incorporated in some models of the 190 scope developed for EVIS EXERA III. In the conventional magnification endoscope (GIF-Q160Z), the user needs to advance the distal end of the endoscope close to the mucosa while controlling the zoom lever on the control section. The dual focus function has enabled the user to switch the zoom mode between wide observation and macroscopic observation with only the touch of a button. This function, combined with the increased focus distance, has facilitated magnified observation. The dual focus function exhibits its benefits when used in combination with the brighter second-generation NBI.

 Video clips to accompany this book can be found in the online material at www.wiley.com/go/cohen/NBI

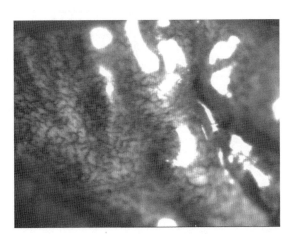

Figure 2.1 The 415-nm narrowband image of human tongue mucosa. The 415-nm narrowband image reflects the fine capillary pattern on the mucosa, which is hard to visualize under conventional white light. (Copyright K. Gono.)

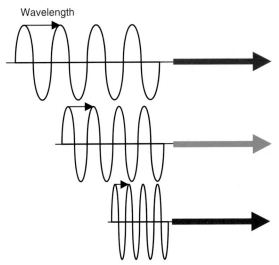

Figure 2.2 Wavelength and related color. Wavelength is defined as the distance from peak to peak in each wave. Longer wavelengths have a reddish appearance while shorter wavelengths have a bluish appearance. (Copyright K. Gono.)

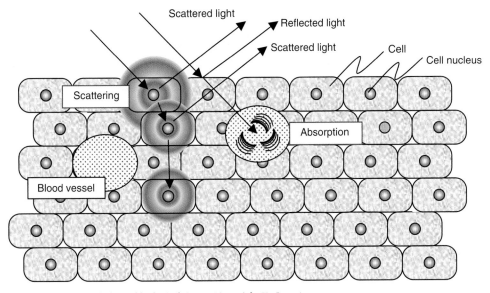

Figure 2.3 Interaction between light and biological tissue. (Copyright K. Gono.)

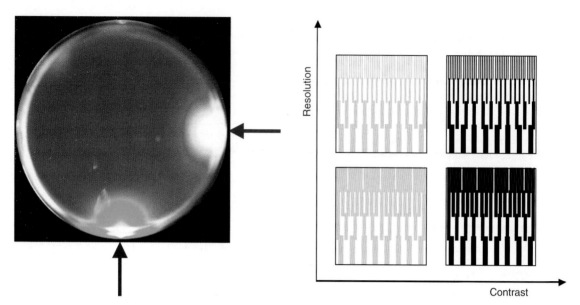

Figure 2.4 Diffusive light propagation in a turbid medium. Red light diffuses widely and deeply in the turbid medium, while blue light does not propagate diffusively. (Copyright K. Gono.)

Figure 2.5 Contrast vs. resolution. Resolution here means the resolution of the CCD used for imaging resolution chart. (Copyright K. Gono.)

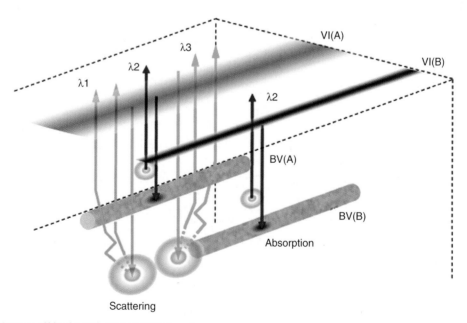

Figure 2.6 Contrast of blood vessel. (Copyright K. Gono.)

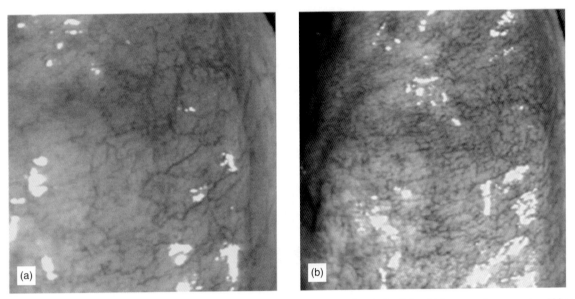

Figure 2.7 Blood vessels of human tongue: (a) image under conventional broadband blue light; (b) image under narrowband blue light. (Copyright K. Gono.)

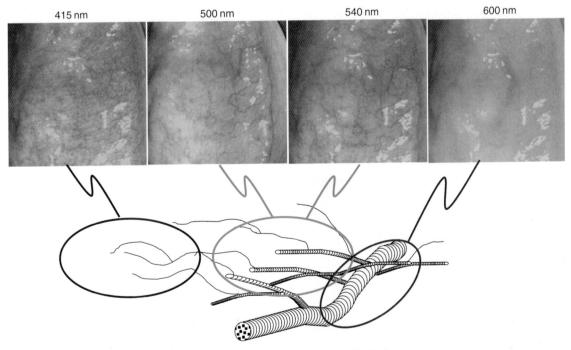

Figure 2.8 Endoscopic images of human hypoglottis mucous membrane. (Copyright K. Gono.)

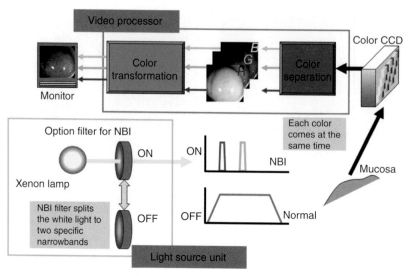

Figure 2.9 Structure of NBI system. (Copyright K. Gono.)

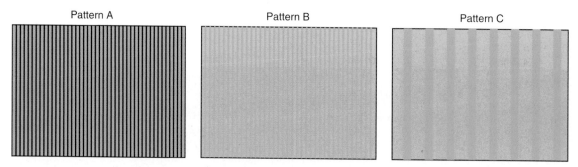

Figure 2.10 Human visual perception of black and white pattern and color pattern. (Copyright K. Gono.)

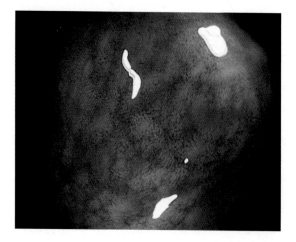

Figure 2.11 Appearances of endoscopic findings on NBI endoscopy EXCERA III. Fine superficial capillaries appear brown whereas the deeper vessels appear cyan in color. (Image courtesy of Jonathan Cohen, NYU Langone Medical Center.)

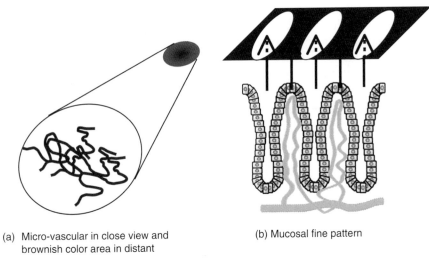

(a) Micro-vascular in close view and brownish color area in distant

(b) Mucosal fine pattern

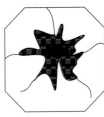

(c) SCJ

Figure 2.12 Application of NBI: (a) microvasculature in close-up view and brownish color in distant view; (b) mucosal fine pattern; (c) squamo-columnar junction. (Copyright K. Gono.)

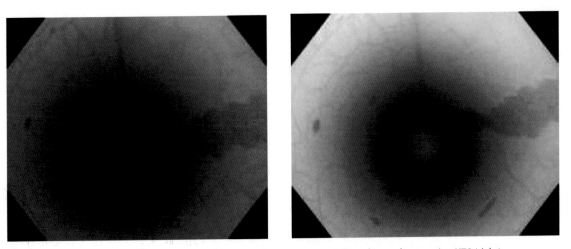

Figure 2.13 Difference in brightness of test models between first-generation (left) and second-generation NBI (right).

3 Getting started with narrowband imaging

Neil Gupta, Ajay Bansal, and Prateek Sharma

Introduction

The advent of novel endoscopic imaging modalities, including electronic image enhancement technologies such as narrowband imaging (NBI), represents an immense improvement over the current standard white light endoscopy. NBI uses a filter within the endoscopy processor that narrows the spectrum of light to blue light (440–460 nm) and green light (540–560 nm). This results in improved visualization of the superficial details of the gastrointestinal mucosa. The detailed mechanisms of this technology are discussed elsewhere. However exciting the new technology, there will be a significant but not insurmountable learning curve associated with familiarizing oneself with the detailed mucosal features that can be visualized with NBI and interpretation of findings. The following sections introduce the endoscopist to the basic use of NBI, but the only way to improve recognition of patterns is initial training and then regular performance of NBI endoscopy with ongoing self-directed feedback.

NBI endoscopes

NBI endoscopes are similar to currently used endoscopes, with the same tactile feel except for the novel functions of various buttons on the endoscope. They can be used with the current generation of standard processors that are capable of providing high-resolution, high-definition endoscopy. NBI-capable endoscopes function similarly to conventional endoscopes, differing only in ability to activate the NBI feature and the quality of the image obtained with NBI. NBI endoscopes have a few specific features that the user needs to be acquainted with (Figure 3.1). This chapter refers primarily to the 190 series EVIS EXCERA III system utilized in the United States and the 290 series EVIS LUCERA ELITE system utilized in Europe. By the switch of a button, it can convert white light images to NBI images and vice versa. Depress another switch (dual focus capability) and the image can be digitally enhanced to provide precise focusing at a very shallow depth of field that is immune to slight extrinsic motion, thereby allowing better visualization of detailed surface patterns at a specific point in the gastrointestinal tract. Finally, another switch and the image can be digitally magnified. Each press of the switch changes the magnification, with a maximum magnification of 1.5×. The magnification function in endoscopes is identical to the optical and digital zoom functions of commercially available cameras: the quality of a magnified image will be maintained by the optical zoom when a new set of lenses come into play, while the digital zoom will artificially magnify the already captured image.

Preparing the patient

During regular white light endoscopy, macroscopic abnormalities are examined, whereas during NBI, the mucosal pattern and subtle changes are sought. Observing these finer minute details of the mucosa and the blood vessels with NBI requires a great deal of patient cooperation, much more so than with standard white light endoscopy. This requires a well-trained and experienced nurse or anesthetist who can keep the patient adequately sedated throughout the entire duration of the procedure. This may seem like a minor issue but, occasionally, agitation on the part of the patient makes it harder to maintain the NBI image in focus and prolongs the procedure. Effective communication with the sedation staff is key to ensure adequate sedation and cooperation of the patient.

Cap-assisted endoscopy

Affixing a cap to the distal tip of the endoscope can help the endoscopist inspect areas of the gastrointestinal tract closely with NBI (Figure 3.2). The cap is a distal attachment (Olympus, disposable distal attachment, D-201-x, with variable models for each endoscope size) that is transparent and maintains a distance of 2–3 mm between the mucosa and the tip of the endoscope. This helps obtain a well-focused image. Secondly, it helps keep the area of the mucosa in the field of vision for the details to be evaluated by the endoscopist. Finally, the cap helps maintain scope stability on the area of interest while examining it in detail with NBI. The cap will give the tip of the endoscope a wider dimension that may sometimes make esophageal and cecal intubation tricky at first, but with practice and patience, the endoscope with the fitted cap can be advanced throughout the entire gastrointestinal tract with fair ease. The procedure can be performed without a cap but the mucosal and vascular details may be difficult to appreciate, especially when starting.

Preparing the esophagus

A major challenge in performing and evaluating the esophagus is that of mucus/oral secretions within the esophagus that may interfere with obtaining clear images. This can be tackled by adequate washes with water to clear the surface of the mucosa. If water rinses do not eliminate the mucus, then 10–20 mL of 50% *N*-acetylcysteine can be sprayed with the help of the spray catheter or flushed into the esophagus through the working channel of the endoscope to clear the mucus. It is critical that the esophagus is as clean as possible before detailed inspection is carried out.

Peristalsis of the esophagus can make the performance of NBI difficult as the image can move in and out of focus. The cap technique may help with this. Also, use of an anti-peristaltic agent may diminish esophageal motility but has to be balanced against the potential side effects of the drug. At present, we do not use any anti-peristaltic agent in our practice. One such agent is butylscopolamine, which has been approved for use in Europe and has been extensively used with confocal endoscopy, which requires an immobile esophagus [1]. Butylscopolamine has a similar mechanism of action to scopolamine but a much shorter half-life (20 min vs. 2–3 hours with scopolamine). The potential side effects are primarily anticholinergic, such as glaucoma exacerbation, urinary retention, blurry vision, dry mouth, and confusion, but such significant side effects related to the drug have not been reported. With time and experience, esophageal motility may prove to be a minor issue with NBI. Nevertheless, the effect of this drug on visualization during NBI has never been studied.

Examining the esophagus

Initially, a high-resolution white light examination should be performed to identify any visible lesions such as nodules, ulcers, and plaques. All these lesions will be highlighted during NBI but their visualization under white light may help the endoscopist perform a more focused NBI examination. Another reason for a thorough examination under white light is to ensure that no obvious lesions are missed since we are all familiar with white light and using NBI will definitely have a learning curve to appreciate things. During this part of the procedure with white light, the mucosal surface should be thoroughly washed using multiple rinses of water to expedite the subsequent NBI portion that is more technically challenging. An important issue is that all biopsies should be deferred to the end of the procedure, as presence of blood will interfere with the NBI examination.

Once the white light examination of the esophagus, stomach and duodenum is performed in the standardized manner, the user switches to NBI. This is accomplished by pushing a button on the top of the handle of the endoscope. The duodenum, antrum, body and fundus can then be examined followed by gradual withdrawal from the stomach until the circular pattern of the cardia (Figure 3.3) at the gastroesophageal junction is visualized. While focusing on this cardiac pattern and taking a cue by the proximal margin of the gastric folds, the endoscopist will notice a distinct change in the mucosal pattern that should coincide very closely with the end of the gastric folds. In a patient with Barrett's esophagus (BE), this change in the mucosal pattern would be a transition into a ridge/villous pattern, suggestive of intestinal metaplasia. The identification of the proximal margin of the gastric folds is the traditional way of identifying the distal aspect of the BE segment. However, in fact, although not formally reported, the change in the mucosal pattern from circular to ridge/villous may be better at identifying the extent of the BE segment distally.

The first step is to examine the entire BE segment looking for macroscopic lesions not visualized on while light endoscopy and making a note of the abnormality by describing the level in centimeters and clock position in the esophagus. This will help in revisiting the lesions for subsequent biopsies. This initial NBI examination should be performed with the dual focus set to the "far" mode and without digital magnification. Under white light blood appears red, but during NBI it looks pitch black and hence a biopsy prior to a complete NBI examination will affect the assessment of the patterns adversely due to the introduction of blood. After the initial overview examination of BE is completed, then is the time to pay attention to the mucosal and vascular details that are seen due to the contrast provided by NBI in the "near" mode of the dual focus function of the endoscope and, if needed, by activating digital magnification. Mentally, the examiner should try to focus on the two aspects of the examination: mucosal surface and vascular pattern. Finding an abnormal mucosal pattern should prompt search for abnormal vascular patterns and vice versa and it is possible that, in the same area, either one of the patterns is clearer and distinct from the other. Every abnormal area should be noted in terms of location and biopsied separately to permit later correlation and mapping of the extent of dysplasia. After the NBI examination is complete, targeted as well as random biopsies can be obtained.

Examining the stomach, duodenum, and colon

The stomach, duodenum, and colon can all be examined under NBI. This kind of examination mainly takes advantage of the contrast afforded by the NBI image to facilitate detection of abnormalities that might appear subtle on white light examination. Similar to examination in the esophagus, the "far" mode without digital magnification is used to conduct the initial examination and detect subtle lesions. After the initial detection of these abnormalities, the "near" mode and/or digital magnification can be used to conduct a closer examination of the detailed mucosal and vascular patterns of the abnormality. In the duodenum and colon, the novice quickly learns to recognize the appearance of bilious fluid and residual stool as pink in color. The limitations of poor colon preparation create the same difficulties for an NBI examination as with a standard colonoscopy. Similar to the esophagus, gastrointestinal motility can be an issue. The use of a cap and anti-peristaltic agents are two options to help with this problem.

Surface patterns observed by NBI

The following sections discuss the patterns of NBI in BE patients as an example of how specifically NBI is applied in the gastrointestinal tract. The reader is referred to individual chapters for detailed NBI patterns of the esophagus, stomach and colon, and for preliminary data supporting the utility of this imaging modality in detecting lesions and making endoscopic diagnoses in these organs.

Normal patterns

What are the "normal" patterns visualized in a BE segment without dysplasia? The intestinal metaplasia within a BE segment appears as a regular ridge/villous pattern (Figure 3.4). This appears as alternate longitudinal bands of dark and light areas. Some areas of the BE segment appear to have a circular pattern and these areas have a higher likelihood of harboring cardiac-type mucosa [2]. On NBI, the normal vascular pattern in BE comprises regularly branching, uniformly organized small vessels. This should be differentiated from the larger-caliber palisading vessels in the distal esophagus that are usually well visualized under white light examination.

Abnormal patterns

Knowing the normal patterns will help the endoscopist diagnose abnormal lesions. The most worrisome pathology in flat BE mucosa is high-grade dysplasia (HGD)/esophageal adenocarcinoma (EAC). This is manifested by irregular mucosal patterns characterized by patterns of varying shapes and lengths distributed unevenly, giving a nonuniform look to the mucosa (Figure 3.5). This is obviously a subjective description and is the primary reason for initial training. The BE segment may need to be examined multiple times before the beginner achieves a reasonable degree of skill at detecting the most clinically relevant lesions of HGD/early EAC. Numerous examples of both nondysplastic and dysplastic Barrett's appearance on NBI can be found within this book.

The vascular pattern is comparatively harder to decipher than the mucosal pattern, presumably because the process of angiogenesis may result in various sizes and shapes of vessel formation. Nevertheless, abnormal vascularity appears as increased numbers of tortuous, dilated, corkscrew-type small blood vessels of varying caliber. Others have described abnormal vascularity in multiple ways, with two descriptions that particularly correlate well with the presence of HGD: spiral vessels of varying caliber and small isolated blood vessels [3].

Learning to use NBI

Several training modules have been developed and used in prior studies evaluating the performance of NBI in diagnosing colon polyp histology. Classroom-type training programs, varying in length from 20 min to 4 hours, have been found to be effective in teaching experienced academic endoscopists, endoscopy trainees, and non-endoscopy medical trainees [4–6]. Self-directed, computer-based training modules, ranging from 15 to 20 min in length, have also been found to be effective in teaching academic endoscopists, endoscopy trainees, non-endoscopy medical trainees, and community endoscopists [7–9]. Self-directed computer modules combined with both self-directed and expert-provided ongoing feedback have been found to be effective [10,11].

While there have been several studies evaluating training programs for teaching NBI for diagnosing colon polyps, there are few data on other applications such as BE and gastric and duodenal indications. A randomized controlled trial comparing classroom-type training with self-directed computer-based training of NBI for diagnosing BE-associated neoplasia found no difference between the two groups, but also found that neither group performed very well after training [12]. With regard to the stomach, a web-based training module combined with ongoing self-directed feedback was effective in teaching NBI for diagnosing gastric lesions [13]. As one can see, many questions remain regarding how to learn to use NBI. The optimal training method, learning curve duration, and whether training requirements are different based on the disease and the clinical application have all yet to be clearly determined.

What is clear is that every person learns differently. Some may learn better with continued instruction from a teacher whereas others learn better by self-directed methods. Some individuals learn quickly and some slowly. As a result, many options for NBI training have been created and are available. These run the gamut of training program types, including classroom-type programs (available through endoscopy medical societies and postgraduate training programs), self-directed computer programs (some available through the internet and industry), and several image/video atlases including this book. Endoscopists looking to implement NBI in their practice should identify the training resources that best fit their learning preferences and utilize them as they use NBI.

 Video clips to accompany this book can be found in the online material at www.wiley.com/go/cohen/NBI

The following videos relate specifically to this chapter:
Video 11 NBI patterns in a patient with nondysplastic Barrett's esophagus
Video 13 NBI detection of focal dysplasia in Barrett's esophagus using cap examination

References

1 Kiesslich R, Gossner L, Goetz M *et al.* In vivo histology of Barrett's esophagus and associated neoplasia by confocal laser endomicroscopy. *Clin Gastroenterol Hepatol* 2006;4:979–87.

2 Sharma P, Bansal A, Mathur S *et al.* The utility of a novel narrow band imaging endoscopy system in patients with Barrett's esophagus. *Gastrointest Endosc* 2006;64:167–75.

3 Kara MA, Ennahachi M, Fockens P, ten Kate FJ, Bergman JJ. Detection and classification of the mucosal and vascular patterns (mucosal morphology) in Barrett's esophagus by using narrow band imaging. *Gastrointest Endosc* 2006;64:155–66.

4 Raghavendra M, Hewett DG, Rex DK. Differentiating adenomas from hyperplastic colorectal polyps: narrowband imaging can be learned in 20 minutes. *Gastrointest Endosc* 2010;72:572–6.

5 Dai J, Shen YF, Sano Y *et al.* Evaluation of narrow-band imaging in the diagnosis of colorectal lesions: is a learning curve involved? *Dig Endosc* 2013;25:180–8.

6 Rogart JN, Jain D, Siddiqui UD *et al.* Narrow-band imaging without high magnification to differentiate polyps during real-time colonoscopy: improvement with experience. *Gastrointest Endosc* 2008;68:1136–45.

7 Rastogi A, Rao DS, Gupta N *et al.* Impact of a computer-based teaching module on characterization of diminutive colon polyps by using narrow-band imaging by non-experts in academic and community practice: a video-based study. *Gastrointest Endosc* 2014;79:390–8.

8 Sinh P, Gupta N, Rao DS *et al.* Community gastroenterologists can learn diminutive colon polyp histology characterization with narrow band imaging by a computer-based teaching module. *Dig Endosc* 2015;27:374–80.

9 Ignjatovic A, Thomas-Gibson S, East JE *et al.* Development and validation of a training module on the use of narrow-band imaging in differentiation of small adenomas from hyperplastic colorectal polyps. *Gastrointest Endosc* 2011;73:128–33.

10 Singh R, Bhat YM, Thurairajah PH *et al.* Is narrow band imaging superior to high-definition white light endoscopy in the assessment of diminutive colorectal polyps? *J Gastroenterol Hepatol* 2013;28:472–8.

11 Patel SG, Rastogi A, Austin G *et al.* Gastroenterology trainees can easily learn histologic characterization of diminutive colorectal polyps with narrow band imaging. *Clin Gastroenterol Hepatol* 2013;11:997–1003.e1.

12 Daly C, Vennalaganti P, Soudagar S, Hornung B, Sharma P, Gupta N. Randomized controlled trial of self-directed vs in-classroom didactic teaching of narrow band imaging in diagnosing Barrett's esophagus associated neoplasia. *Gastrointest Endosc* 2016;83:101–6.

13 Dias-Silva D, Pimentel-Nunes P, Magalhaes J *et al.* The learning curve for narrow-band imaging in the diagnosis of precancerous gastric lesions by using Web-based video. *Gastrointest Endosc* 2014;79:910–20; quiz 983-e1, 983-e4.

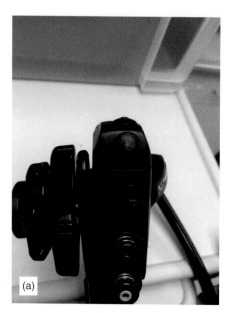
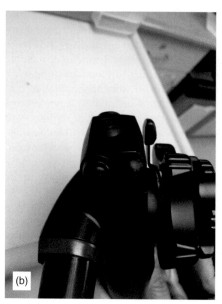

Figure 3.1 Handle of an Olympus 190 series endoscope (GIF-HQ190) illustrating the multiple control buttons: (a) buttons 1 and 2 on the front; (b) button 3 on the top and buttons 4 and 5 on the back.

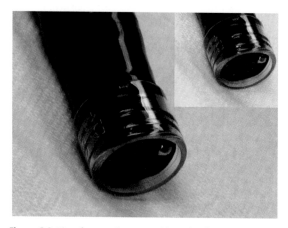
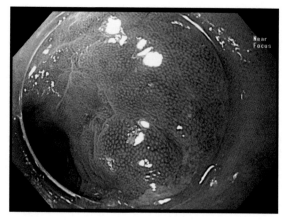

Figure 3.2 Tip of an endoscope with a distal attachment cap placed on the tip.

Figure 3.3 Cardia of the stomach seen with NBI (near focus) illustrating the circular mucosal pattern.

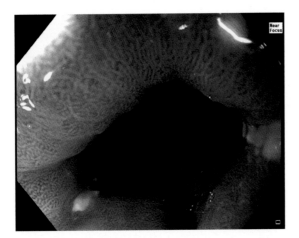

Figure 3.4 Nondysplastic Barrett's esophagus seen with NBI (near focus) illustrating the ridged/villous mucosal pattern.

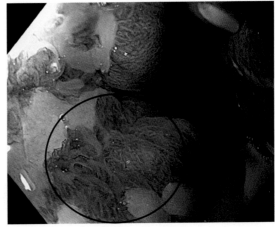

Figure 3.5 Barrett's esophagus with high-grade dysplasia seen with NBI illustrating the irregular mucosal and irregular vascular patterns.

PART 2

Application of High-Resolution Endoscopy and NBI in Diagnosis and Therapy

SECTION 1
Pharynx and Esophagus

4 | Detection of superficial cancer in oropharyngeal and hypopharyngeal mucosal sites and the value of NBI in qualitative diagnosis

Manabu Muto, Atsushi Ochiai, and Shigeaki Yoshida

Why is diagnostic examination of the pharynx necessary?

The clinical care of the pharynx is generally carried out by otolaryngologists. For this reason, many gastrointestinal physicians do not fully inspect and make diagnoses in the area of the oropharynx and hypopharynx during routine endoscopy. At the same time, it has been recognized difficult to detect an early cancer in oropharyngeal and hypopharyngeal mucosal sites, because most cancers in this region are found in an advanced stage, with a number of symptoms such as dysphagia and severe pain. The organ of the pharynx is essential to life by transferring food and liquid, and by breathing and phonation. Once the cancer is found to be progressing, patients lose these functions and their quality of life becomes remarkably poor. Needless to say, detection of cancer at an early stage is very much appreciated.

Narrowband imaging (NBI) is a new technology in the field of gastrointestinal endoscopy. Since we first reported the value of NBI in combination with magnifying endoscopy for the detection of cancer in oropharyngeal and hypopharyngeal mucosal sites, its importance in the diagnosis of oropharyngeal and hypopharyngeal mucosal sites has become increasingly recognized [1]. In other words, the detection of cancer in oropharyngeal and hypopharyngeal mucosal sites at early stages using upper gastrointestinal endoscopy has gained momentum. Indeed, the diagnosis of cancer at an early stage is expected to contribute to patient quality of life and improve prognosis by enabling minimally invasive therapy to spare organs and thereby preserve function.

Cancer in the area of the pharynx and its risk factors

According to the GLOBOCAN 2012 report by the International Agency for Research on Cancer (http://globocan
.iarc.fr/Pages/fact_sheets_population.aspx), new cancer cases in Japan exceeded 14,067,894 in all areas [2]. The number of new cases of cancer in the area of lip, oral cavity and pharynx was 314,106 (2.2% of total cases), that is, approximately half the number of cases of gastric cancer (631,293, 8.5% of total cases). Most of the cancers generated in oropharyngeal and hypopharyngeal mucosal sites are squamous cell carcinoma. Alcohol and smoking have been recognized as two major risk factors for cancers at these sites, as well as in the esophagus. A recent study has pointed to a critical role for acetaldehyde, generated by the metabolism of alcohol, in promoting carcinogenesis. In particular, in Asian people including the Japanese there is a genetic polymorphism in aldehyde dehydrogenase type 2 (ALDH2), an enzyme responsible for the elimination of acetaldehyde. Heterozygotes for the inactive gene (ALDH2-2) have a higher risk of carcinogenesis when they keep drinking [3]. In other words, those individuals with a tendency to blush when drinking (flushing response) are at higher risk for esophageal and pharyngeal cancer.

Superficial cancer in oropharyngeal and hypopharyngeal mucosal sites

Current guidelines for head and neck cancer do not include an exact definition of superficial cancer [4]. In Japan, where there is a high incidence of squamous cell

Comprehensive Atlas of High-Resolution Endoscopy and Narrowband Imaging, Second Edition. Edited by Jonathan Cohen.
© 2017 John Wiley & Sons, Ltd. Published 2017 by John Wiley & Sons, Ltd.
Companion website: www.wiley.com/go/cohen/NBI

carcinoma, the guideline for esophageal cancer considers a cancer invading up to the submucosa as "superficial cancer" and a cancer invading beneath the muscularis propria as "advanced cancer" [5]. Among superficial cancers, one invading up to the epithelium or lamina propria mucosae without lymph node involvement or metastasis is defined as "cancer in early stage." There is no definition of invasion in the field of pharyngeal cancer except for carcinoma in situ (Tis) that reflects pathologic invasion. In 2001, according to statistics from Japan's Head and Neck Cancer Society (with 29 hospitals), carcinoma in situ accounted for only one case among 218 cases of hypopharyngeal cancer and no cases among all cases of oropharyngeal cancer [6]. Accordingly, it is recognized as extremely difficult to detect carcinoma in situ in oropharyngeal and hypopharyngeal mucosal sites. Generally, carcinoma in situ is recognized as a tumor with no risk of lymph node metastasis. When prognosis is taken into consideration, a definition linked to lymph node metastasis should be necessary. Histologic diagnosis in this area should be studied further. Therefore in this chapter, high-grade intraepithelial neoplasia as defined in the World Health Organization (WHO) classification is regarded as "carcinoma in situ" and a cancer slightly invasive beneath epithelium as "superficial cancer" (Figures 4.1–4.4).

Diagnosis of superficial cancer in oropharyngeal and hypopharyngeal mucosal sites by NBI

It is now safe to say that the era of gastrointestinal endoscopy has changed from realistic diagnosis with white light and dye to the diagnosis of biological change using special light observation. For neoplastic lesions in particular, diagnosis previously relied on observation of the enlargement between the lesion and the surrounding area, along with the appearance of reddening. Now using the properties of special light, the rationale of diagnosis has been changing, supported by the observation of biological change. NBI employs selectively filtered light at 415 nm wavelength that is well absorbed by hemoglobin. NBI therefore provides endoscopic images that show fine capillary patterns and detailed changes in the mucosal surface, especially when combined with high-resolution imaging and magnification (Figures 4.5–4.9).

We have studied NBI images of superficial head and neck cancer with regard to aspects of "visibility" and "character of image" in combination with magnified endoscopy [7,8]. In terms of visibility, NBI displays cancerous areas as brownish in color, so that a border between the lesion and the normal mucosa can be clearly

identified. In contrast, it is difficult to identify the border under normal white light observation. NBI clearly displays abnormal angiogenesis in a speckled appearance that is distinctively found in the lesion. On histology, this abnormal angiogenesis is similar to the morphological changes of intrapapillary capillary loop (IPCL) within squamous epithelium used to improve diagnosis in the esophagus, as described in detail in Chapter 5 [9].

Prospective randomized study has shown NBI to be superior in the detection and characterization of superficial head and neck cancer compared with conventional white light endoscopy [10].

Change in color-defining areas at NBI observation (brownish area)

Superficial cancer tends to be displayed as brownish areas at NBI observation. Superficial cancer with reddening can be identified under normal white light observation. However, NBI can display the border between a lesion and normal mucosa whether reddening is present or not. The surface of normal squamous epithelium is seen as whitish with luster. In contrast, NBI displays lesions with tumorous change as brownish in color and shows a clear border between the lesion and the normal surrounding mucosa.

Benign lesions such as inflammation and basal cell hyperplasia often appear as a slight extension and generation of subtle vessels, but its interspersion do not comprise a well-demarcated area. For example, a lesion with an abnormal change in IPCL but more diffuse interspersion is less likely to be cancerous. Conversely, a lesion that is seen as occupying a wide area but with a blurry IPCL change and a ground-glass appearance also tends to have a benign etiology such as inflammation.

Change in IPCL shape

The size of the IPCL in normal epithelium is about 10 μm; however, its size increases to 100 μm in cases of cancerous lesions. IPCL changes by extension, prolongation and meandering. Extension and prolongation reach to the surface of epithelium so that they are clearly observed endoscopically. The number of vessels also increases within the lesion and beneath the epithelium. However, there are multiple patterns of change in IPCL shape even within a lesion. Within carcinoma in situ, there are multiple patterns in angiogenesis among lesions. IPCL patterns in the esophagus have been studied for their relationship to cancer invasion and histological staging (discussed in Chapter 5). However, the oropharynx and hypopharynx would tend to be different from the esophagus because the muscularis mucosae does not exist in the pharyngeal area. Further study is needed regarding the implications of IPCL patterns in the pharynx.

Video clips to accompany this book can be found in the online material at www.wiley.com/go/cohen/NBI

The following videos relate specifically to this chapter:

Video 1 NBI examination of the oropharynx

Video 2 Benign lesion, hyperplasia

Video 3 Neoplastic lesion, low-grade intraepithelial neoplasia

Video 4 Diagnosis of superficial squamous cell carcinoma

Video 5 Pharyngeal squamous cell carcinoma, type V IPCL pattern

Video 6 Hyperplastic changes following radiation and chemotherapy

Video 7 Inflammatory change

Video 8 Residual carcinoma, coexisting with hyperplastic change post radiation and chemotherapy

References

1 Muto M, Nakane M, Katada C *et al.* Squamous cell carcinoma in situ in oropharyngeal and hypopharyngeal mucosal sites. *Cancer* 2004;101:1375–81.

2 Foundation for Promotion of Cancer Research. *Cancer Statistics in Japan 2003*, pp. 46–47, 2004 (only available in Japanese).

3 Yokoyama A, Kato H, Yokoyama T *et al.* Genetic polymorphisms of alcohol and aldehyde dehydrogenases and glutathione S-transferase M1 and drinking, smoking, and diet in Japanese men with esophageal squamous cell carcinoma. *Carcinogenesis* 2002;23:1851–9.

4 Japan Society of Head and Neck Cancer. *Clinical Guideline for Head and Neck Cancer*, 3rd version. Kanehara Shuppan, Tokyo, 2001 (only available in Japanese).

5 Japan Esophageal Society. *Clinical Guideline for Esophageal Cancer*, 9th version. Kanehara Shuppan, Tokyo, 1999 (only available in Japanese).

6 Japan Society for Head and Neck Cancer Registry Committee. Report of Head and Neck Cancer Registry of Japan: clinical statistics of registered patients, 2001. *Jpn J Head Neck Cancer* 2005;31:60–80.

7 Muto M, Ugumori T, Sao Y *et al.* Narrow band imaging combined with magnified endoscopy for the cancer at the head and neck region. *Dig Endosc* 2005;17:S23–S24.

8 Muto M, Katada C, Sano Y *et al.* Narrowband imaging: a new diagnostic approach to visualize angiogenesis in the superficial neoplasm. *Clin Gastroenterol Hepatol* 2005;3:S16–S20.

9 Inoue H, Honda T, Nagai K *et al.* Ultra-high magnification endoscopic observation of carcinoma in situ of the oesophagus. *Dig Endosc* 1997;9:16–18.

10 Muto M, Minashi K, Yano T *et al.* Early detection of superficial squamous cell carcinoma in the head and neck region and esophagus by narrow band imaging: a multicenter randomized controlled trial. *J Clin Oncol* 2010;28:1566–72.

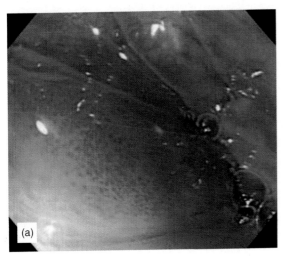 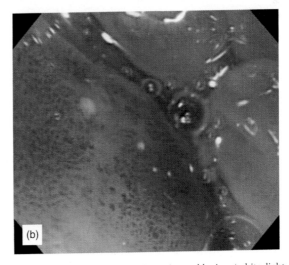

Figure 4.1 Carcinoma in situ in left piriform sinus. (a, b) Lesion in left piriform sinus shows intensive reddening (white light observation). (continued)

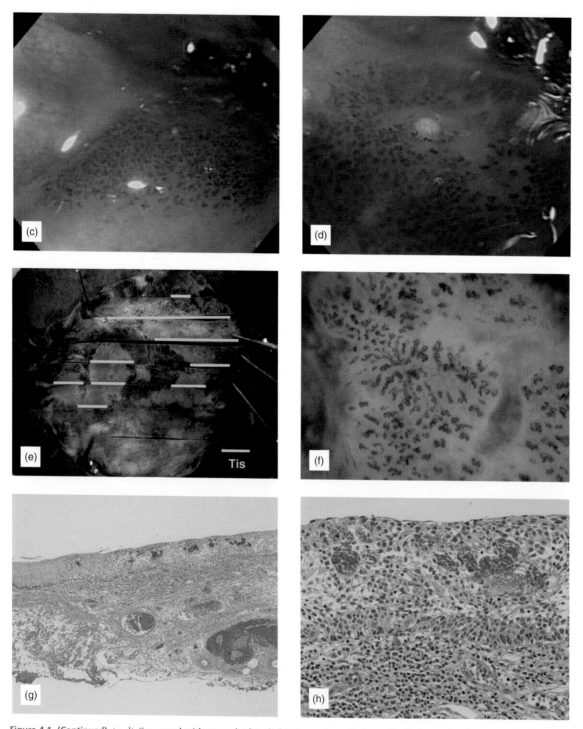

Figure 4.1 (Continued) (c, d) Compared with normal white light observation, the lesion is displayed clearly as a brownish area by NBI. Intensive speckle-like angiogenesis is clearly seen by NBI combined with zoom endoscopy. (e) Iodide-dyed specimen obtained by endoscopic resection under general anesthesia. Carcinoma in situ is identified in area not stained by iodide. (f) Stereomicroscopic view of angiogenesis in area not stained by iodide, which represents the mucosal lesion and which appears as a "pinky" color. Angiogenesis clearly extends unevenly and displays a meandering serpiginous shape. (g, h) H&E view of specimen obtained by endoscopic mucosal resection (EMR). (g) Low magnification of squamous cell carcinoma in situ. (h) High magnification extended IPCL is identified within carcinoma in situ. (Copyright M. Muto, A. Ochiai, and S. Yoshida.)

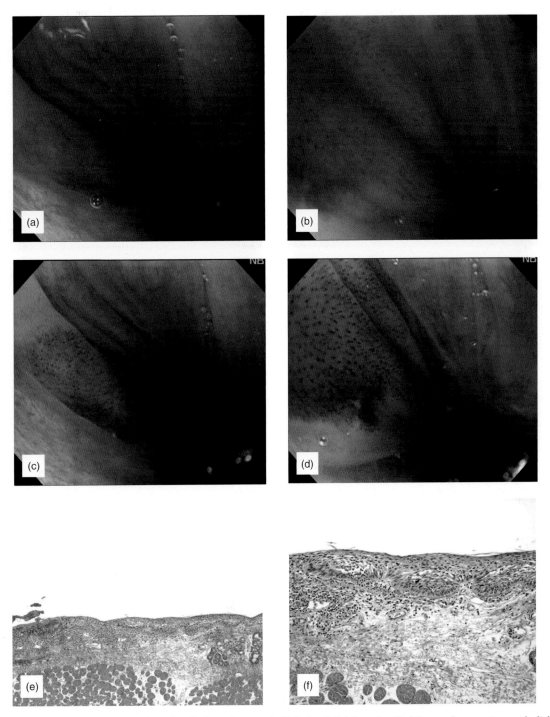

Figure 4.2 Carcinoma in situ in left lateral wall of oropharynx. (a, b) Lesion in left lateral wall of the oropharynx. Area with slight reddening can be identified but it is hard to identify its dimensions. Melanotic change is observed to some extent. It is a general tendency to see this in the area around superficial cancers in the head and neck. Slight dot-type reddening identified by zoom endoscopy. (c, d) Compared with white light observation, this lesion can be clearly identified using NBI as a brownish area. In particular, the border of the melanosis is clearly seen. NBI frequently displays melanotic change as brownish areas. In such cases, careful observation is needed. Zoom endoscopy clearly shows extension and prolongation of angiogenesis. (e, f) H&E view of specimen obtained by EMR. (e) Low magnification of squamous carcinoma in situ. (f) High magnification: melanin pigment is identified to some extent. (Copyright M. Muto, A. Ochiai, and S. Yoshida.)

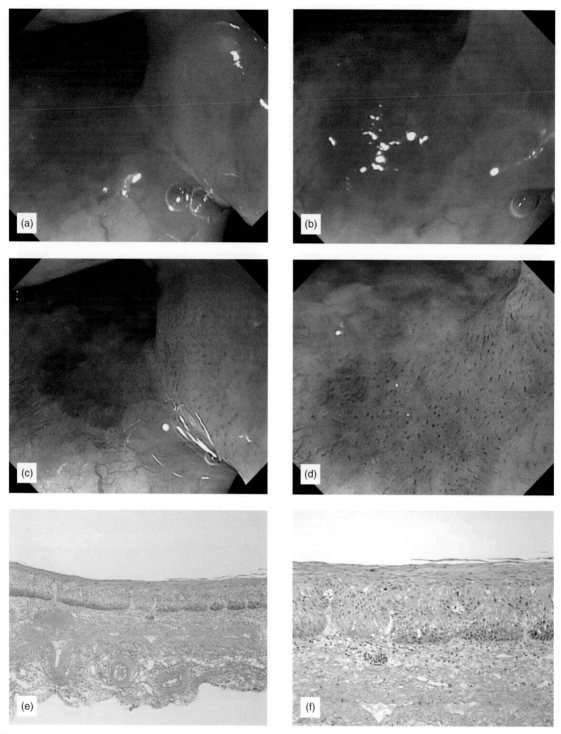

Figure 4.3 Carcinoma in situ at right side of vallecula epiglottica. (a, b) Lesion at right side of vallecula epiglottica. Vanishing vessels, slight reddening in the area and whitish mucosa at right base of tongue are identified. Reddening with luster in the area of vessel vanishes on zoom endoscopic view. (c, d) Area displayed in brown by NBI matches with area of vanished vessels on right side of vallecula epiglottica. At the right base of the tongue, a short slight whitish elevation is identified. Dot-like angiogenesis in a brownish area is identified under zoom endoscopy. (e, f) H&E view of specimen obtained by EMR. (e) Low magnification of squamous carcinoma in situ within epithelium. (f) High magnification. (Copyright M. Muto, A. Ochiai, and S. Yoshida.)

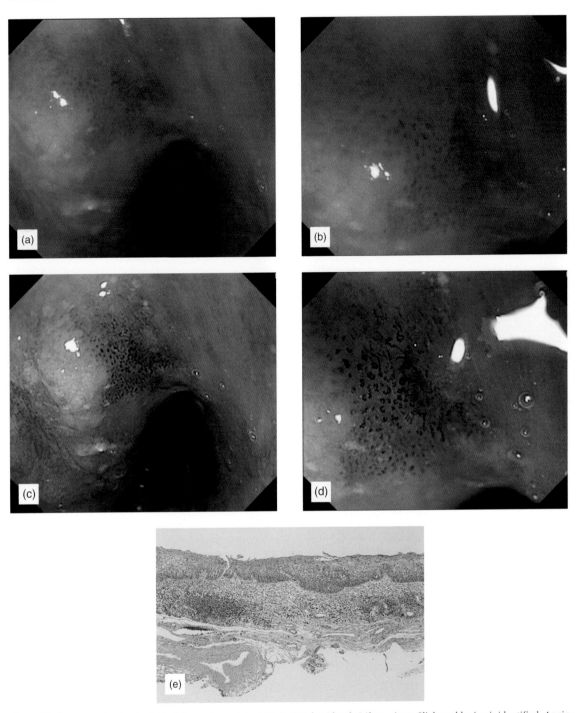

Figure 4.4 Carcinoma in situ in right piriform sinus. (a, b) Lesion at right side of piriform sinus. Slight reddening is identified. Angiogenesis and vessel extension in reddening area is identified under zoom endoscopy. (c, d) Lesion is clearly identified as a brownish area by NBI. Uneven prolongation and extension colored brown are identified under zoom endoscopy. (e) H&E view of specimen obtained by EMR. Squamous carcinoma in situ. The lesion is 5 mm in diameter and stays within the epithelium. (Copyright M. Muto, A. Ochiai, and S. Yoshida.)

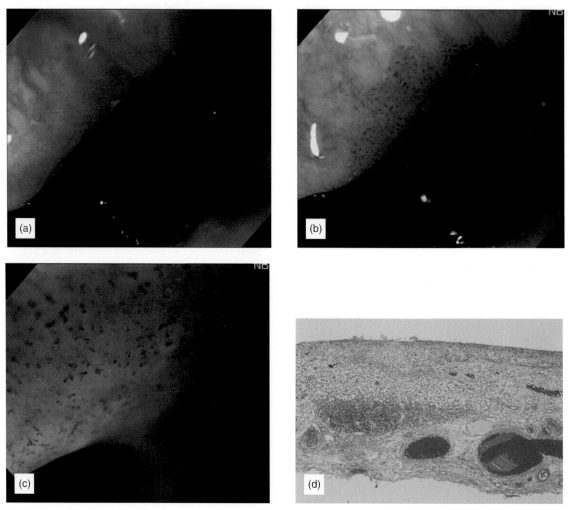

Figure 4.5 Superficial cancer in right piriform recess. Comparison between normal white light and NBI observation. (a) Lesion in right piriform recess is difficult to identify with normal white light observation. (b) Brownish area clearly separated by border is seen by NBI observation. (c) Uneven angiogenesis identified in brownish area under zoom endoscopy. (d) H&E view of specimen obtained by EMR. Squamous carcinoma in situ slightly invading beneath epithelium. Depth of tumor is 200 μm from the surface. (Copyright M. Muto, A. Ochiai, and S. Yoshida.)

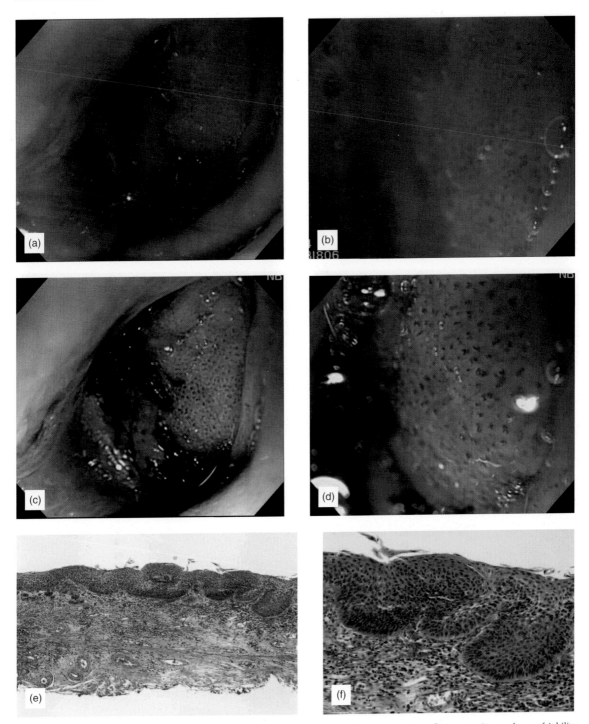

Figure 4.6 Carcinoma in situ in right piriform sinus. (a) Lesion in right piriform sinus. Short flat protrusion and easy friability. (b) Angiogenesis is identified under zoom endoscopy. (c) Identification of brownish area is difficult by NBI, but intensive dot-like pattern is seen. (d) Uneven angiogenesis with prolongation and extension (like frog eggs) are identified under zoom endoscopy. (e, f) H&E view of specimen obtained by EMR. (e) Squamous carcinoma in situ within epithelium. (f) High cell density. Angiogenesis is not remarkable. (Copyright M. Muto, A. Ochiai, and S. Yoshida.)

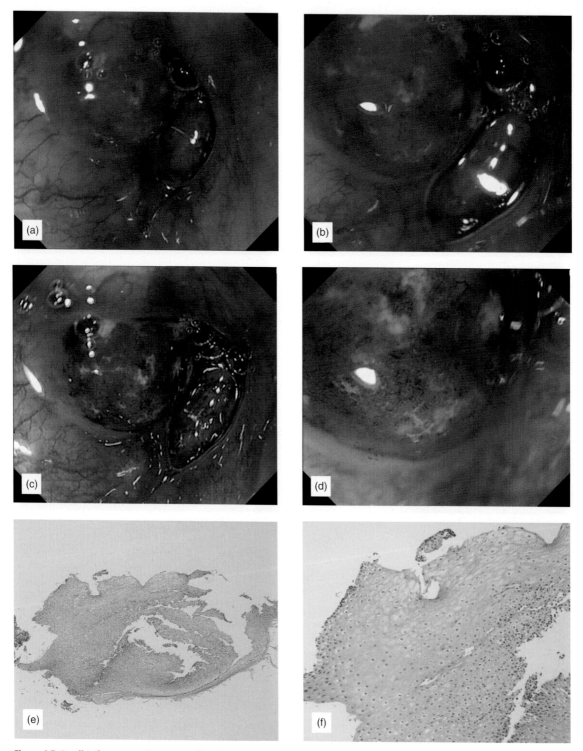

Figure 4.7 Small inflammatory lesion in vallecula epiglottica. (a) Slight reddening with vanishing vessel identified by normal white light observation. (b) Only reddening and erosion are identified under zoom endoscopy. (c) Color change to brown is identified by NBI. (d) Angiogenesis is not identified under zoom endoscopy. (e, f) H&E view of specimen. Concluded to be squamous epithelium with inflammatory infiltration. (Copyright M. Muto, A. Ochiai, and S. Yoshida.)

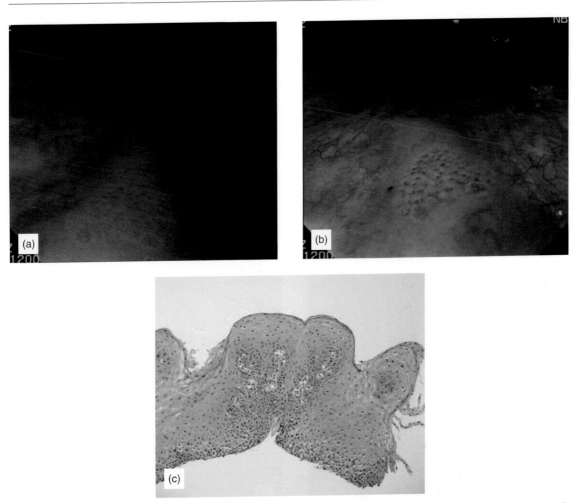

Figure 4.8 Small lesion in posterior wall of oropharynx. (a) Dimple-like lesion with rough surface somehow identified. (b) Dimple-like lesion with rough surface is identified by NBI. Difference from surrounding normal mucosa is not remarkable. Only shows slight thickness. (c) H&E view of specimen. Concluded to be squamous epithelium with low-grade papilla-like growth. (Copyright M. Muto, A. Ochiai, and S. Yoshida.)

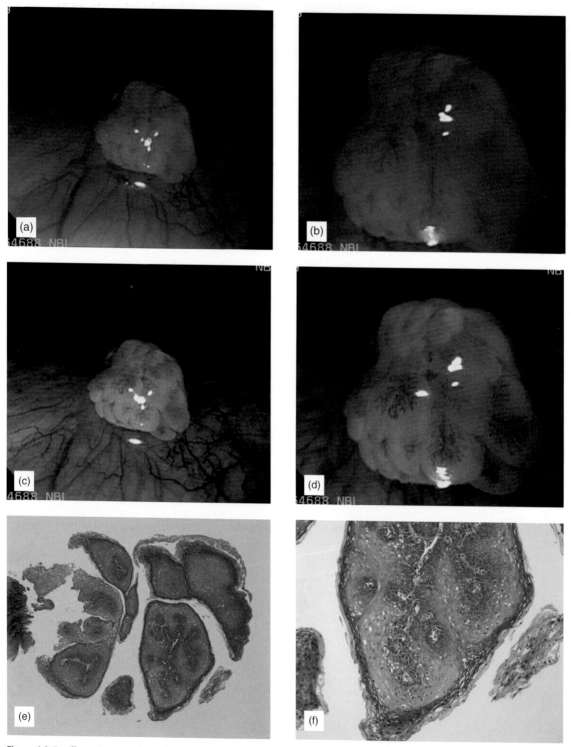

Figure 4.9 Papilloma in posterior wall of oropharynx. (a) Whitish pine-cone-like elevated lesion is identified. (b) Surface pattern and slight prolongation is identified under zoom endoscopy. (c) Papillary pattern is clearly identified from distance. Angiogenesis with prolongation inside papilloma slightly identified. (d) Fern-leaf-like prolonged angiogenesis is identified within papillary pattern under zoom endoscopy. (e, f) H&E view of specimen. Papillary propagation in squamous epithelium. Concluded to be a papilloma. (Copyright M. Muto, A. Ochiai, and S. Yoshida.)

5

Magnifying endoscopic diagnosis of tissue atypia and cancer invasion depth in the area of pharyngoesophageal squamous epithelium by NBI enhanced magnification image: IPCL pattern classification

Robert Bechara and Haruhiro Inoue

Background

Pharyngeal and esophageal squamous neoplasms are usually asymptomatic, with symptom development occurring only at advanced stages. As a result, over 50% of patients have advanced disease at presentation, limiting the possibility of curative endoscopic resection [1]. To improve the prognosis of these neoplasms, two strategies must be applied. First is early detection prior to the development of invasive disease, and second is curative resection with endoscopic mucosal resection (EMR)/endoscopic submucosal dissection (ESD) [2–4]. Therefore, training in meticulous endoscopic examination is essential for early detection of these subtle lesions. A well-trained endoscopist able to detect 1-mm lesions is unlikely to overlook those 5–10 mm in size, thus maximizing the opportunity for curative endoscopic resection. This was well illustrated in a large series of flat pharyngeal neoplasia. It was found that all lesions measuring less than 5 mm and 90% of lesions measuring 5–10 mm in were carcinoma in situ [5]. Once a lesion is detected, accurate endoscopic characterization is required to ensure selection of the appropriate treatment. For mucosal cancer (stage T1a), the risk of lymph node metastasis is exceedingly rare and current guidelines recommend endoscopic resection [6,7]. Generally, excisional biopsy is performed for mucosal lesions 2 mm and smaller, EMR for lesions greater than 2 mm and up to 2 cm, and ESD for lesions greater than 2 cm. Comprehensive treatment with chemoradiation/surgery is suggested for neoplasms with submucosal invasion of 200 μm (sm2) or more due to the significant risk of lymph node metastasis [8,9]. With careful endoscopic examination, early detection of pharyngoesophageal neoplasia is maximized. This leads to increased curative endoscopic resection of superficial pharyngoesophageal neoplasia, resulting in improved patient outcomes.

Since the pharynx and esophagus possess stratified squamous epithelium and lack a glandular epithelium, they do not exhibit a pit pattern as seen in the stomach and colon. However, the squamous epithelium microvasculature can be examined with magnifying endoscopy, allowing the identification and classification of the intrapapillary capillary loops (IPCLs). The IPCLs demonstrate characteristic changes that result from tissue atypia and depth of neoplastic invasion [10,11]. With a tissue diagnosis of low-grade intraepithelial neoplasia (Vienna classification category 3), close surveillance is recommended, whereas with high-grade intraepithelial neoplasia (Vienna classification category 4) the recommendation is for endoscopic resection. This illustrates the importance of an accurate endoscopic tool that can distinguish subtle changes in a lesion that reflect the degree of tissue atypism, as the clinical management may vary significantly.

Comprehensive Atlas of High-Resolution Endoscopy and Narrowband Imaging, Second Edition. Edited by Jonathan Cohen.
© 2017 John Wiley & Sons, Ltd. Published 2017 by John Wiley & Sons, Ltd.
Companion website: www.wiley.com/go/cohen/NBI

Magnifying endoscopy of normal esophageal mucosa

The superficial mucosal and submucosal microvasculature in the normal esophagus is illustrated in Figure 5.1. In esophageal mucosa without magnification, branching vessels are observed immediately above the muscularis mucosae. The IPCLs, which arise perpendicularly from the branching vessels, are barely visible with nonmagnifying white light endoscopy (WLE) (Figure 5.5). However, with a magnifying endoscope such as the GIF-Q290Z with magnification up to 80× (Olympus Medical Systems, Tokyo, Japan), the IPCLs can be identified as red dots with standard WLE, and as well-defined tiny brown loops with narrowband imaging (NBI). Thus, with magnifying NBI (M-NBI) the pharyngoesophageal microvasculature can be clearly visualized, with the deeper branching vessels appearing green and the superficial IPCLs as brown loops (Figure 5.5).

Magnifying endoscopy and the IPCL classification

With the early detection of pharyngoesophageal neoplasia, there is increased opportunity for endoscopic curative treatment. This is because neoplasms limited to the mucosa can be treated with EMR/ESD as they generally have minimal risk of lymph node metastasis. As previously mentioned, changes in IPCL type reflect tissue atypia and depth of neoplastic invasion, making the IPCL classification an extremely useful adjunct for lesion characterization and estimation of invasion depth.

In pharyngoesophageal squamous cell carcinoma, four characteristic IPCL changes are observed: dilation, tortuosity, irregular caliber, and form variation (Figure 5.3). These changes occur progressively, reflecting changes in the inflammation–dysplasia–carcinoma sequence. The characterization of a lesion is performed in a stepwise fashion. First, a lesion is detected as reddened area or Lugol-void lesion with WLE or as brownish area when viewed with NBI. Thus, nonmagnifying endoscopy allows for general morphologic characterization (Paris classification, color and alterations in surface contour with insufflation). Second, the lesion is examined with M-NBI to evaluate the IPCL pattern (Figure 5.2). With the recently upgraded NBI system, a xenon lamp results in a brighter image than its predecessor. As a result, the IPCLs are easier to observe and classify. Specifically, the IPCLs can be classified from type I (normal mucosa) to type Vn (carcinoma with deep submucosal invasion) (Figures 5.2–5.15). Based on the four characteristic changes in IPCLs (dilation, tortuosity, irregular caliber,

and form variation), the five basic types of IPCLs are as follows.

- *Type I*: normal pattern.
- *Type II*: have one to two out of the four characteristic changes, with elongation and/or dilatation commonly seen.
- *Type III*: minimal changes, but differ from type I as they have a brownish color under NBI and are Lugol-negative.
- *Type IV*: have three out of four changes.
- *Type V*: IPCLs have all four characteristic changes indicating carcinoma.

Recently, we introduced a simplified clinical classification system (Figure 5.16) based on the original IPCL classification. Clinically, the IPCL classification is simplified into three groups: group 1 comprise non-neoplastic lesions (IPCL I, II) that do not require resection or regular surveillance; group 2 comprise borderline lesions (IPCL III, IV) that require close surveillance or resection (depending on collateral morphologic assessment); and group 3 lesions comprise neoplastic lesions (IPCL V) that warrant treatment. Group 3 is further subclassified into group 3A (IPCL V1–V3), which have an invasion depth of intramucosal/sm1 and can be resected endoscopically, and group 3B, which have an invasion depth greater than 200 µm (Vn) and warrant non-endoscopic treatment [12].

Assessing depth of invasion of superficial carcinoma

With standard WLE, estimation of invasion depth is based on the Paris classification, color, and alterations in surface contour with insufflation. M-NBI provides additional reliable information to improve characterization and evaluation of invasion depth. Invasion depth is reflected in the IPCLs by the distortion and eventual destruction of the regular IPCL loop structure. With IPCL type V, all four characteristic findings (dilation, tortuosity, irregular caliber, and form variation) are seen and advance from V1 to Vn according to invasion from the mucosa and superficial submucosa (m1–m3/sm1) to deep submucosa (sm2 and greater). IPCL type V1 (group 3A) lesions correspond to carcinoma confined to the epithelium (m1, Category 5.1 Vienna classification). IPCL type V2 lesions correspond to carcinoma confined to the lamina propria (m2, Category 5.1 Vienna classification). Thus, in IPCL types V1–V2 loop structure is conserved while elongation of deformed IPCLs is seen in type V2. IPCL type V3 corresponds to carcinoma confined to the muscularis mucosa with or without slight invasion into the submucosa (m3/sm1). In type V3, irregular IPCLs are identified with partially destroyed loop structure. IPCL type Vn (group 3B) corresponds to carcinoma with deeper invasion into the submucosa (sm2 or greater, Category 5.2 Vienna classification). In type Vn, newly formed abnormal vessels are identified with at least three times the caliber seen in IPCL types V1–V3, with complete destruction of the original loop structure [13]. Thus, using M-NBI in conjunction with other morphologic features, mucosal carcinoma in situ can be strongly suspected when the following four conditions are met:

1 well-demarcated margins;
2 loss of visibility of the green branching vessels in the lesion;
3 marginal elevation of peripheral mucosa;
4 change in vascular pattern to IPCL types IV, V1 and V2.

Whenever all four criteria are met, carcinoma in situ is strongly suspected (Category 4.2 Vienna classification) [14].

Differences in IPCL patterns between mucosal and submucosal cancer

For purely mucosal lesions which correspond to IPCL type II (group 1) to type V2 (group 3A) morphologic changes of the IPCLs occur in the vertical plane, conserving the IPCL loop structure. On the other hand, irregularly arranged IPCLs in m3/sm1 involve the advanced destruction of the original IPCL and run in a horizontal plane (Figures 5.9–5.11). In IPCL type Vn, the IPCL loop structure is completely destroyed, and new large-caliber tumor vessels run horizontally (Figures 5.9 and 5.12). Thus, IPCL types V1 and V2, which correspond to m1/m2 lesions respectively, exhibit changes in structure that occur vertically, while IPCL types V3 and Vn, which correspond to m3/sm1 and >sm2, respectively, exhibit changes that occur horizontally. The endoscopic distinction between IPCL types V3 and Vn is made based on the difference in vessel caliber. Specifically, the caliber of the new tumor vessels, IPCL type Vn, is approximately three times larger than that of IPCL type V3 [13].

In a recent study examining early esophageal squamous neoplasms, 446 IPCL type V lesions were identified. These were then subclassified as IPCL type V1 (185), type V2 (109), type V3 (104), and type Vn (48). The endoscopic and pathologic diagnoses were analyzed [15]. The sensitivity and specificity of IPCL type V1–V2 for invasion confined to the epithelium/lamina propria (m1/m2) was 89.5% and 79.6%, respectively. The sensitivity and specificity of IPCL type V3 for invasion confined to the muscularis mucosa or slight submucosal invasion (m3/sm1) was 58.7% and 83.8%, respectively. The sensitivity and specificity of IPCL type Vn for deeper invasion (sm2/sm3) was 55.8% and 98.6%, respectively. Thus although

considered specific markers for m3/sm1 and >sm2 lesions, respectively, the low sensitivity of IPCL type V3 and Vn implies that these vascular changes are not high prevalence markers. Therefore, if muscularis mucosa or submucosal invasion is suspected based on tumor morphology, but IPCL types V3 or Vn are not seen, then further evaluation with endoscopic ultrasound (EUS) should be considered to better define depth of invasion.

The pink–silver sign

Neoplastic pharyngoesophageal lesions do not stain with Lugol, but rather display a color change after Lugol application, initially appearing yellow and pink 2–3 min later. This is not observed in noncancerous lesions or in low-grade intraepithelial neoplasia. This color change phenomenon has been termed the "pink color sign" (PCS) and was demonstrated to be sensitive and specific for high-grade intraepithelial neoplasia and invasive cancer [16]. Application of NBI to lesions that display the PCS results in a metallic silver appearance that in some cases can be easier to detect than the PCS. In addition, this "metallic silver sign" (MSS) was shown to have an exceptional diagnostic accuracy of 98.4% in cancerous lesions [17]. The MSS can be recognized approximately 7 min after Lugol staining. This time can be shortened by spraying of sodium thiosulfate solution immediately after Lugol staining. The combination of PCS and MSS is called the "pink–silver sign" (Figures 5.11 and 5.12).

Minute lesions

Detection of diminutive pharyngoesophageal lesions is just as important as detection of larger lesions, if not more so. These smaller lesions offer the greatest opportunity for curative endoscopic resection. When the mucosa is observed under white light, particular care should be taken to identify reddened areas. These can be particularly subtle and easily overlooked if a thorough examination is not performed. The application of NBI allows these subtle reddened areas to become easily identified as brown spots (Figures 5.13 and 5.14). Thus, with the application of NBI, even minute lesions are more readily detected. In a recent series, minute pharyngeal lesions were diagnosed in 93 of approximately 3000 patients that were examined by M-NBI [18]. Of the 93 lesions (all IPCL type IV) that were measured, 62 were approximately 1 mm, 17 were 1–2 mm, and three were greater than 2.1 mm in size. Of the 79 lesions with available histology, five lesions were histologically diagnosed as high-grade dysplasia, 39 as low-grade dysplasia, and 39 as nondysplastic lesions. There were no mucosal or submucosal cancers. This study demonstrated the feasibility of minute lesion detection, in addition to the clinical importance, as some of the minute lesions harbored high-grade dysplasia, which if not resected would likely continue along the dysplasia–carcinoma sequence.

Conclusions

In the pharyngoesophageal squamous epithelium, M-NBI allows detailed examination of the microvasculature. The IPCLs display characteristic changes that reflect tissue atypia and neoplastic invasion depth. With use of the IPCL classification as an adjunct to other measures (i.e., morphologic characteristics observed on conventional endoscopy or EUS), it allows the characterization, prediction of depth of invasion, and accurate stratification of squamous pharyngoesophageal lesions into three management-based groups. As a result of its effectiveness and ease of application, the IPCL classification has been an invaluable tool in daily clinical practice.

 Video clips to accompany this book can be found in the online material at www.wiley.com/go/cohen/NBI

The following videos relate specifically to this chapter:
Video 9 Superficial squamous cell cancer, IIc+IIa
Video 10 Detection and cap EMR of minute focus of early squamous cancer (HGD)
Video 21 Normal squamous esophageal mucosa
Video 22 Esopahgeal squamous high-grade intraepithelial neoplasia

References

1 Rustgi AK, El-Serag HB. Esophageal carcinoma. *N Engl J Med* 2014;371:2499–509.
2 Ono H, Kondo H, Gotoda T *et al.* Endoscopic mucosal resection for treatment of early gastric cancer. *Gut* 2001;48:225–9.
3 Inoue H, Takeshita K, Hori H, Muraoka Y, Yoneshima H, Endo M. Endoscopic mucosal resection with a cap-fitted panendoscope for esophagus, stomach, and colon mucosal lesions. *Gastrointest Endosc* 1993;39:58–62.
4 Inoue H. Magnification endoscopy in the esophagus and stomach. *Dig Endosc* 2001;13:S40–S41.
5 Momma K, Fujiwara J. Endoscopic diagnosis of superficial pharyeal cancer. *J Jpn Soc Gastroenterol* 2009;106:1299–305.
6 Evans JA, Early DS, Chandraskhara V *et al.* The role of endoscopy in the assessment and treatment of esophageal cancer. *Gastrointest Endosc* 2013;77:328–34.
7 Kuwano H, Nishimura Y, Oyama T *et al.* Guidelines for diagnosis and treatment of carcinoma of the esophagus April 2012 edited by the Japan Esophageal Society. *Esophagus* 2015;12:1–30.
8 Ancona E, Rampado S, Cassaro M *et al.* Prediction of lymph node status in superficial esophageal carcinoma. *Ann Surg Oncol* 2008;15:3278–88.
9 Endo M, Yoshino K, Kawano T, Nagai K, Inoue H. Clinicopathologic analysis of lymph node metastasis in surgically resected superficial cancer of the thoracic esophagus. *Dis Esophagus* 2000;13:125–9.
10 Inoue H, Honda T, Nagai K *et al.* Ultra-high magnification endoscopic observation of carcinoma in situ of the esophagus. *Dig Endosc* 1997;9:16–18.
11 Inoue H, Honda T, Yoshida T *et al.* Ultra-high magnification endoscopy of the normal esophageal mucosa. *Dig Endosc* 1996;8:134–8.
12 Inoue H, Kaga M, Ikeda H *et al.* Magnification endoscopy in esophageal squamous cell carcinoma: a review of the intrapapillary capillary loop classification. *Ann Gastroenterol* 2015;28:41–8.
13 Santi EG, Inoue H, Ikeda H *et al.* Microvascular caliber changes in intramucosal and submucosally invasive esophageal cancer. *Endoscopy* 2013;45:585–8.
14 Schlemper RJ, Riddell RH, Kato Y *et al.* The Vienna classification of gastrointestinal epithelial neoplasia. *Gut* 2000;47:251–5.
15 Sato H, Inoue H, Ikeda H *et al.* Utility of intrapapillary capillary loops seen on magnifying narrow-band imaging in estimating invasive depth of esophageal squamous cell carcinoma. *Endoscopy* 2015;47:122–8.
16 Ishihara R, Yamada T, Iishi H *et al.* Quantitative analysis of the color change after iodine staining for diagnosing esophageal high-grade intraepithelial neoplasia and invasive cancer. *Gastrointest Endosc* 2009;69:213–18.
17 Maselli R, Inoue H, Ikeda H *et al.* The metallic silver sign with narrow-band imaging: a new endoscopic predictor for pharyngeal and esophageal neoplasia. *Gastrointest Endosc* 2013;78:551–3.
18 Kumamoto T, Sentani K, Oka S, Tanaka S, Yasui W. Clinicopathological features of minute pharyngeal lesions diagnosed by narrow-band imaging endoscopy and biopsy. *World J Gastroenterol* 2012;18:6468–74.

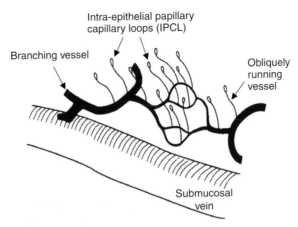

Figure 5.1 Schematic of the pharyngoesophageal microvasculature. Superficial blood vessels in the esophageal mucosa consist of branching vessels that sit above the muscularis mucosa and run horizontally. The IPCLs originate from these branching vessels and run vertically (perpendicular to the lamina propria) extending into the intraepithelial papilla.

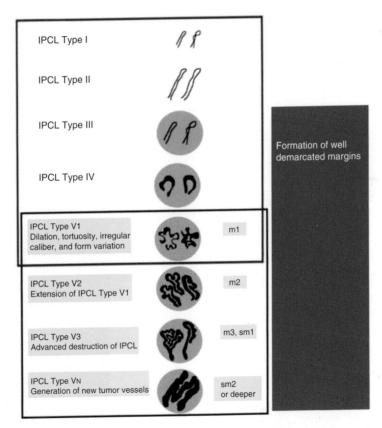

Figure 5.2 IPCL classification. IPCL classification from IPCL type I to type V1 is used for the tissue characterization of flat lesions (red outline). IPCL type V1 to type Vn reflects cancer infiltration depth (blue outline). IPCL type III (group 2) corresponds to borderline lesions that include esophagitis and low-grade intraepithelial neoplasia. In IPCL type IV (group 2), high-grade intraepithelial neoplasia can occur. For type III and type IV IPCLs (group 2), EMR/ESD can be considered depending on morphologic assessment. EMR/ESD is suggested for IPCL types V1 and V2 (group 3A) as they are definite m1 or m2 carcinoma. Diagnostic/therapeutic EMR/ESD should be applied to type V3 (group 3A) lesions, which correspond to m3/sm1 carcinoma. In IPCL type Vn (group 3B) the cancer is associated with sm2 invasion or worse and surgical/chemoradiation treatment is recommended.

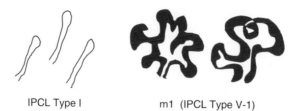

IPCL Type I   m1 (IPCL Type V-1)

Figure 5.3 The IPCL pattern in normal mucosa vs carcinoma in situ (m1). In normal epithelium, IPCLs are observed as a smooth-running small-diameter capillary vessels (IPCL type I/group 1). In carcinoma in situ, IPCLs demonstrate characteristic changes. For m1 lesions (carcinoma in situ) the IPCL pattern displayed is IPCL type V1 (group 3A), which exhibit four characteristic changes: dilation, tortuosity, irregular caliber, and form variation. (Copyright H. Inoue, M. Kaga, Y. Sato, S. Sugaya, and S. Kudo.)

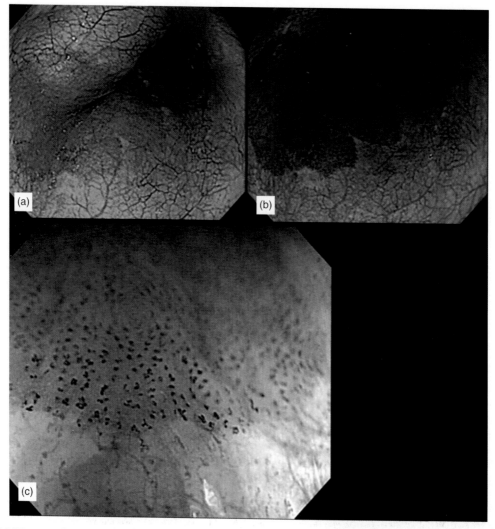

Figure 5.4 Microvasculature of esophageal mucosa in a Paris 0–IIb lesion. (a) Nonmagnifying WLE image showing branching vessels of the normal mucosa and a demarcated reddened area. (b) Nonmagnifying NBI image showing branching vessels of the normal mucosa and a well-demarcated brownish lesion with IPCLs visible as tiny brown dots. (c) M-NBI showing IPCL type V1 (group 3A). Proximal to the lesion normal mucosa with IPCL type 1 (group 1) can be seen. Note the contrast in vessel caliber between IPCL types 1 and V1 (V1 has approximately three times larger caliber) and the slight loss in visibility of the branching vessels in the lesion compared with the adjacent normal mucosa. (Copyright H. Inoue.)

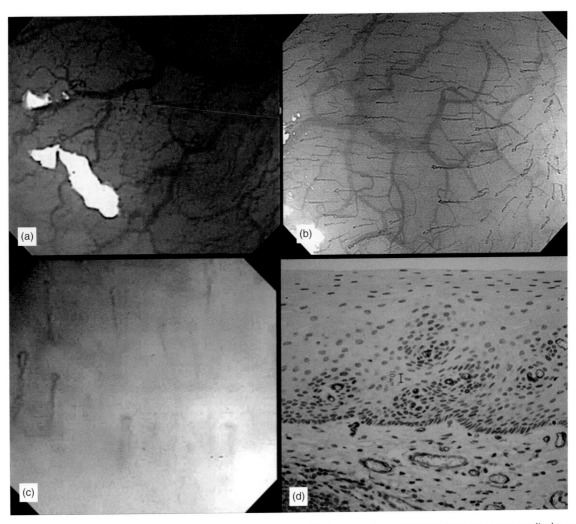

Figure 5.5 Normal mucosa displaying IPCL type I (group 1). (a) Magnifying observation with WLE. The IPCLs run perpendicular to the branching vessel and are observed as red dots with approximately 80× magnification. (b) M-NBI image of IPCL type 1 (group 1). Branching vessels located at the surface of muscularis mucosa are seen as a green vascular network running horizontally. The IPCLs are observed as tiny brown vessels running vertically in the epithelium. (c) WLE image with 150× magnification using prototype Endocytoscope (GIF-Y0001, Olympus Medical Systems, Tokyo, Japan). IPCLs are seen as red loops. (d) Histopathologic image of normal esophageal mucosa with CD34 staining. The IPCLs are seen extending into the epithelium from the branching vessels, which are just above the muscularis mucosa. (Copyright H. Inoue, M. Kaga, Y. Sato, S. Sugaya, and S. Kudo.)

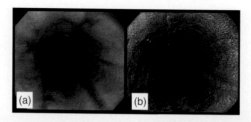

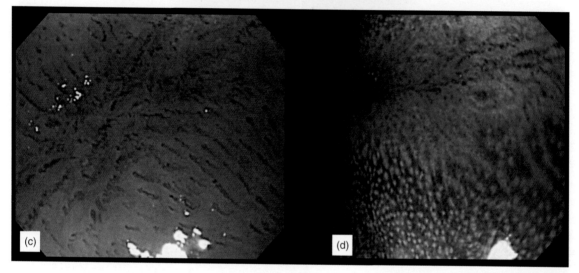

Iodine staining + potassium thiosulfate

Figure 5.6 Gastroesophageal reflux disease displaying IPCL type II (group 1). (a) Nonmagnifying WLE showing Los Angeles classification grade D esophagitis. (b) Nonmagnifying WLE with Lugol staining clearly delineating the eroded mucosa. (c) Magnifying WLE showing IPCL lengthening (engorgement). Important to note the IPCLs are running in the normal vertical axis. The central area of the erosion contains mild degrees of tortuosity. These are mild changes and the lesion margins are not well demarcated (in contrast to neoplastic lesions that are well demarcated). (d) Magnifying WLE with Lugol staining further demonstrating the indistinct margins. (Copyright H. Inoue, M. Kaga, Y. Sato, S. Sugaya, and S. Kudo.)

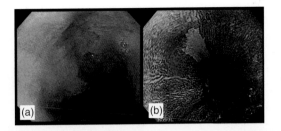

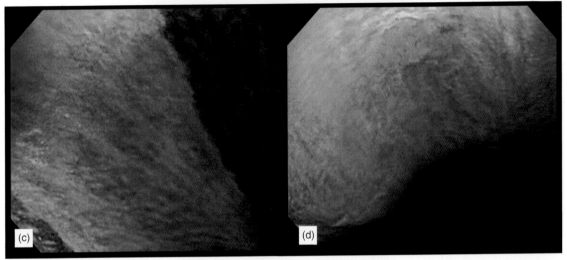

Iodine staining + potassium
thiosulfate

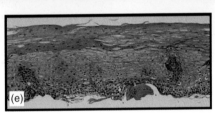

Figure 5.7 Chronic esophagitis displaying IPCL type III (group 2). Although a clearly demarcated Lugol-void lesion is recognized, no changes in IPCLs are seen, indicating lack of proliferating neoplastic vessels. (a) Nonmagnifying WLE image showing a reddened mucosal area. (b) The same area after Lugol staining showing Lugol-void lesion. (c) WLE close-up view of Lugol-void lesion. (d) Magnifying endoscopic view of the same area after application of sodium thiosulfate to the Lugol-stained area. No vessel proliferation was observed. (e) Histopathologic image of biopsy specimen from the Lugol-void lesion, showing diagnosis of chronic esophagitis. (Copyright H. Inoue, M. Kaga, Y. Sato, S. Sugaya, and S. Kudo.)

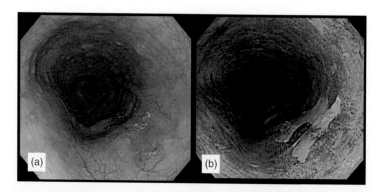

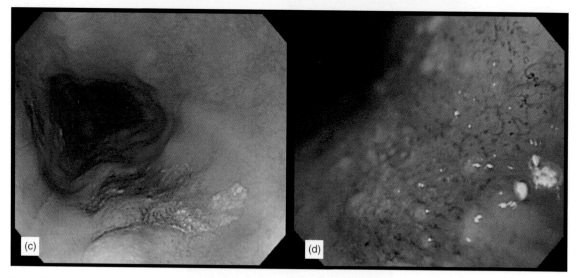

Figure 5.8 A Paris 0–IIb esophageal lesion displaying IPCL type IV (group 2). (a) A subtle erosion is observed on the surface mucosa. (b) With Lugol staining, it is shown as a Lugol-void area with a well-defined margin. (c) Under NBI imaging the lesion displays the MSS. (d) On M-NBI, the changes were consistent with IPCL type IV (group 2).

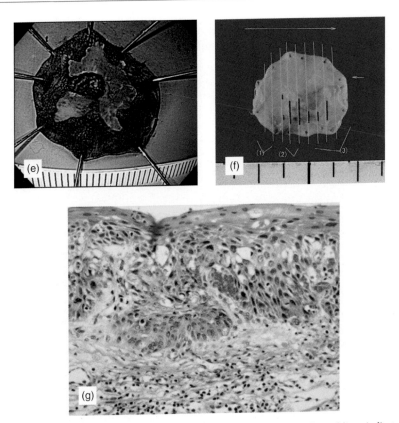

Figure 5.8 (Continued) (e) EMR is performed. Lugol-void area was resected en bloc. (f) The red lines indicate distribution of m1 cancer. IPCL type IV often includes high-grade dysplasia and m1 cancer as in this case. (g) Histopathologic image of the lesion. It was diagnosed as noninvasive high-grade intraepithelial neoplasia. (Copyright H. Inoue, M. Kaga, Y. Sato, S. Sugaya, and S. Kudo.)

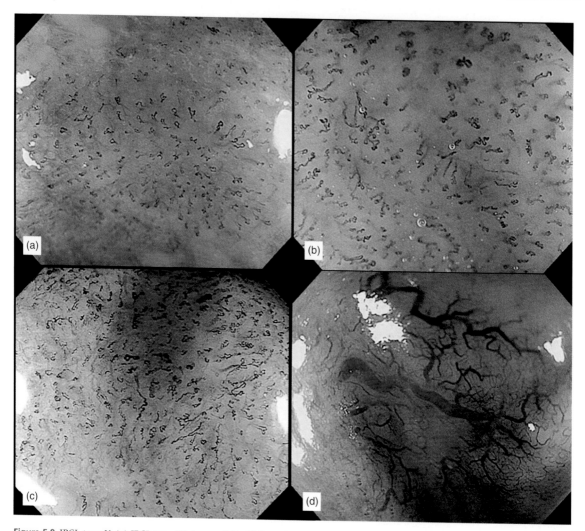

Figure 5.9 IPCL type V. (a) IPCL type V1 (group 3A). All four characteristic changes are seen (dilation, tortuosity, irregular caliber, and form variation), corresponding to carcinoma confined to epithelium (m1). (b) IPCL type V2 (group 3A). Elongation of deformed IPCLs with conserved loop structure, corresponding to carcinoma confined to lamina propria (m2). (c) IPCL type V3 (group 3A). IPCLs with partially destroyed loop structure are identified, corresponding to carcinoma limited to the muscularis mucosa with or without slight invasion into the submucosa (m3/sm1). (d) IPCL type Vn (group 3B). Newly formed abnormal vessels with completely destroyed loop structure, corresponding to deep invasion into submucosa (sm2 or greater). (Copyright H. Inoue.)

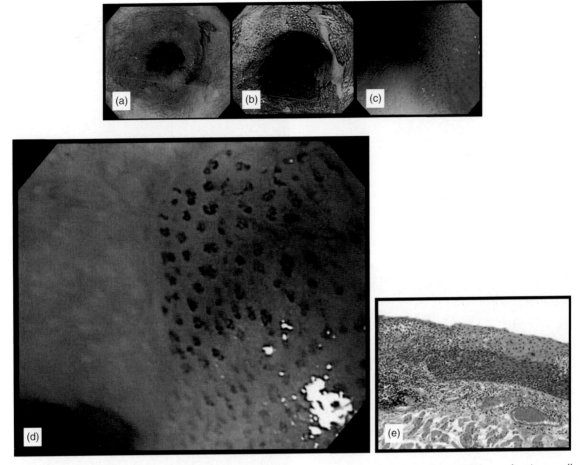

Figure 5.10 An esophageal Paris 0–IIc lesion displaying IPCL type V1 (group 3A). (a) Nonmagnifying WLE image showing a well-demarcated reddened lesion with slight depression. (b) With Lugol staining, the lesion is observed as a Lugol-void area, which corresponds to the reddened area in (a). (c) With magnifying WLE, the reddened area is further examined and IPCLs are seen as red dots. (d) M-NBI showing IPCL type V1 (group 3A). The lesion is diagnosed as a definite m1 and an ESD is performed. (e) Histopathologic diagnosis on the ESD sample is m1. (Copyright H. Inoue, M. Kaga, Y. Sato, S. Sugaya, and S. Kudo.)

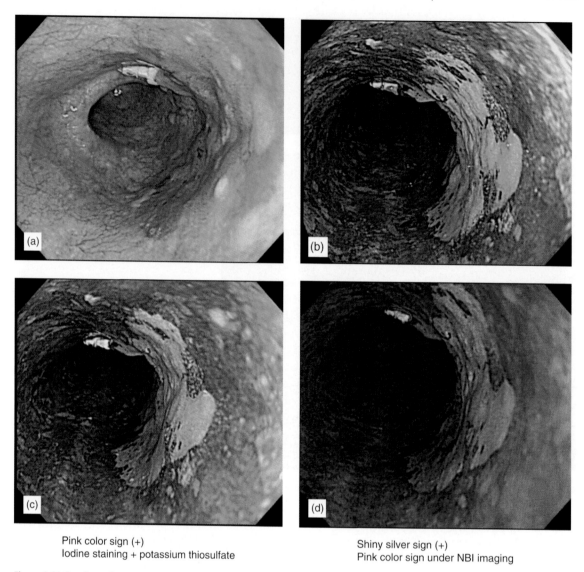

Pink color sign (+)
Iodine staining + potassium thiosulfate

Shiny silver sign (+)
Pink color sign under NBI imaging

Figure 5.11 Esophageal Paris 0–IIa + 0–IIc lesion with IPCL types V1–V3 (group 3A). (a) WLE image with the lesion extending from 1 to 5 o'clock. Nonmagnifying morphology is indicative of deeper than m2 invasion. There was no hard nodule, which would suggest sm2 infiltration. Therefore, the nonmagnification diagnosis was m3/sm1 infiltration. (b) WLE Lugol staining shows a clearly delineated Lugol-void lesion. (c) WLE 2–3 min after Lugol application displaying the pink color sign. (d) NBI image showing MSS.

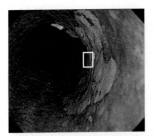

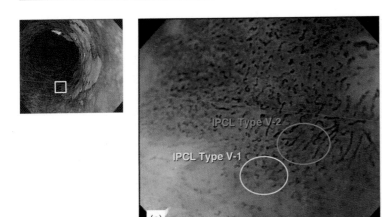

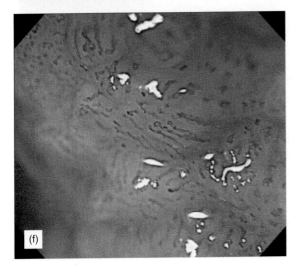

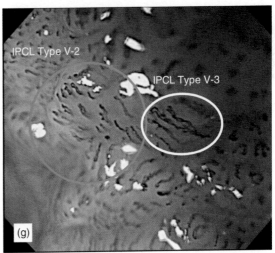

Figure 5.11 (Continued) (e) On M-NBI, IPCL type V1 is observed at the margin of the lesion (yellow circle) and corresponds to m1 invasion depth. The change of IPCL type V2 is observed proximal to the distal margin and corresponds to m2 invasion depth (green circle). (f, g) Within the center of the lesion, IPCL types V2 and V3 are observed (green and white circles, respectively). Note the contrast between white light (f) and NBI (g) images. (continued)

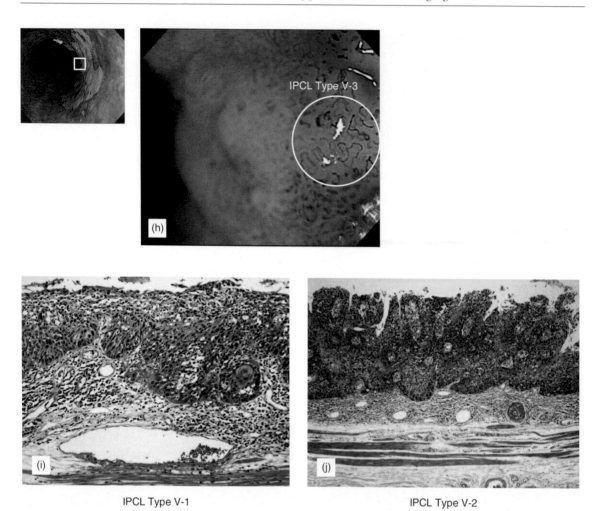

IPCL Type V-1 IPCL Type V-2

Figure 5.11 (Continued) (h) Near the central part of the lesion IPCL type V3 can be seen. These are irregular and deformed IPCLs are seen running transversely (white circle). (i) Histopathology of the margin of the lesion recognized as IPCL type V1, with m1 invasion depth corresponding with (e). (j) Histopathologic specimen showing that most of the lesion is infiltrated as deeply as m2, but there are some areas with invasion very close to the muscularis mucosae and may be diagnosed as m3. (Copyright H. Inoue, M. Kaga, Y. Sato, S. Sugaya, and S. Kudo.)

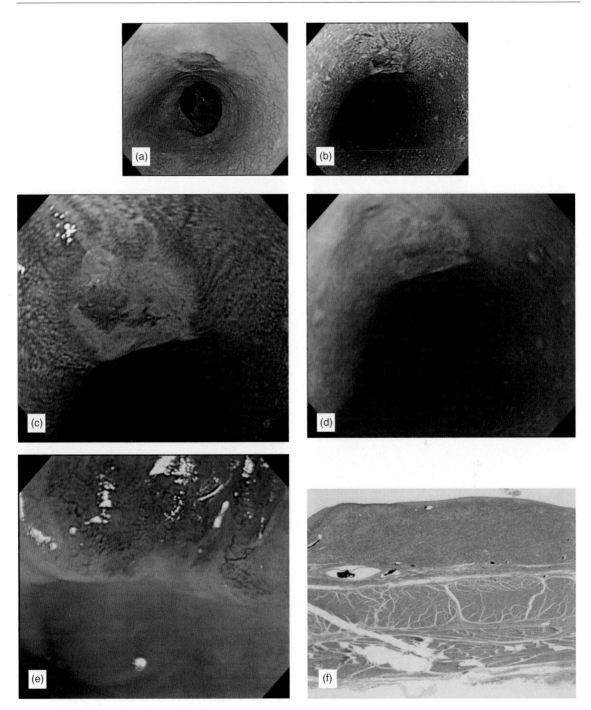

Figure 5.12 Esophageal Paris 0–III lesion displaying IPCL type Vn (group 3B). (a) With WLE, submucosal invasive cancer is suspected due to central excavation with marginal uplift. (b) With WLE and Lugol staining, the area of exposed cancer is seen as Lugol-negative. The area of marginal uplift is Lugol-positive as is an area of depression due to regenerating epithelium after previous biopsy. (c) WLE a few minutes after Lugol. The exposed tumor displays the PCS. (d) NBI a few minutes thereafter displaying MSS, corresponding to the PCS seen under WLE. Together, both (c) and (d) are called the "pink–silver sign." (e) M-NBI showing new large-diameter tumor vessels Vn (new tumor vessel), which are usually running in the horizontal plane. The lesion was diagnosed as sm massive cancer as Vn was found extensively in the lesion. (f) Histopathologic specimen showing squamous cancer, sm2 invasion. (Copyright H. Inoue, M. Kaga, Y. Sato, S. Sugaya, and S. Kudo.)

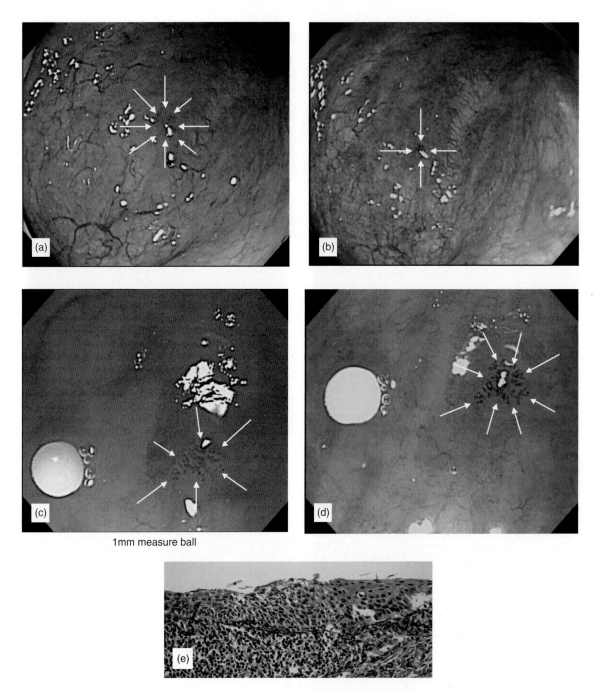

1mm measure ball

Figure 5.13 A 1-mm cancerous lesion in the posterior pharynx. (a) The lesion is observed as a small red spot with WLE. (b) Under NBI, it is recognized as a brown spot (white arrows). (c) Magnification WLE. The white measuring ball has diameter of 1 mm. The lesion (white arrows) is 1 mm in size. (d) M-NBI of lesion showing IPCL type IV (group 3A). (e) Histopathologic specimen showing carcinoma in situ. (Copyright H. Inoue, M. Kaga, Y. Sato, S. Sugaya, and S. Kudo.)

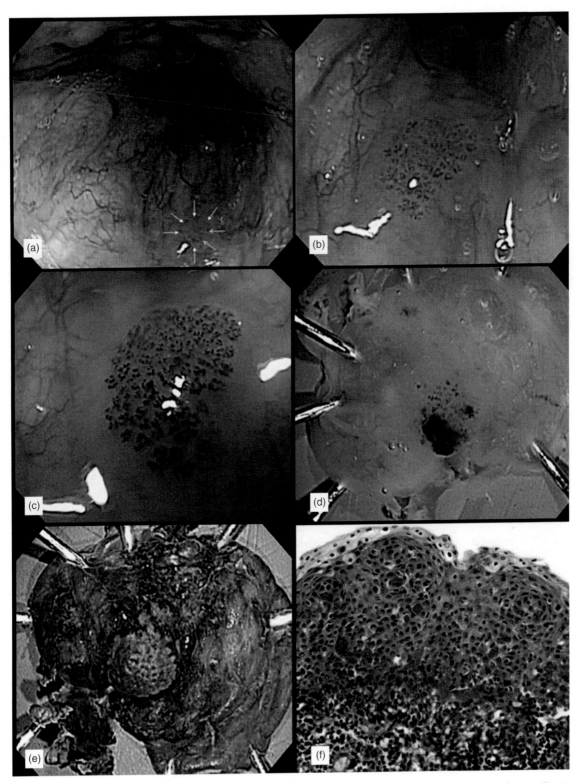

Figure 5.14 A 3-mm cancerous lesion of pharynx. (a) The lesion again is a small reddened area with WLE. (b) With magnification WLE it is more apparent as a red patch. (c) M-NBI showing IPCL V1 (group 3A). (d) Gross specimen. (e) Gross specimen after Lugol stain. (f) Histopathologic specimen showing carcinoma in situ. (Copyright H. Inoue.)

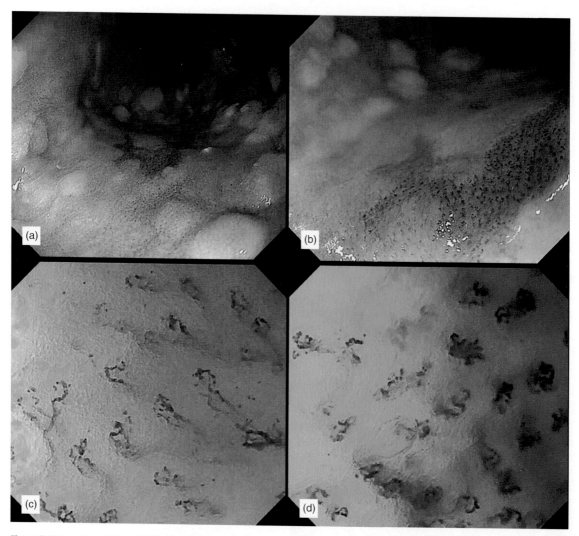

Figure 5.15 Esophageal Paris 0–IIb lesion displaying IPCL type IV/V1 (group 3A). (a) Nonmagnifying NBI showing a well-demarcated brownish lesion. (b) M-NBI showing IPCL type IV/V1 (group 3A). (c) IPCL type IV (group 3A) can be seen in great detail with a prototype Endocytoscope GIF-Y0002, which has up to 380× magnification and NBI. Note that individual red blood cells (approximate diameter 8 μm) can be seen coursing through the IPCLs. (d) Endocytoscopic image with NBI showing IPCL type V1 (group 3A). (Copyright H. Inoue.)

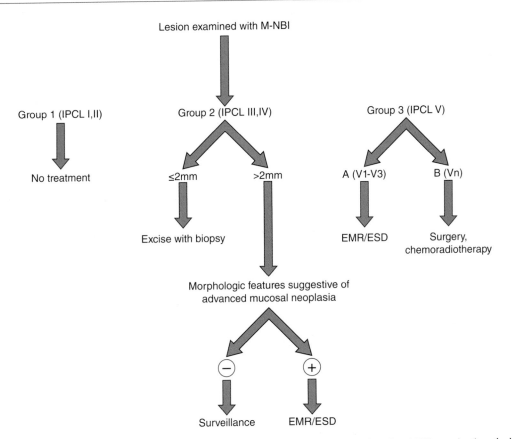

Figure 5.16 Suggested general treatment algorithm using simplified IPCL classification. Based on the M-NBI examination, the lesions can be categorized as group 1, 2 or 3. Group 1 are benign and require no treatment. For lesions in group 2, which correspond to low-grade or high-grade intraepithelial neoplasia, based on their size and collateral morphologic assessment, either surveillance or resection is suggested. Group 3 comprises two subgroups, group 3A which are endoscopically resectable cancers while group 3B are cancers that require more extensive treatment with chemoradiation/surgery. Note that if muscularis mucosa or submucosal invasion is suspected based on tumor morphology, but IPCL types V3 or Vn are not seen, further evaluation with EUS should be performed to define depth of invasion.

6

Applications of NBI HRE and preliminary data: Barrett's esophagus and adenocarcinoma

Anne-Fré Swager, Prateek Sharma, Jacques J. Bergman, and Wouter L. Curvers

Barrett's esophagus and esophageal adenocarcinoma

Barrett's esophagus (BE) is a known precursor lesion of esophageal adenocarcinoma (EAC), a cancer with a steeply rising incidence [1,2]. In BE the lining of the esophageal wall changes from squamous to columnar epithelium, caused by chronic exposure to gastric esophageal reflux. BE is defined as the endoscopic presence of columnar lined epithelium in the distal esophagus and histologic presence of intestinal metaplasia (IM) [3]. Carcinogenesis in BE is not fully unraveled but is believed to occur through a stepwise pattern from low-grade dysplasia (LGD) to high-grade dysplasia (HGD) to adenocarcinoma. Advanced EAC has a dismal prognosis; only 50% of symptomatic patients are eligible for treatment with curative intent. Therefore, the cascade of mucosal changes creates a window of opportunity for early detection of neoplastic lesions, which is of great importance since early-stage lesions can be treated endoscopically with excellent prognosis.

Current guidelines recommend surveillance of Barrett's patients using white light endoscopy (WLE) to obtain targeted biopsies from suspicious lesions, followed by random four-quadrant biopsies for every 2 cm of the Barrett's segment [4]. However, most early neoplastic lesions are subtle and often difficult to see with standard endoscopy. Furthermore, random biopsy protocols are hampered by sampling error that compromises the effectiveness of endoscopic BE surveillance. Advanced imaging techniques may improve the recognition of early neoplastic lesions and potentially make random biopsies obsolete, leading to more cost-effective BE surveillance.

High-resolution endoscopy, chromoendoscopy, and narrowband imaging

High-definition (HD) video endoscopes are equipped with charge coupled devices and have high-quality image sensors delivering clear and high-resolution images with minimal halation and image noise. Most experts advise the use of HD endoscopes for the inspection of BE during endoscopic surveillance. Detailed inspection of the superficial mucosal and vascular patterns (i.e., "mucosal morphology") could be achieved by high-resolution magnification endoscopy, which is technically demanding. In the latest HD gastroscopes (GIF-HQ190, Olympus Inc., Tokyo, Japan) "dual focus" has been introduced that allows easy switching from normal to near focus for detailed inspection of the mucosal morphology (Figures 6.2–6.5). Magnification endoscopy, in combination with chromoendoscopy, has been shown to improve the detection of IM (and to a lesser extent of early neoplasia) in BE [5].

Chromoendoscopy is a technique in which dyes are sprayed on the mucosal surface in order to enhance the detection and/or delineation of early neoplastic lesions. Chromoendoscopy is associated with some important limitations: (i) it requires the use of dyes and spraying catheters and lengthens the total procedure time; (ii) the technique is operator-dependent and requires experience for optimal results; (iii) dye may not spread evenly across the mucosa; (iv) switching between the white light view and the enhanced pattern chromoendoscopy view is impossible; and (v) mucosal morphology consists of both the mucosal and the vascular patterns, of which the latter may be obscured by the use of stains.

Narrowband imaging (NBI) is an endoscopic imaging technique that enhances the mucosal surface contrast without the use of dyes. The technique utilizes differences in wavelength, providing contrast and enhancing visualization of mucosal morphology and vascular patterns. Depending on the endoscopy system, both WLE and NBI can be used in multiple modes: overview, magnification, and near focus.

In general the overview mode is used for the detection of suspicious areas while the near focus or magnification mode is used for the characterization or delineation of areas of interest. In this chapter the potential applications of NBI during BE endoscopy will be discussed as follows: (i) characterization or differentiation of IM and neoplasia; (i) detection of BE neoplasia; (iii) delineation of neoplastic lesions; and (iv) follow-up after endoscopic therapy.

The American Society for Gastrointestinal Endoscopy (ASGE) has published recommendations through the "Preservation and Incorporation of Valuable Endoscopic Innovations" (PIVI) process regarding the performance characteristics that would be required for an imaging technology to be used in BE. This was done specifically to eliminate the need for random biopsies during endoscopic surveillance of patients with nondysplastic BE. The suggested thresholds were a per-patient sensitivity of 90% or more and a negative predictive value of 98% or more for detecting HGD or EAC as compared to the current standard protocol (WLE and targeted plus random biopsies every 2 cm), and a specificity of 80% of more [6].

Characterization of mucosal morphology in Barrett's esophagus

Intestinal metaplasia

Different classification systems for grading mucosal morphology (i.e., mucosal and vascular patterns) with NBI have been proposed [7–10] (Figure 6.1). Goda et al. [9] presented a complex categorization that focused on recognition of IM in columnar-lined esophagus. The accuracy of NBI for the differentiation of IM was assessed by a systematic review with a total of 338 areas with histologically proven IM that were evaluated with NBI. Sensitivities of 77–100%, specificities of 79–94% and overall accuracies of 88–96% were reported [11]. Furthermore, a meta-analysis found comparably high sensitivity and low specificity in a pooled per-lesion analysis (respectively 95% and 65%) [12].

Early neoplasia

More clinically relevant is the characterization of HGD/EAC in BE. Table 6.1 lists several different classification systems for the characterization of early neoplasia in BE with NBI [7,8,10]. Mucosal patterns of neoplastic lesions with NBI are shown in Figures 6.2, 6.5 and 6.6 Kara et al. [7] designed a relatively simple classification with regular versus irregular mucosal and vascular pattern, the so-called Amsterdam 1 classification. The classification of Sharma et al. [8] (Kansas classification) shows resemblance in the vascular pattern, but divided mucosal pattern into the categories ridged/villous, circular, and irregular/distorted. Another classification is designed by Singh et al. [10] (Nottingham classification) who combined sets of mucosal and vascular types in four different categories with descriptions similar to those described by Kara and Sharma. The potential limiting factor for use of these classifications in daily practice is their complexity. Therefore, a simplified consensus-driven NBI classification was developed by Alvarez Herrero et al. [13] (Amsterdam 2 classification), which was based on the similarities between the previously mentioned classifications.

A pooled analysis of five studies on the accuracy of NBI for differentiation of HGD/EAC from LGD or non-dysplastic BE resulted in a sensitivity of 97%, specificity of 94%, and overall accuracy of 96% [11]. A meta-analysis by Mannath et al. [12] reported high numbers for the identification of neoplasia, with per-lesion sensitivity and specificity of 96% and 94%, respectively.

In order to investigate the external validity of the initial positive results, several interobserver studies were

Table 6.1 Classification systems of mucosal morphology for characterizing neoplasia in Barrett's esophagus with NBI.

Mucosal morphology	Classifications			
	Amsterdam 1	Amsterdam 2	Kansas	Nottingham
Mucosal pattern	Regular/flat/irregular	Regular/irregular	Circular/ridge/villous/ irregular/distorted	Round oval pits (type A) Villous/ridge/linear pits (type B) Absent pits (type C) Distorted pits (type D)
Vascular pattern	Regular/irregular	Regular/irregular	Normal/abnormal	Regular microvasculature (types A + B + C) Irregular microvasculature (type D)
Abnormal blood vessels	Absent/present	—	—	—

performed [14–18]. These studies reported disappointing moderate to fair interobserver agreements and no significant differences in diagnostic accuracy and agreement between experienced and inexperienced assessors were found [13–15]. An important limitation of the above-mentioned studies was the use of still images. Therefore, Baldaque Silva *et al.* [14,15] used videos in an attempt to optimally replicate daily endoscopic practice. However, interobserver agreement and accuracy were similar or lower compared with the above-mentioned interobserver studies.

In a multicenter randomized controlled trial performed by expert endoscopists, NBI was used for characterization of suspicious areas detected with WLE and/ or autofluorescence endoscopy [19]. In this real-time NBI evaluation of areas suspicious for neoplasia, 17% of lesions containing HGD/EAC were misclassified as nondysplastic. These real-life results confirmed the disappointing results from the above-mentioned interobserver studies [19].

In conclusion, although initial studies showed promising results for NBI characterization of neoplasia, succeeding validation studies were disappointing. Current classification systems cannot therefore be implemented in daily clinical practice. However, an international working group on Barrett's esophagus (BING) has presented preliminary results on a consensus-driven classification that may improve some of the shortcomings described. Using these BING criteria, especially for high-confidence readings, dysplasia could be identified with high accuracy (92%), sensitivity (91%), specificity (93%), positive predictive value (89%), and negative predictive value (95%) and showed substantial interobserver agreement ($\kappa = 0.681$) [20].

Detection of intestinal metaplasia and early neoplasia

Intestinal metaplasia

At present only one study has investigated the detection of IM using a randomized crossover protocol that compared NBI-targeted biopsies with HD-WLE including standard Seattle protocol biopsies [21]. The results showed no difference in detection of IM between HD-WLE with four-quadrant biopsies and NBI but the latter required significantly fewer biopsies (mean 3.6 per patient with NBI vs. mean 7.6 per patient with HD-WLE). The majority of the IM-specific patterns (e.g., ridge/ villous mucosal) seen with NBI contained IM on histology (sensitivity 94%, specificity 87%). These results from three tertiary BE referral centers seem promising in regard to a more cost-effective biopsy protocol for the detection of IM in columnar-lined epithelium of the distal esophagus, but need to be confirmed in a community practice setting.

Early neoplasia

The hallmark of BE surveillance is the detection of early neoplasia, and for this indication NBI may potentially have the largest impact on improving current clinical practice. Figures 6.2–6.5 and 6.7–6.8 show several examples of subtle lesions within the Barrett's segment on examination with WLE and NBI.

In an unblinded prospective cohort study, it was aimed to compare the Seattle protocol with a targeted biopsy protocol with HD-WLE and NBI. The esophagus was mapped in fixed areas which were examined by one endoscopist first with HD-WLE followed by NBI. Subsequently all areas were biopsied according to the Seattle protocol [22]. NBI had a higher sensitivity for the detection of HGD/EAC than HD-WLE (89% vs. 79%, respectively). The authors concluded that the targeted protocol with HD-WLE and NBI was superior over the random biopsy protocol. However, the sequential and unblinded design hampers good comparison between WLE and NBI and may have considerably biased the outcomes.

In a randomized crossover study with 28 patients comparing HD-WLE followed by NBI with HD-WLE followed by chromoendoscopy, most lesions were detected by HD-WLE and NBI did not significantly increase the number of HGD/EAC cases. However, the study may have been underpowered to detect relevant differences [23].

A more recent prospective, blinded, tandem endoscopy study conducted by Wolfsen *et al.* [24] evaluated 65 patients with previously detected dysplasia with standard resolution WLE (SR-WLE) followed by HD-WLE plus NBI by another endoscopist. Lesions detected with SR-WLE were disclosed for biopsy after NBI-targeted biopsies were obtained. NBI detected a higher grade of dysplasia in more patients compared with SR-WLE (18% vs. 0%; $P < 0.001$) and in 57% of the patients dysplasia was found with NBI compared to 43% with SR-WLE. Additionally, less biopsies needed to be sampled with NBI (NBI 4.7 vs. SRE 8.5; $P < 0.001$). However, this study has some important limitations that may have biased the results. First, during the HD-WLE plus NBI procedure the BE was inspected twice: once with HD-WLE endoscopy and once with NBI. Second, the HD-WLE plus NBI procedures were performed by two endoscopists with extensive experience in NBI and early BE neoplasia, whereas the SR-WLE was performed by general endoscopists with less experience in this field. Third, approximately half of the patients targeted with NBI showing dysplasia contained only indefinite for dysplasia or LGD.

Sharma *et al.* [21] performed a randomized controlled trial comparing HD-WLE plus the standard Seattle biopsy protocol to NBI-targeted biopsies in patients with BE. Patients were randomized to undergo upper endoscopy with either HD-WLE or NBI (without examination with HD-WLE) on day 1 and returned for the alternative procedure performed by a different endoscopist within 3–8 weeks. With NBI more patients with any dysplasia (LGD/HGD/EAC) were detected compared with HD-WLE (39 vs. 32 patients, respectively), which was not a statistically significant difference. An important limitation is that only 14 patients were diagnosed with HGD/EAC and therefore no conclusion can be drawn from this study on the detection performance of NBI for early neoplasia.

A recent ASGE meta-analysis concluded that in a pooled analysis of nine NBI studies, the PIVI thresholds were met [25]. This study and the AGA white paper reached the same conclusion: in the hands of endoscopists consistently achieving the PIVI thresholds, the use of NBI-assisted targeted biopsies is appropriate [26]. However, in all other cases, the current random biopsy protocol should still be performed.

In conclusion, random biopsy sampling still remains the standard of care, whereby experienced endoscopists are endorsed to perform NBI-targeted biopsies. Larger cohort studies in non-academic centers will need to investigate if NBI-targeted biopsies could replace random biopsy sampling.

Delineation of neoplastic lesions and follow-up after radiofrequency ablation

The zoom or magnification endoscope (GIF-Q240Z, Olympus Inc., Tokyo, Japan) works through optical magnification and can be used for delineation of lesions prior to endoscopic resection [7,8,16,25]. The NBI near-focus function is the newest development implemented in the most recent endoscopy systems (NBI EVIS EXERA II 180 and III 190, Olympus Inc., Tokyo, Japan). Near-focus enables more detailed visualization of the mucosal surface by just a click of a button and is therefore a useful tool in distinguishing minute differences in the epithelium (Figure 6.6) [24,26]. Utilizing the near-focus or magnification function for interrogation of the mucosa is technically demanding and generally not applied in BE surveillance outside tertiary referral centers. To our knowledge no formal studies have examined the use of NBI for delineation of early neoplastic lesions in BE. However, in our experience, NBI is superior to HD-WLE for this purpose. Detailed inspection with NBI allows identification of the demarcation line (Figure 6.6), determining subtle differences in mucosal and vascular patterns and slight elevations. In the hands of endoscopists

who are experienced in treatment of BE neoplasia, NBI can be used to determine the differences between transition zones from normal to dysplastic mucosa in order to facilitate lesion delineation, like the delineation performed for resection of early gastric neoplasia [27–29].

NBI is considered a promising technique in the follow-up of BE patients being treated with radiofrequency ablation. Although we have demonstrated that NBI cannot reliably predict the presence or absence of IM at the neosquamo-columnar junction, NBI may allow the detection of small residual islands of Barrett's mucosa that are easily overlooked with HD-WLE [28,30]. Recent studies suggest that detailed inspection with NBI of the neosquamous epithelium after endoscopic therapy is probably more useful than obtaining random biopsy specimens [31].

Conclusion and future perspectives

NBI is one of the most widely studied imaging techniques for BE. Since it is a simple and user-friendly technique, it is a promising system for the detection of neoplasia during BE surveillance. However, no consensus has been reached on the different NBI classification systems for grading mucosal morphology. However, an international working group on BE (BING) has developed a consensus-driven classification that may improve some of the shortcoming of currently proposed criteria. Furthermore, NBI has not yet proven to be accurate enough as a neoplasia characterization and detection tool, in order to potentially replace random biopsy sampling by NBI-targeted sampling.

Currently the most important clinical applications of NBI in BE are as an auxiliary delineation tool prior to resection of neoplastic lesions and for inspection of neosquamous epithelium after radiofrequency ablation.

 Video clips to accompany this book can be found in the online material at www.wiley.com/go/cohen/NBI

The following videos relate specifically to this chapter:
Video 12 Measuring hiatal hernia and Barrett's landmarks
Video 13 NBI detection of focal dysplasia in Barrett's esophagus using cap examination
Video 14 Band EMR of focal high-grade dysplasia in Barrett's
Video 15 Radiofrequency ablation of Barrett's tongues
Video 16 Barrett's cap EMR of high-grade dysplasia
Video 23 Barrett's high-grade intraepithelial neoplasia
Video 24 Barrett's carcinoma of the gastroesophageal junction
Video 25 Long-segment Barrett's esophagus with low-grade dysplasia
Video 26 NBI in a patient with C9M9 Barrett's esophagus

References

1 Post PN, Siersema PD, Van Dekken H. Rising incidence of clinically evident Barrett's oesophagus in The Netherlands: a nation-wide registry of pathology reports. *Scand J Gastroenterol* 2007;42:17–22.

2 Pohl H, Sirovich B, Welch HG. Esophageal adenocarcinoma incidence: are we reaching the peak? *Cancer Epidemiol Biomarkers Prev* 2010;19:1468–70.

3 Wang KK, Sampliner RE. Updated guidelines 2008 for the diagnosis, surveillance and therapy of Barrett's esophagus. *Am J Gastroenterol* 2008;103:788–97.

4 Spechler SJ, Sharma P, Souza RF, Inadomi JM, Shaheen NJ. American Gastroenterological Association medical position statement on the management of Barrett's esophagus. *Gastroenterology* 2011;140:1084–91.

5 Bruno MJ. Magnification endoscopy, high resolution endoscopy, and chromoscopy: towards a better optical diagnosis. *Gut* 2003;52(Suppl 4):iv7–11.

6 Sharma P, Savides TJ, Canto MI et al. The American Society for Gastrointestinal Endoscopy PIVI (Preservation and Incorporation of Valuable Endoscopic Innovations) on imaging in Barrett's esophagus. *Gastrointest Endosc* 2012;76:252–4.

7 Kara MA, Ennahachi M, Fockens P, ten Kate FJ, Bergman JJ. Detection and classification of the mucosal and vascular patterns (mucosal morphology) in Barrett's esophagus by using narrow band imaging. *Gastrointest Endosc* 2006;64:155–66.

8 Sharma P, Bansal A, Mathur S et al. The utility of a novel narrow band imaging endoscopy system in patients with Barrett's esophagus. *Gastrointest Endosc* 2006;64:167–75.

9 Goda K, Tajiri H, Ikegami M, Urashima M, Nakayoshi T, Kaise M. Usefulness of magnifying endoscopy with narrow band imaging for the detection of specialized intestinal metaplasia in columnar-lined esophagus and Barrett's adenocarcinoma. *Gastrointest Endosc* 2007;65:36–46.

10 Singh R, Anagnostopoulos GK, Yao K, Yao K et al. Narrowband imaging with magnification in Barrett's esophagus: validation of a simplified grading system of mucosal morphology patterns against histology. *Endoscopy* 2008;40:457–63.

11 Curvers WL, van den Broek FJ, Reitsma JB, Dekker E, Bergman JJ. Systematic review of narrow-band imaging for the detection and differentiation of abnormalities in the esophagus and stomach (with video). *Gastrointest Endosc* 2009;69:307–17.

12 Mannath J, Subramanian V, Hawkey CJ, Ragunath K. Narrow band imaging for characterization of high grade dysplasia and specialized intestinal metaplasia in Barrett's esophagus: a meta-analysis. *Endoscopy* 2010;42:351–9.

13 Alvarez Herrero L, Curvers WL, Bansal A et al. Zooming in on Barrett oesophagus using narrow-band imaging: an international observer agreement study. *Eur J Gastroenterol Hepatol* 2009;21:1068–75.

14 Baldaque Silva F, Dinis-Ribeiro M, Vieth M et al. Endoscopic assessment and grading of Barrett's esophagus using magnification endoscopy and narrow-band imaging: accuracy and interobserver agreement of different classification systems (with videos). *Gastrointest Endosc* 2011;73:7–14.

15 Baldaque Silva F, Marques M, Lunet N et al. Endoscopic assessment and grading of Barrett's esophagus using magnification endoscopy and narrow band imaging: impact of structured learning and experience on the accuracy of the Amsterdam classification system. *Scand J Gastroenterol* 2013;48:160–7.

16 Curvers WL, Bohmer CJ, Mallant-Hent RC et al. Mucosal morphology in Barrett's esophagus: interobserver agreement and role of narrow band imaging. *Endoscopy* 2008;40:799–805.

17 Curvers WL, Baak L, Kiesslich R et al. Chromoendoscopy and narrow-band imaging compared with high-resolution magnification endoscopy in Barrett's esophagus. *Gastroenterology* 2008;134:670–9.

18 Singh M, Bansal A, Curvers WL et al. Observer agreement in the assessment of narrowband imaging system surface patterns in Barrett's esophagus: a multicenter study. *Endoscopy* 2011;43:745–51.

19 Curvers WL, Alvarez Herrero L, Wallace MB et al. Endoscopic tri-modal imaging is more effective than standard endoscopy in identifying early-stage neoplasia in Barrett's esophagus. *Gastroenterology* 2010;139:1106–14.

20 Alsop BR, Bergman JJ, Goda K et al. Development and validation of a NBI classification system for the prediction of dysplasia in Barrett's esophagus (BE): consensus results from an International Working Group. *Gastroenterology* 2015;148(Suppl 1):S-91.

21 Sharma P, Hawes RH, Bansal A et al. Standard endoscopy with random biopsies versus narrow band imaging targeted biopsies in Barrett's oesophagus: a prospective, international, randomised controlled trial. *Gut* 2013;62:15–21.

22 Jayasekera C, Taylor AC, Desmond PV, Macrae F, Williams R. Added value of narrow band imaging and confocal laser endomicroscopy in detecting Barrett's esophagus neoplasia. *Endoscopy* 2012;44:1089–95.

23 Kara MA, Peters FP, Rosmolen WD et al. High-resolution endoscopy plus chromoendoscopy or narrow-band imaging in Barrett's esophagus: a prospective randomized crossover study. *Endoscopy* 2005;37:929–36.

24 Wolfsen HC, Crook JE, Krishna M et al. Prospective, controlled tandem endoscopy study of narrow band imaging for dysplasia detection in Barrett's esophagus. *Gastroenterology* 2008;135:24–31.

25 Thosani N, Abu Dayyeh BK, Sharma P *et al.* ASGE Technology Committee systematic review and meta-analysis assessing the ASGE Preservation and Incorporation of Valuable Endoscopic Innovations thresholds for adopting real-time imaging-assisted endoscopic targeted biopsy during endoscopic surveillance. *Gastrointest Endosc* 2016;83:684–698e7.

26 Sharma P, Brill J, Canto M *et al.* White Paper AGA: advanced imaging in Barrett's esophagus. *Clin Gastroenterol Hepatol* 2015;13:2209–18.

27 Anagnostopoulos GK, Yao K, Kaye P, Hawkey CJ, Ragunath K. Novel endoscopic observation in Barrett's oesophagus using high resolution magnification endoscopy and narrow band imaging. *Aliment Pharmacol Ther* 2007;26:501–7.

28 Singh R, Shahzad MA, Tam W *et al.* Preliminary feasibility study using a novel narrow-band imaging system with dual focus magnification capability in Barrett's esophagus: is the time ripe to abandon random biopsies? *Dig Endosc* 2013;25(Suppl 2):151–6.

29 Nagahama T, Yao K, Maki S *et al.* Usefulness of magnifying endoscopy with narrow-band imaging for determining the horizontal extent of early gastric cancer when there is an unclear margin by chromoendoscopy (with video). *Gastrointest Endosc* 2011;74:1259–67.

30 Okada K, Fujisaki J, Kasuga A *et al.* Diagnosis of undifferentiated type early gastric cancers by magnification endoscopy with narrow-band imaging. *J Gastroenterol Hepatol* 2011;26:1262–9.

31 Sumiyama K, Kaise M, Nakayoshi T *et al.* Combined use of a magnifying endoscope with a narrow band imaging system and a multibending endoscope for en bloc EMR of early stage gastric cancer. *Gastrointest Endosc* 2004;60:79–84.

32 Alvarez Herrero L, Curvers WL, Bisschops R *et al.* Narrow band imaging does not reliably predict residual intestinal metaplasia after radiofrequency ablation at the neosquamo columnar junction. *Endoscopy* 2014;46:98–104.

33 Phoa KN, Pouw RE, van Vilsteren FG *et al.* Remission of Barrett's esophagus with early neoplasia 5 years after radiofrequency ablation with endoscopic resection: a Netherlands cohort study. *Gastroenterology* 2013;145:96–104.

34 Sharma P, Bergman JJGHM, Goda K *et al.* Development and validation of a classification system to identify high-grade dysplasia and esophageal adenocarcinoma in Barrett's esophagus using narrow band imaging. *Gastroenterology* 2016;150:591–8.

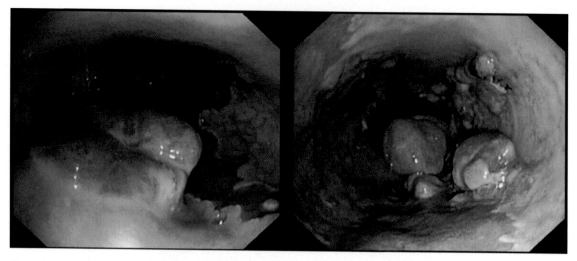

Figure 6.1 Esophageal adenocarcinoma.

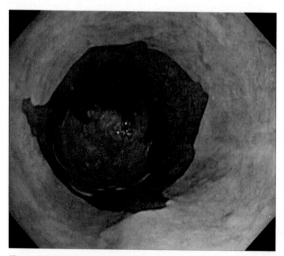

Figure 6.2 Barrett's esophagus.

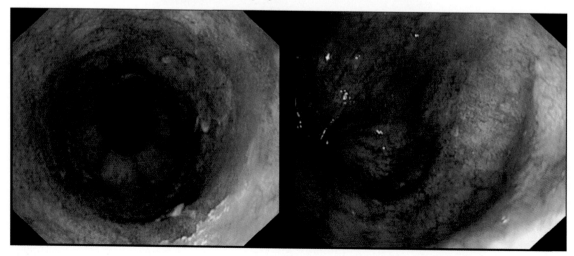

Figure 6.3 Two images with discrete early neoplastic lesions in a BE at the 3 o'clock position.

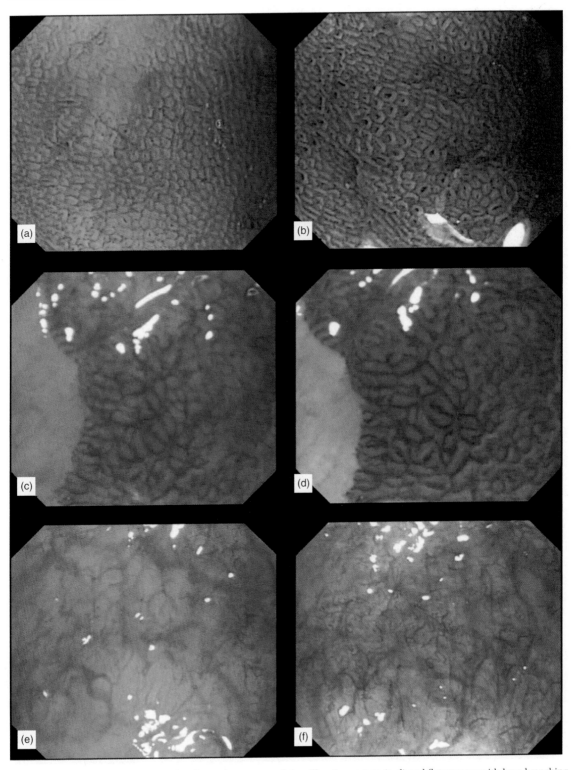

Figure 6.4 Examples of regular mucosal and vascular patterns of the villous/gyrus type (a–d) and flat mucosa with long-branching blood vessels (e and f). All these images contain nondysplastic BE.

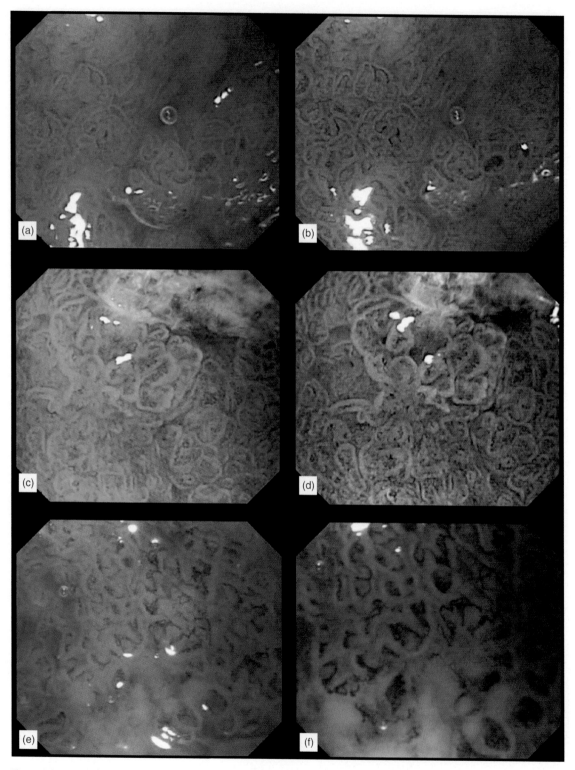

Figure 6.5 Examples of dysplastic BE with irregular and distorted mucosal and vascular patterns (a–d) and abnormal blood vessels (e and f).

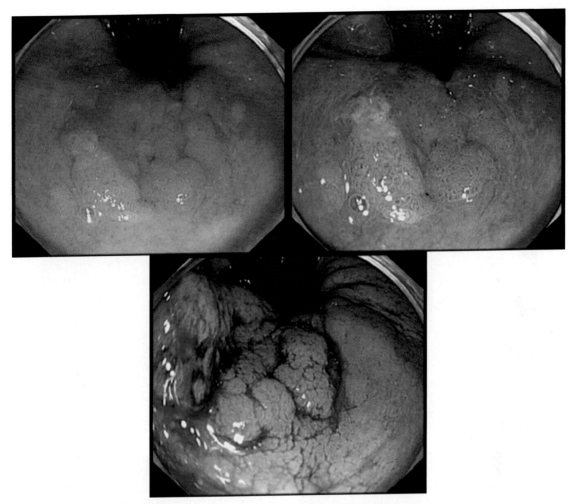

Figure 6.6 Imaging of an early neoplastic lesion in BE using high-resolution endoscopy, narrowband imaging and indigocarmine chromoendoscopy.

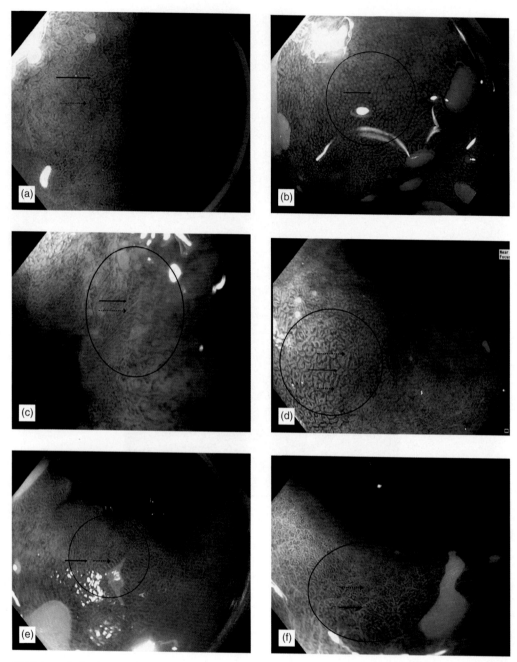

Figure 6.7 High-resolution images of nondysplastic BE using NBI. (a) Note the presence of circular mucosal patterns (solid arrow) that are arranged in an orderly fashion and blood vessels that clearly follow the mucosal architecture (dashed arrow). (b) Note the presence of circular mucosal patterns that are arranged in an orderly fashion and blood vessels that clearly follow the normal architecture of mucosa (solid arrow). (c) Note the presence of circular mucosal patterns (solid arrow) that are arranged in an orderly fashion and blood vessels that clearly follow the architecture of the mucosal ridges (dashed arrow). (d) Note the presence of ridge/villous mucosal patterns (solid arrow) that are arranged in an orderly fashion and blood vessels that are arranged in a regular fashion between the mucosal ridges (dashed arrows). (e) Note the presence of circular mucosal patterns (solid arrow) that are arranged in an orderly fashion and blood vessels that follow the architecture of the mucosa (dashed arrow). (f) Note the presence of circular (solid black arrow) and ridge/villous (red arrow) mucosal patterns arranged in an orderly fashion and blood vessels that follow the mucosal ridge architecture (dashed arrow). *Source*: Sharma *et al.* [34]. Reproduced with permission of Elsevier.

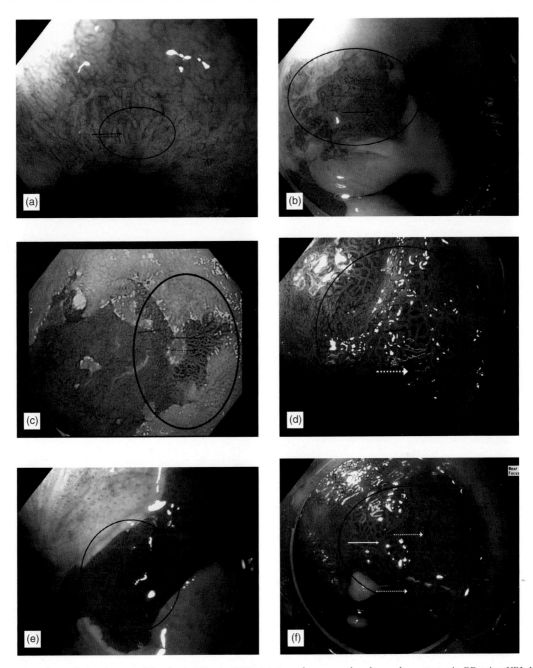

Figure 6.8 High-resolution images of dysplastic BE using NBI. (a) Irregular mucosal and vascular patterns in BE using NBI. Note the irregular mucosal pattern (black arrow) and vascular pattern (red arrow). (b) Irregular mucosal and vascular patterns in BE using NBI. Note the irregular mucosal pattern (black arrow) and vascular pattern (red arrow). The vessels do not follow the normal architecture of the mucosa. (c) Irregular mucosal and vascular patterns in BE using NBI. Note the irregular mucosal pattern (solid black arrow) and vascular pattern (dashed arrow). In contrast, red arrow shows area on the mucosa where vessels are arranged in a regular fashion that follow the normal architecture of the mucosa. (d) Irregular mucosal and vascular patterns in BE using NBI. Note the irregular mucosal and vascular patterns (dashed arrow). The focally or diffusely distributed vessels do not follow the normal architecture of the mucosa. (e) Irregular mucosal and vascular patterns in BE using NBI. Note the irregular mucosal and vascular patterns (solid arrow), while the dashed arrow in contrast shows regularly arranged mucosal and vascular pattern. (f) Irregular mucosal and vascular patterns in BE using NBI. Note the irregular mucosal pattern (solid arrow) and vascular patterns (dashed arrows). *Source*: Sharma *et al.* [34]. Reproduced with permission of Elsevier.

SECTION 2
Stomach and Duodenum

7 Clinical application of magnification endoscopy with NBI in the stomach and the duodenum

Kenshi Yao, Takashi Nagahama, Fumihito Hirai, Suketo Sou, Toshiyuki Matsui, Hiroshi Tanabe, Akinori Iwashita, Philip Kaye, and Krish Ragunath

Introduction

Currently, within the stomach and the duodenum, there is no evidence to demonstrate the clinical usefulness of narrowband imaging (NBI) during non-magnifying endoscopic observation for the purpose of detecting abnormal pathology. However, several clinical applications are possible if NBI is applied to the magnification endoscopy technique in the stomach and the duodenum. Hence, in this chapter, we describe the clinical usefulness of magnification endoscopy when used in conjuction with NBI.

Basic principles for the analysis of magnified endoscopic findings

When analyzing the magnified endoscopic findings, there are two distinctly different anatomic findings which need to be examined [1]:
1 the subepithelial microvascular (MV) architecture;
2 the mucosal microsurface (MS) structure.
We should analyze these findings independently. By white light alone, only the MV architecture can be noted, but when we utilize NBI both the MV architecture and the MS structure can be visualized.

Magnification endoscopy procedure

The preparation of the patient for magnification endoscopy is the same as that for standard endoscopy. The endoscopy procedures described and illustrated in this chapter were performed using a high-resolution magnifying upper gastrointestinal endoscope (GIF-Q240Z,

Olympus, Tokyo, Japan) and the Olympus EVIS LUCERA SPECTRUM system. The structure-enhancement function of the video processor is set at a level of 4, 6, or 8 (level 4 or 6 for non-magnified observation and level 8 for magnified observation). Prior to endoscopy, a black soft hood (MB-162, Olympus, Tokyo) is attached to the tip of the scope (Figure 7.1) to enable the endoscopist to fix the focal distance at 3 mm between the tip of the scope and the mucosal surface at maximal magnification [2]. In practice, when a lesion on the gastric mucosa is found during non-magnifying observation, visualization of the lesion is immediately zoomed up to maximal magnification, and then the tip of the scope is allowed to contact the mucosa immediately after reaching the maximal magnification level. In this system, one can easily change the light source to either white light or NBI by using a button on the handle of the scope.

The stomach

In the stomach, the NBI technique is only useful when applied to magnification endoscopy. From a technical point of view, the mucosal image obtained by NBI when observing without magnification is too dark and noisy for meaningful investigation because the lumen of the stomach is large.

Normal gastric mucosa (Figures 7.2 and 7.3)
Basically, magnified endoscopy of normal gastric mucosa without pathologic change (e.g., *Helicobacter pylori* infection) produces different findings depending on which part of the stomach is being viewed, i.e., the gastric body or the gastric antrum [3–5].

Comprehensive Atlas of High-Resolution Endoscopy and Narrowband Imaging, Second Edition. Edited by Jonathan Cohen.
© 2017 John Wiley & Sons, Ltd. Published 2017 by John Wiley & Sons, Ltd.
Companion website: www.wiley.com/go/cohen/NBI

With regard to the MV architecture in the normal gastric body (Figure 7.2a), this shows a honeycomb-like subepithelial capillary network (SECN) pattern with collecting venules (CVs) (Figure 7.2b). More precisely, a polygonal loop of subepithelial capillary surrounds each gastric pit and these loops form a honeycomb-like network beneath the epithelium and converge onto a CV. By magnification with NBI, the MS structure becomes evident, namely the pits demonstrate a round or oval shape (Figure 7.2c). If there is no pathologic change such as *H. pylori* gastritis in the mucosa, both the MV architecture and the MS structure constantly show a regular shape and arrangement [6–8].

On the other hand, the gastric antrum demonstrates distinctly different magnified endoscopic findings from those of the gastric body. In the MV architecture, the antral mucosa depicts a coil-shaped SECN (Figure 7.3b) [3]. CVs are rarely observed on the mucosal surface in the gastric antrum because anatomically the CV is thought to be located in a deeper part of the lamina propria in the gastric antrum than in the gastric body [5]. With regard to the MS structure of the gastric antrum, it also shows a quite different pattern from that of the gastric body. According to the classical convention, the gastric pits are thought to be round, but this idea is not correct. The pits demonstrate a linear or reticular pattern. Each coil-shaped subepithelial capillary is located in an apical part which is separated by a linear or reticular crypt opening [3]. This characteristic MV architecture together with the MS structure can be clearly visualized when NBI is applied to magnification endoscopy (Figure 7.3c).

Chronic gastritis

Magnification endoscopy has also been reported to be useful for identifying *H. pylori*-associated gastritis and gastric atrophy (Figure 7.4) [6–8]. Briefly, the magnified endoscopic findings in the gastric body mucosa have been categorized into four types: type 1, honeycomb-like SECN with regular arrangement of CVs and regular round pits; type 2, honeycomb-like SECN with regular round pits, but loss of CVs; type 3, loss of normal SECN and CVs, with enlarged white pits surrounded by erythema; and type 4, loss of normal SECN and round pits together with an irregular arrangement of CVs [7]. Type 1 pattern is highly predictive for normal gastric mucosa with negative findings for *H. pylori* infection. Type 2 or 3 pattern is predictive for *H. pylori*-infected stomach, while type 4 pattern is predictive for gastric atrophy. This classification was made through modification of the original findings of both Yagi *et al.* [6] and Nakagawa *et al.* [8].

Uedo *et al.* [9] reported an interesting concept and new application of NBI with magnifying endoscopy for the diagnosis of gastric intestinal metaplasia (Figure 7.5). They indicated that a distinctive finding called "light blue crest" (LBC) was a good indicator of histologic intestinal metaplasia, which is a risk factor for the development of differentiated (intestinal)-type gastric cancer. The LBC was defined as a fine blue–white line on the crests of the epithelial surface or gyri as visualized by magnification endoscopy with NBI. This appearance is speculated to be caused by reflection of the short and narrow wavelength light (400–430 nm) at the surface of the ciliated tissue structure, i.e., the brush border in the gastric intestinal metaplasia and the duodenum. Current applications of this finding have not yet been established, but it could play a key role in the approach to the pathogenesis of chronic metaplastic gastritis as visualized by endoscopy.

Early gastric cancer

In 2001–2002, we published the first reports of unique magnified endoscopic findings based on MV architecture characteristics for early gastric cancer [2,3]. These findings differed depending on the histologic type, namely differentiated carcinoma (intestinal type) or undifferentiated carcinoma (diffuse type) (Table 7.1).

With regard to differentiated carcinoma (Figure 7.6), briefly, the surrounding noncancerous mucosa showed an SECN which was regular in both shape and arrangement. In contrast, the regular SECN pattern had disappeared at the margin of the carcinoma and instead microvessels which were irregular in both shape and arrangement had proliferated within the cancerous mucosa (irregular microvascular pattern, IMVP). In addition, a clear demarcation line (DL) could be noted between the cancerous and the noncancerous mucosa. The presence of a DL and the disappearance of the regular SECN pattern were explained by the histologic findings in which cancerous tissue replaces noncancerous tissue when it extends horizontally.

Microvessels irregular in both shape and arrangement are thought to be tumorous vessels that have proliferated within the carcinomatous interstitial tissue, which shows irregularity in its histologic findings. These findings were thought to be useful in clinical practice for making a correct diagnosis between superficial cancer and focal gastritis [10] and for determining the margin of the carcinoma

Table 7.1 Magnified endoscopic findings characteristic for early gastric cancer.

Differentiated carcinoma (intestinal type)
1 Disappearance of regular SECN pattern
2 A demarcation line (DL)
3 Irregular microvascular pattern (IMVP)
Undifferentiated carcinoma (diffuse type)
1 Reduced MV pattern

prior to endoscopic resection [11,12]. On the other hand, with regard to undifferentiated carcinoma, the cancerous mucosa only showed reduced density of the SECN pattern (Figure 7.7). Other examples of how the information from high-resolution endoscopy (HRE) NBI with magnification can be used to differentiate between cancer and berign gastritis, as well as detect neoplasm invisible on standard endoscopy, are shown in Figures 7.8–7.11.

The duodenum

Normal duodenal mucosa

By magnification endoscopy, finger- or leaf-like villi with a smooth surface that is regular in arrangement can be observed. NBI enables the endoscopist to obtain a clear view of the LBC at the edge of the villi and the intravillous capillary loop network (Figure 7.12).

Celiac disease

Magnification endoscopy can enable the endoscopist to not only detect villous atrophy [13] but also assess the degree of villous atrophy [14]. A scoring system (Z score) was proposed for grading the appearance of villous atrophy: Z1 for normal mucosa, Z2 for blunted villi, Z3 for markedly blunted villi (with ridges and pits), and Z4 for flat mucosa [14]. This scoring system seemed to be well correlated with histologic assessment of villous atrophy. It was suggested that if we applied NBI to this magnification endoscopy, this grading system may remain accurate without the necessity for dye spraying, since NBI can optically enhance both the MS structure and the MV architecture. Celiac disease is one of the promising indications for magnification endoscopy with NBI, as well illustrated by Figures 7.13–7.15.

Conclusion

Numerous findings by magnification endoscopy with NBI are still under investigation. Nevertheless, the most important advantage of this technique is that it can visualize both the MV architecture and the MS structure without the need to introduce any artificial materials (such as dye) into the human body. In the near future, magnification endoscopy with NBI is expected to be practiced as a standard endoscopy technique that is quick, safe, and accurate for making a precise diagnosis of gastrointestinal pathology.

Acknowledgment

We wish to thank Miss Katherine Miller (Royal English Language Centre, Fukuoka, Japan) for revising the English.

 Video clips to accompany this book can be found in the online material at www.wiley.com/go/cohen/NBI

The following videos relate specifically to this chapter:
Video 27 Normal stomach
Video 28 Systematic white light EGD examination
Video 29 Systematic NBI H190 EGD examination
Video 30 Gastric body: gastritis
Video 31 Gastric body: early gastric cancer, type IIb, differentiated type
Video 32 Gastric angle: early gastric cancer, type IIb, differentiated to undifferentiated type
Video 33 Gastric body: early gastric cancer, type IIc, differentiated type
Video 34 Gastric cardia: early cancer, type IIc, undifferentiated type
Video 35 Low-grade gastric dysplasia
Video 36 NBI detection of poorly differentiated superficial gastric cancer not seen on white light
Video 37 Endoscopic submucosal dissection of superficial gastric cancer
Video 40 Normal duodenum
Video 41 Duodenal AVMs
Video 42 Saline injection polypectomy of sessile duodenal adenoma
Video 43 Large duodenal adenoma in patient with familial adenomatous polyposis
Video 76 Normal ileum with stool mimicking a lesion

References

1 Yao K, Iwashita A. Clinical application of zoom endoscopy for the stomach [Japanese with English abstract]. *Gastroenterol Endosc* 2006;48:1091–101.
2 Yao K, Oishi T, Matsui T, Yao T, Iwashita A. Novel magnified endoscopic findings of microvascular architecture in intramucosal gastric cancer. *Gastrointest Endosc* 2002;56:279–84.
3 Yao K, Oishi T. Microgastroscopic findings of mucosal microvascular architecture as visualized by magnifying endoscopy. *Dig Endosc* 2001;13:S27–S33.
4 Yao K. Gastric microvascular architecture as visualized by magnifying endoscopy: body mucosa and antral mucosa without pathological change demonstrate two different patterns of microvascular architecture. *Gastrointest Endosc* 2004;59:596–7.
5 Gannon B. The vasculature and lymphatic drainage. In: Whitehead R, ed. *Gastrointestinal and Oesophageal Pathology*. Edinburgh: Churchill Livingstone, 1995, pp. 129–99.
6 Yagi K, Nakamura A, Sekine A. Characteristic endoscopic and magnified endoscopic findings in the normal stomach without *Helicobacter pylori* infection. *J Gastroenterol Hepatol* 2002;17:39–45.

7 Anagnostopoulos GK, Yao K, Kaye P *et al.* High-resolution magnification endoscopy can reliably identify normal gastric mucosa, *Helicobacter pylori*-associated gastritis, and gastric atrophy. *Endoscopy* 2007;39:1–6.

8 Nakagawa S, Kato M, Shimizu Y *et al.* Relationship between histopathologic gastritis and mucosal microvascularity: observation with magnifying endoscopy. *Gastrointest Endosc* 2003;58:71–5.

9 Uedo N, Ishihara R, Iishi H *et al.* A new method of diagnosing gastric intestinal metaplasia: narrow band imaging with magnifying endoscopy. *Endoscopy* 2006;38:819–24.

10 Yao K, Iwashita A, Kikuchi Y *et al.* Novel zoom endoscopy technique for visualizing the microvascular architecture in gastric mucosa. *Clin Gastroenterol Hepatol* 2005;3:S23–S26.

11 Yao K, Yao T, Iwashita A. Determining the horizontal extent of early gastric carcinoma: two modern techniques based on differences in the mucosal microvascular architecture and density between carcinoma and non-carcinomatous mucosa. *Dig Endosc* 2002;14:S83–S87.

12 Yao K, Kikuchi Y, Tanabe H *et al.* Novel zoom endoscopy technique for visualizing the microvascular architecture of early gastric cancer enables the precise margin of the cancer to be determined thereby allowing successful resection by the endoscopic submucosal dissection method. *Endoscopy* 2004;36:A6.

13 Siegel LM, Stevens PD, Lightdale CJ *et al.* Combined magnification endoscopy with chromoendoscopy in the evaluation of patients with suspected malabsorption. *Gastrointest Endosc* 1997;46:226–30.

14 Badreldin R, Barrett P, Wooff DA, Mansfield J, Yiannakou Y. How good is zoom endoscopy for assessment of villous atrophy in coeliac disease? *Endoscopy* 2005;37:994–8.

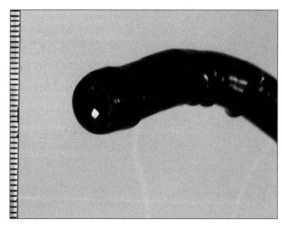

Figure 7.1 A black soft hood mounted at the tip of the scope. (Copyright K. Yao, T. Nagahama, F. Hirai, S. Sou, T. Matsui, H. Tanbe, A. Iwashita, P. Kaye, and K. Ragunath.)

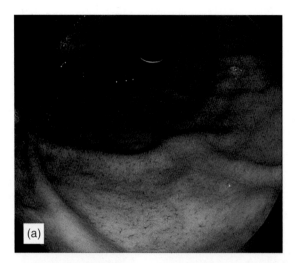

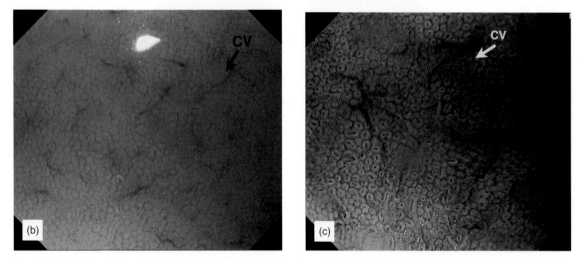

Figure 7.2 Normal gastric body mucosa. (a) Non-m-magnified endoscopic view. (b) Magnified endoscopic findings by white light. A honeycomb-like SECN pattern with CV (arrow) can be noted. (c) Magnified endoscopic findings by NBI. In addition to the micro-vasculature, a round or oval pit pattern becomes evident. The MV architecture and MS structure appear regular in both shape and arrangement in the normal gastric body mucosa. (Copyright K. Yao, T. Nagahama, F. Hirai, S. Sou, T. Matsui, H. Tanbe, A. Iwashita, P. Kaye, and K. Ragunath.)

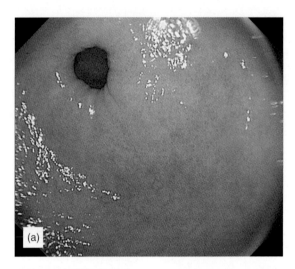

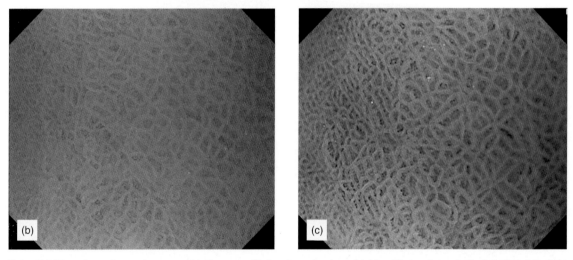

Figure 7.3 Normal gastric antral mucosa. (a) Non-magnified endoscopic view. (b) Magnified endoscopic findings by white light. A coil-shaped SECN pattern is present. (c) Magnified endoscopic findings by NBI. Both the coil-shaped SECN pattern and the reticular MS structure are clearly demonstrated by NBI. (Copyright K. Yao, T. Nagahama, F. Hirai, S. Sou, T. Matsui, H. Tanabe, A. Iwashita, P. Kaye, and K. Ragunath.)

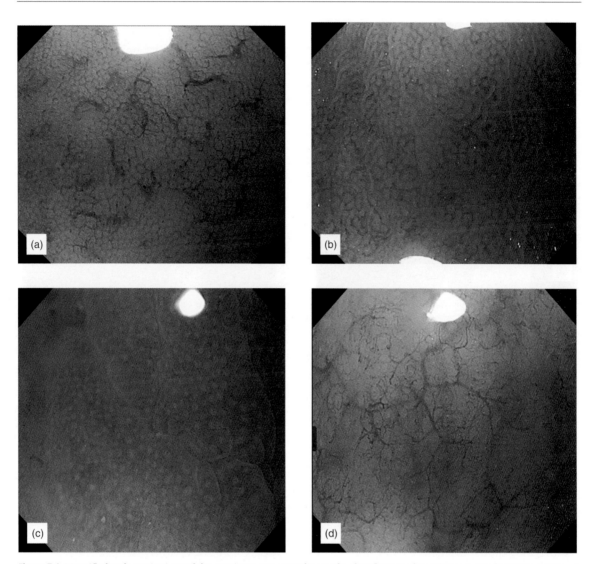

Figure 7.4 Magnified endoscopic views of the gastric mucosa according to the classification of *H. pylori*-associated gastritis. (a) Type 1: honeycomb-like SECN with regular arrangement of CVs and regular round pits. (b) Type 2: honeycomb-like SECN with regular round pits, but loss of CVs. (c) Type 3: loss of normal SECN and CVs, with enlarged white pits surrounded by erythema. (d) Type 4: loss of normal SECN and round pits, together with an irregular arrangement of CVs. (Copyright K. Yao, T. Nagahama, F. Hirai, S. Sou, T. Matsui, H. Tanabe, A. Iwashita, P. Kaye, and K. Ragunath.)

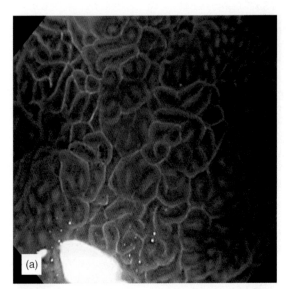

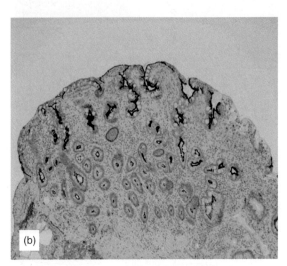

Figure 7.5 (a) Magnified endoscopic findings of LBC in the gastric antral mucosa. LBC is clearly visualized as blue–white lines on the epithelial edge or surface by magnification with NBI. (b) Histologic findings of a biopsy specimen from the area positive for LBC (immunostain, CD10). The epithelial surface with intestinal metaplasia and goblet cells is strongly stained by CD10. (The images of Figure 7.5a and 7.5b were kindly provided by Dr N. Uedo, Osaka Medical Center for Cancer and Cardiovascular Diseases, Osaka, Japan.) (Copyright K. Yao, T. Nagahama, F. Hirai, S. Sou, T. Matsui, H. Tanabe, A. Iwashita, P. Kaye, and K. Ragunath.)

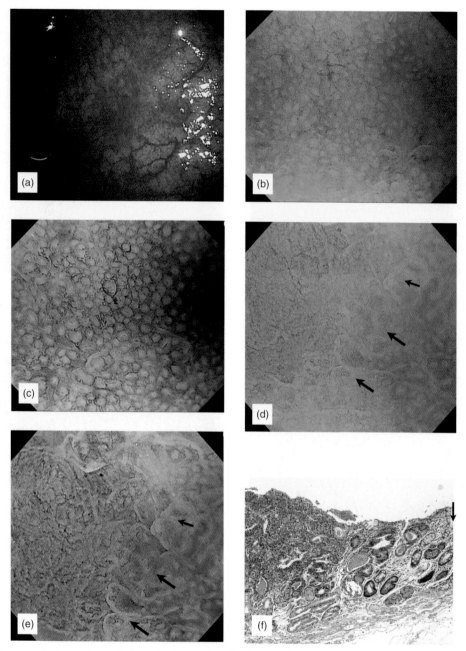

Figure 7.6 An example of an early gastric cancer in the gastric cardia. (a) On ordinary white light endoscopy, a flat reddened mucosal lesion can be noted. (b) Magnification endoscopy with white light shows a regular SECN pattern of the noncancerous surrounding mucosa. (c) With NBI, the regular shape and arrangement of the capillaries together with the pit pattern become evident. (d) At the margin of the carcinoma, white light magnification endoscopy shows a DL (arrows). At that location, the regular SECN pattern has disappeared and, instead, microvessels which are irregular in both shape and arrangement can be seen to have proliferated within the cancerous mucosa. (e) When the white light imaging is changed to NBI, the characteristic findings for differentiated carcinoma, such as the presence of a DL (arrows) and an irregular microvascular pattern (IMVP), become distinct. (f) Histologic findings (H&E stain) of the endoscopically resected specimen demonstrate well-differentiated adenocarcinoma replacing the noncancerous tissue. Arrow shows the histologic margin between cancerous and noncancerous tissues. (Copyright K. Yao, T. Nagahama, F. Hirai, S. Sou, T. Matsui, H. Tanabe, A. Iwashita, P. Kaye, and K. Ragunath.)

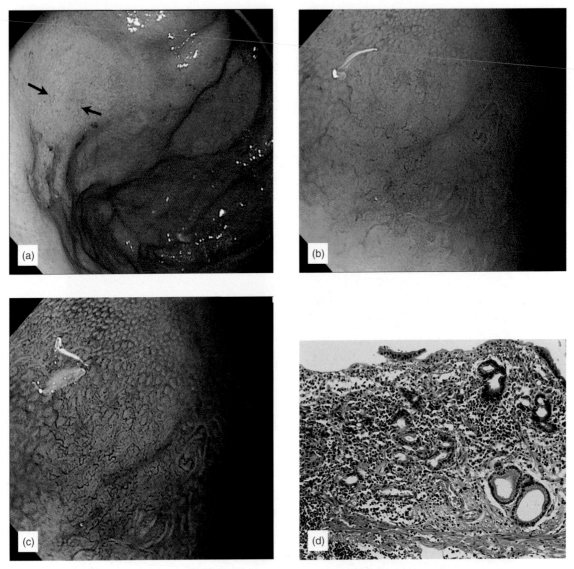

Figure 7.7 An example of early gastric cancer of undifferentiated type in the gastric fundus. (a) Ordinary white light endoscopic view shows a pale mucosal area (arrows) with ulceration. (b) Magnification endoscopic findings of that pale mucosa only show loss of the regular SECN pattern. (c) With NBI, flat mucosa with loss of the regular SECN is easily visualized. (d) Histopathologic findings (H&E stain) demonstrate that poorly differentiated adenocarcinomatous cells are infiltrating within the lamina propria without any proliferation of interstitial tissue and that they are destroying the noncancerous interstitial tissues. (Copyright K. Yao, T. Nagahama, F. Hirai, S. Sou, T. Matsui, H. Tanabe, A. Iwashita, P. Kaye, and K. Ragunath.)

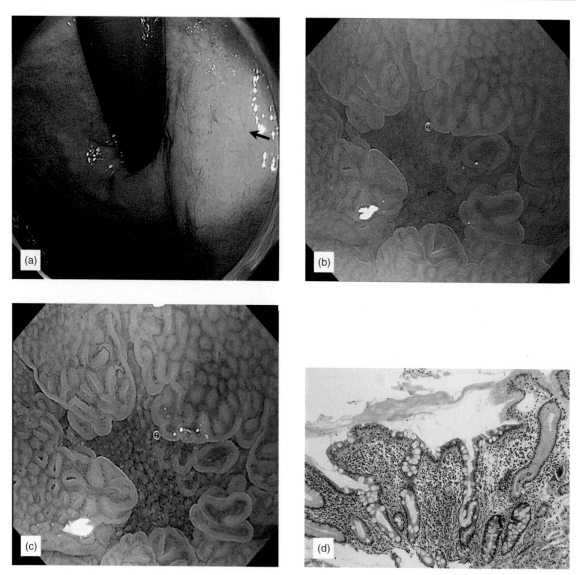

Figure 7.8 How to make a correct diagnosis by magnification endoscopy: Case 1, a focal mucosal lesion due to gastritis. (a) A slightly reddened depressed lesion with an irregularly shaped margin can be noted within the upper part of the gastric body. (b) When we observe this lesion at maximal magnification with white light, some of the MV network within the depressed part becomes visible. However, it is difficult to determine whether or not the shape and the arrangement of the microvessels are regular by these findings alone. (c) When we switch from white light to NBI, both the MV network and the pit pattern prove to be regular in both shape and arrangement. Accordingly, these findings are compatible with chronic focal gastritis. (d) Histopathologic findings demonstrate only chronic gastritis with intestinal metaplasia. (Copyright K. Yao, T. Nagahama, F. Hirai, S. Sou, T. Matsui, H. Tanabe, A. Iwashita, P. Kaye, and K. Ragunath.)

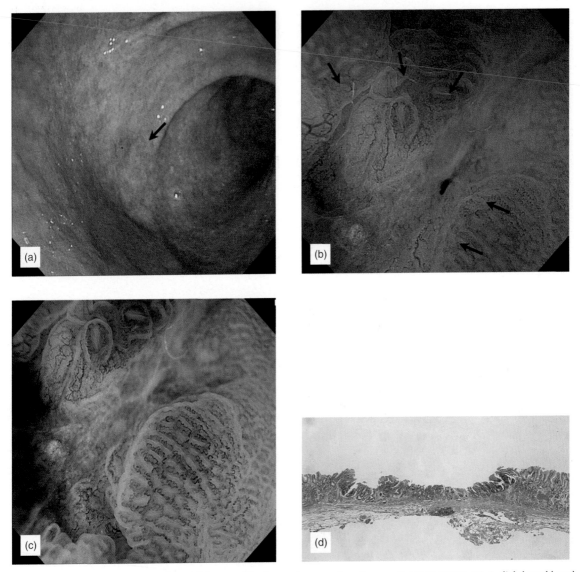

Figure 7.9 How to make a correct diagnosis by magnification endoscopy: Case 2, a small gastric cancer. (a) A slightly reddened depressed lesion with an irregularly shaped margin can be detected within the gastric antrum. (b) When we magnify this lesion, an IMVP can be identified within the depressed part (arrows). (c) With NBI, the distinct morphology of each of the microvessels can be observed in higher contrast than with white light. In addition, the mucosal surface of the depressed part depicts unevenness. (d) Histopathologic findings of the endoscopically resected specimen represent a well-differentiated adenocarcinoma restricted to the mucosa. (Copyright K. Yao, T. Nagahama, F. Hirai, S. Sou, T. Matsui, H. Tanabe, A. Iwashita, P. Kaye, and K. Ragunath.)

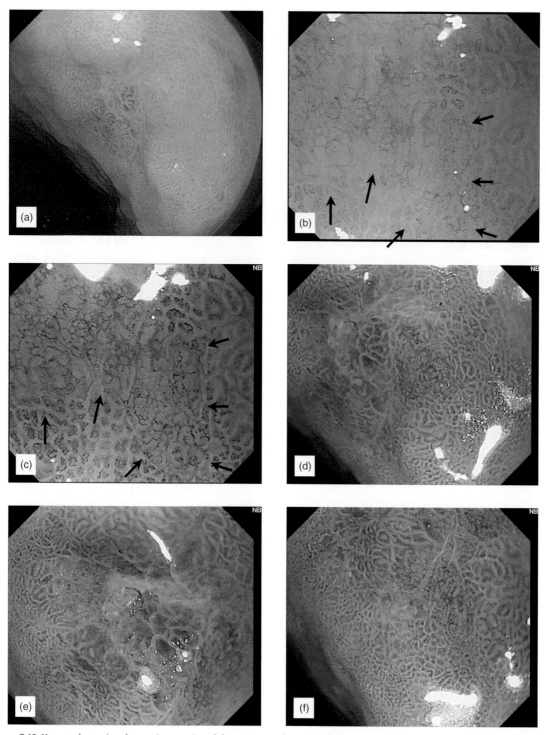

Figure 7.10 How to determine the precise margins of the carcinoma for successful resection by the endoscopic submucosal dissection (ESD) method. (a) A small, poorly demarcated mucosal lesion can be noted in the gastric body. (b) By magnification with white light, there is a DL; furthermore, in this location, the regular SECN pattern has disappeared and instead microvessels which are irregular in both shape and arrangement can be seen to have proliferated. (c) With NBI, these magnified endoscopic findings characteristic for differentiated carcinoma become easy to identify.(d–f) Once these magnified endoscopic findings characteristic for carcinoma are verified, all the margins of the carcinoma can be determined even at weak magnification by endoscopic findings alone. (continued)

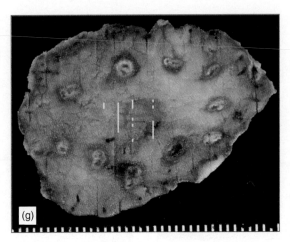

Figure 7.10 (Continued) (g) According to the histologic investigation, the area of the carcinoma was reconstructed on the specimen which was resected by the ESD method. We can see that the reconstructed area is well correlated with that determined by magnification endoscopy with NBI. (Copyright K. Yao, T. Nagahama, F. Hirai, S. Sou, T. Matsui, H. Tanabe, A. Iwashita, P. Kaye, and K. Ragunath.)

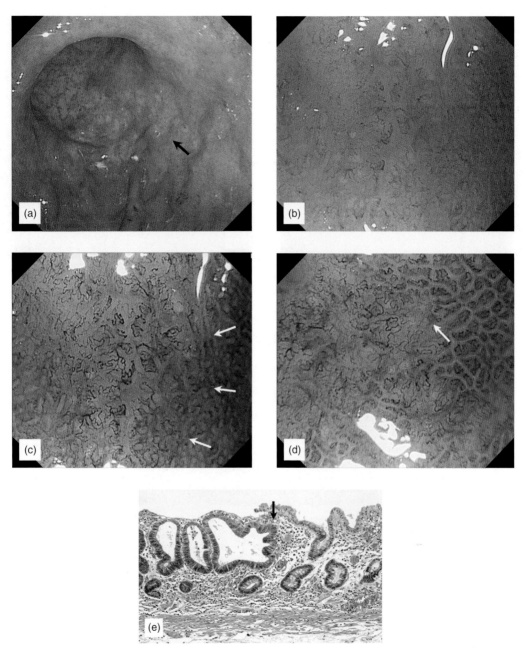

Figure 7.11 How to identify the presence of a carcinoma which does not show any macroscopic findings by ordinary endoscopy (so-called "occult cancer"). (a) One of the multiple random biopsies which were previously taken from the lower gastric body mucosa of the greater curvature was known to have represented well-differentiated adenocarcinoma. However, ordinary endoscopic findings only show multiple healed ulcers on the rough mucosa in the lower gastric body. (b) Instead of taking a second round of multiple biopsies, we scanned this area by weak magnification and successfully found the presence of the carcinoma by identifying an IMVP. (c, d) With NBI, the contrast of microvessels became remarkably high. Such high-contrast images enable the endoscopist to clearly identify a DL (arrows) between the noncancerous and the cancerous mucosa, as well as an IMVP within the cancerous mucosa. These techniques may be useful in helping endoscopists avoid the need to take additional multiple biopsies. (e) Histopathologic findings of the specimen, which was resected by the ESD method, demonstrate well-differentiated adenocarcinoma limited to the mucosa. Arrow shows the margin of the carcinoma. (Copyright K. Yao, T. Nagahama, F. Hirai, S. Sou, T. Matsui, H. Tanabe, A. Iwashita, P. Kaye, and K. Ragunath.)

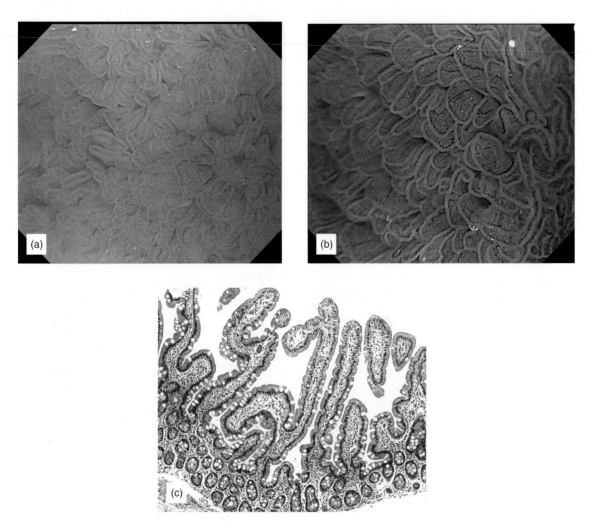

Figure 7.12 The normal duodenal mucosa. (a) Magnified endoscopic findings with white light. The finger- or leaf-like villous formation with a smooth edge is arranged in a regular manner. (b) By NBI, the MS structure of the villi and the MV architecture within the villi become distinct. At the edge of the villi, the LBCs are visualized by NBI. Together, the capillary loops form a regular network underneath the epithelium within the villi (intravillous capillary loop network). (c) Histologic findings of the biopsy specimen show no villous atrophy and no significant inflammatory infiltrate. (Copyright K. Yao, T. Nagahama, F. Hirai, S. Sou, T. Matsui, H. Tanabe, A. Iwashita, P. Kaye, and K. Ragunath.)

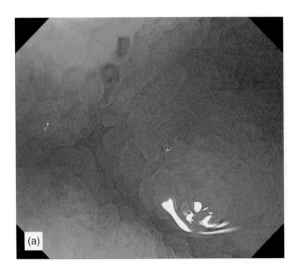
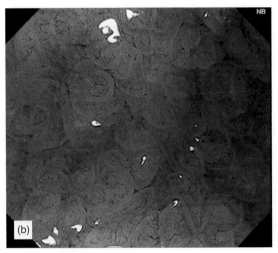

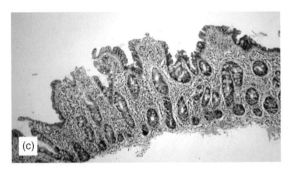

Figure 7.13 Duodenal mucosa in a patient with celiac disease. (a) Magnified endoscopic findings with white light. Blunted villi can be noted. (b) By NBI, the precise morphology of the villi can been seen, i.e., the villi are blunted but the villous structure is preserved. (c) Histologic findings of the biopsy specimen demonstrate duodenal mucosa with mild partial villous atrophy. (Copyright K. Yao, T. Nagahama, F. Hirai, S. Sou, T. Matsui, H. Tanabe, A. Iwashita, P. Kaye, and K. Ragunath.)

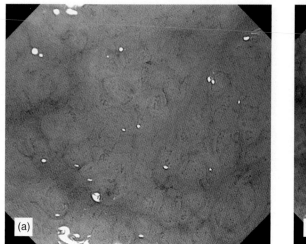

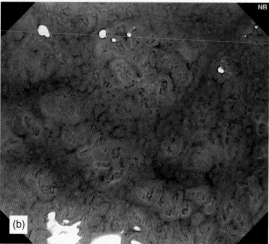

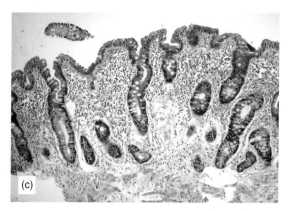

Figure 7.14 Duodenal mucosa in a patient with celiac disease. (a) Magnified endoscopic findings with white light demonstrate that the normal finger- or leaf-like villi have disappeared, but remarkably blunted villi are present. (b) NBI is helpful for visualizing the detailed MS structure, i.e., blunted and broad villi with ridges and crypt openings. (c) Histologic findings of the biopsy specimen represent subtotal villous atrophy and chronic inflammatory infiltration into the epithelium and the lamina propria mucosa. (Copyright K. Yao, T. Nagahama, F. Hirai, S. Sou, T. Matsui, H. Tanabe, A. Iwashita, P. Kaye, and K. Ragunath.)

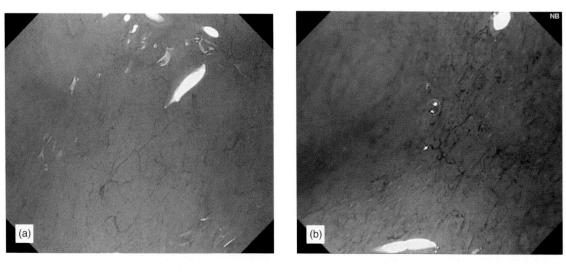

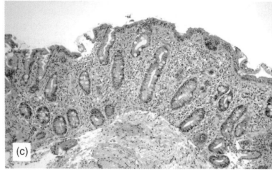

Figure 7.15 The duodenal mucosa in a patient with celiac disease. (a) Magnified endoscopic findings with white light show flat mucosa where the normal villous structure together with the normal microvasculature has disappeared. (b) In addition, NBI is useful for detecting even a small tubular crypt opening on the surface of the flat mucosa. (c) On histologic investigation of the biopsy specimen, it is evident that almost all the villi have disappeared, and only a tubular appearance can be noted. Remarkable infiltration of chronic inflammatory cells into the lamina propria and the epithelium is also present. (Copyright K. Yao, T. Nagahama, F. Hirai, S. Sou, T. Matsui, H. Tanabe, A. Iwashita, P. Kaye, and K. Ragunath.)

8

Magnifying endoscopy with NBI in the diagnosis of superficial gastric neoplasia and its application for endoscopic submucosal dissection

Mitsuru Kaise

Impact of NBI on magnifying endoscopic diagnosis for gastric neoplasia

Although magnifying endoscopic diagnosis for gastric neoplasia has been attempted in the past decades [1], systematic recognition of the magnified gastric surface has been challenging due to the diverse histology of gastric carcinomas, the existence of differences in normal gastric mucosa (Figure 8.1), and various modifications of mucosal structures by atrophy, chronic inflammation, and metaplasia (Figure 8.2). The development of magnifying video-endoscopy combined with narrowband imaging (NBI) has broken this impasse and opened new doors. NBI yields very clear images of fine superficial structure as well as the microvasculature of the gastric mucosa (Figure 8.3) and this has advanced magnifying endoscopic diagnosis to a new level. We have reported that significant correlation between histopathology and microvascular pattern obtained with NBI enables sensitive diagnosis for the existence [2] and extent of superficial gastric cancer, and therefore the modality is applicable for endoscopic submucosal dissection (ESD) [3].

Gastric cancer-specific findings of microvasculature and fine mucosal structure

Gastric cancer in early stages can be endoscopically diagnosed if a target lesion has the following two features: (i) regionality and (ii) cancer-specific findings of microvasculature and fine mucosal structure. Regionality means the presence of a clear border that is recognizable by differences in microvasculature or fine mucosal structure between a target lesion and surrounding reference mucosa (Figure 8.3). Cancerous lesions generally show irregular microvasculature and fine mucosal structure. However, "irregular" is a subjective word, and may be quite variably assessed among endoscopists. We investigated the cancer-specific findings of NBI magnification using objective technical terms [4] and found that the following four features of the microvasculature were cancer-specific (Figure 8.4).

1 *Dilation*: defined as the presence of a group of microvessels whose calibers are twice or more than twice the calibers of surrounding reference microvessels.

2 *Abrupt caliber alteration*: defined as the presence of a group of microvessels whose calibers abruptly become less than half or more than double the original size. Disruption of microvessels is included in this definition.

3 *Heterogeneity in shape*: defined as the presence of a group of microvessels whose shapes are unique and highly variable.

4 *Tortuousness*: defined as the presence of a group of microvessels which are unpredictably twisted or bent.

These features are similarly observed in cancers other than gastric cancer [5], indicating that they are universal in cancerous microvessels.

The cancer-specific findings of fine mucosal structure include the following three features: (i) heterogeneity in shape, (ii) partial or full disappearance, and (iii) micrification (Figure 8.5). Micrification is defined as fine mucosal structure smaller than half of those of surrounding reference mucosa. The cancer-specific findings of fine mucosal structure vary among the different macroscopic appearances of gastric cancer, i.e., 0-I, 0-IIa, 0-IIb, and 0-IIc [6].

Comprehensive Atlas of High-Resolution Endoscopy and Narrowband Imaging, Second Edition. Edited by Jonathan Cohen.
© 2017 John Wiley & Sons, Ltd. Published 2017 by John Wiley & Sons, Ltd.
Companion website: www.wiley.com/go/cohen/NBI

Findings on magnifying endoscopy vary according to macroscopic appearance of gastric cancer

Cancer-specific changes in fine mucosal structure and microvessels observed by NBI magnification vary among the different macroscopic appearances of gastric cancer. Therefore, we show representative endoscopic findings for each type of superficial gastric cancer.

Changes in microvasculature in superficial depressed gastric cancer

Superficial depressed gastric cancer of type 0-IIc often shows partial or full disappearance of fine mucosal structure with cancer-specific microvasculature. Nakayoshi *et al.* [2] proposed a subclassification of microvasculature for predicting the histologic patterns of type 0-IIc gastric cancer. Fine network pattern, in which abundant microvessels are well connected to one another like a mesh, is characteristic of differentiated adenocarcinoma (Figure 8.6a). A corkscrew pattern, in which tortuous microvessels are isolated like a corkscrew, is characteristic of poorly differentiated adenocarcinoma (Figure 8.6b).

Figure 8.7 shows typical findings of type 0-IIc cancer, composed of well-differentiated adenocarcinoma. Fine mucosal structure disappears and microvasculature appears like a fine network (Figure 8.7c,d), indicating that it is a well-differentiated adenocarcinoma. In contrast, a representative case of type 0-IIc cancer demonstrates disappearance of the fine mucosal pattern and corkscrew pattern in microvasculature (Figure 8.8c,d), indicating that the lesion is composed of poorly differentiated adenocarcinoma.

Changes in elevated neoplasias of the stomach

NBI magnification findings of superficial elevated cancer (type 0-IIa) show that the changes in microvasculature are the same as those of superficial depressed cancer (type 0-IIc). However, the visibility of microvessels in superficial elevated cancer is sometimes lacking. Therefore, in these lesions, magnifying endoscopic diagnosis is based on findings of fine mucosal structure. In a representative case of type 0-IIa (Figure 8.9), microvasculature is not observed by NBI magnification. Fine mucosal structure appears heterogeneous in shape, one of the specific findings of gastric cancer, suggesting that this lesion is cancer.

Cancer in hyperplastic polyps (Figure 8.10) can be classified as type 0-I gastric cancer. In this type, micrification of fine mucosal structure is a pivotal cancer-specific finding. Using 64 gastric polyps with or without cancer, we have shown that micrification of fine mucosal structure was highly accurate in discovering the coexistence of cancer (sensitivity 83.3%, specificity 84.6%), but heterogeneity was less accurate (sensitivity 83.3%, specificity 53.8%). The four features of microvasculature that are cancer-specific in type 0-IIc are also less accurate (sensitivity 54.5%, specificity 92.3%).

Application of magnifying endoscopy with NBI for endoscopic resection

The diagnosis of the extent of cancerous infiltration is indispensable for endoscopic or surgical resection of gastric carcinoma. Since around 20% of superficial gastric carcinomas do not exhibit a clear border line, accurate endoscopic diagnosis plays a crucial role for radical cure, especially in endoscopic resection. ESD, a superb method which enables en bloc resection for large lesions or lesions with ulceration, can achieve more radical cure in combination with precise endoscopic diagnosis of the cancerous extent (Figure 8.11). Therefore, we usually perform ESD in combination with magnifying endoscopy with NBI, which allows optical (or endoscopic) and real-time pathology [7].

 Video clips to accompany this book can be found in the online material at www.wiley.com/go/cohen/NBI

The following videos relate specifically to this chapter:

Video 35 Low-grade gastric dysplasia

Video 36 NBI detection of poorly differentiated superficial gastric cancer not seen on white light

Video 37 Endoscopic submucosal dissection of superficial gastric cancer

References

1 Sakaki N, Iida Y, Okazaki Y, Kawamura S, Takemoto T. Magnifying endoscopic observation of the gastric mucosa, particularly in patients with atrophic gastritis. *Endoscopy* 1978;10:269–74.

2 Nakayoshi T, Tajiri H, Matsuda K, Kaise M, Ikegami M, Sasaki H. Magnifying endoscopy combined with narrow band imaging system for early gastric cancer: correlation of vascular pattern with histopathology (including video). *Endoscopy* 2004;36:1080–4.

3 Sumiyama K, Kaise M, Nakayoshi T *et al.* Combined use of a magnifying endoscope with a narrow band imaging system and a multibending endoscope for en bloc EMR of early stage gastric cancer. *Gastrointest Endosc* 2004;60:79–84.

4 Kaise M, Kato M, Urashima M *et al.* Magnifying endoscopy combined with narrow-band imaging for differential diagnosis of superficial depressed gastric lesions. *Endoscopy* 2009;41;310–15.

5 Kumagai Y, Inoue H, Nagai K, Kawano T, Iwai T. Magnifying endoscopy, stereoscopic microscopy, and the microvascular architecture of superficial esophageal carcinoma. *Endoscopy* 2002;34:369–75.

6 Horiuchi H, Kaise M, Inomata H *et al.* Magnifying endoscopy combined with narrow band imaging may help to predict neoplasia coexisting with gastric hyperplastic polyps. *Scand J Gastroenterol* 2013;48:626–32.

7 Kaise M, Kato M, Tajiri H. High definition endoscopy and magnifying endoscopy combined with narrow band imaging in gastric cancer. *Gastroenterol Clin North Am* 2010;39:771–84.

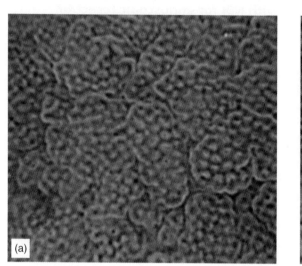
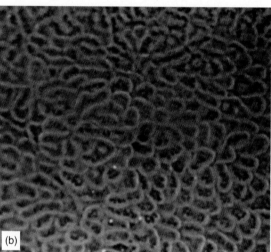

Figure 8.1 Normal mucosal images obtained by magnifying endoscopy with NBI. (a) Mucosal surface of gastric fundic gland showing microvessels surrounding the gland pits and this exhibits a honeycomb pattern. (b) Mucosal surface of pyloric gland showing microvessels in the papillary type pit.

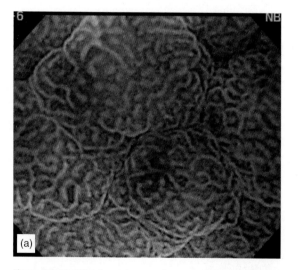
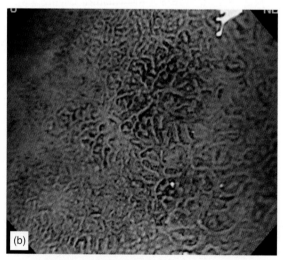

Figure 8.2 Modifications of mucosal structures by atrophy. (a) *H. pylori*-infected fundic mucosa shows round, tubular or gyrus-like pattern of fine superficial structure, which is different from normal fundic mucosa with regular round pit pattern and honeycomb-like microvessels. (b) In *H. pylori*-infected pyloric mucosa, there are various patterns of fine superficial structures, which are invisible in atrophic mucosa. Microvessels surround the various shapes of superficial structure, and the density of microvessel varies from area to area.

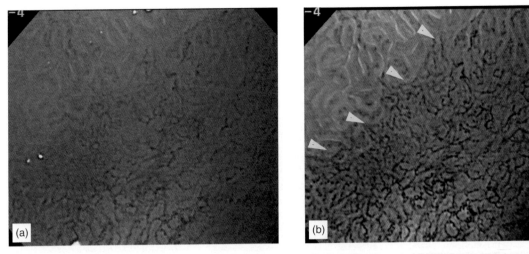

Figure 8.3 Comparison of (a) white light magnifying endoscopy and (b) magnifying endoscopy with NBI. This lesion has clear regionality, well recognized by the presence of a clear border (arrowheads) that is identifiable by the difference in microvasculature or fine mucosal structure between the target lesion and the surrounding reference mucosa.

Cancer-specific findings of microvasculature
1) Dilation; caliber B > 2 x caliber A
2) Abrupt caliber alteration (caliber B > 2 x caliber B') & (caliber B" < caliber B x1/2)
3) Heterogeneity in shape
4) Tortuousness

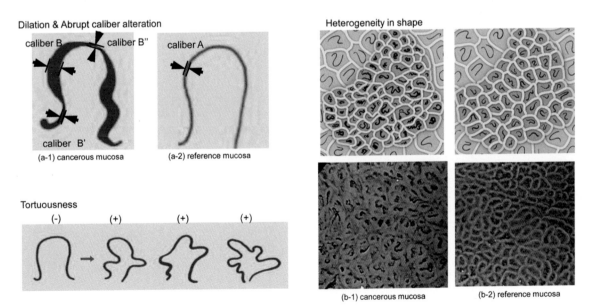

Figure 8.4 Cancer-specific changes in microvasculature: dilation (caliber B > 2× caliber A), abrupt caliber alteration (caliber B > 2× caliber B'; caliber B" < ½ caliber B), heterogeneity in shape, and tortuousness.

<u>Cancer-specific findings of fine mucosal structure</u>
(a) Heterogeneity in shape
(b) Partial or full disappearance
(c) Micrification

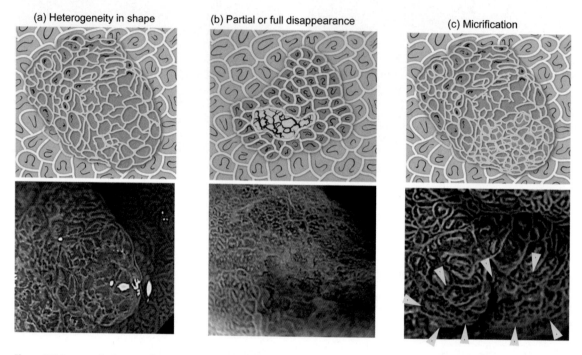

Figure 8.5 Images of microvessels in poorly differentiated (diffuse type) adenocarcinoma. Cancer-specific changes in fine mucosal structure could be expressed by the following three features: (a) heterogeneity in shape; (b) partial or full disappearance; and (c) micrification.

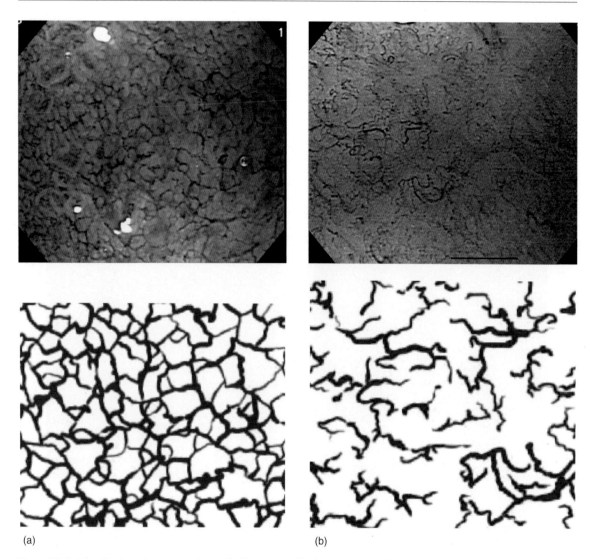

Figure 8.6 Subclassification of microvasculature findings can predict histologic type of adenocarcinoma. (a) Fine network pattern like a mesh, in which abundant microvessels connect with one another, is characteristic of differentiated adenocarcinoma. (b) Cork-screw pattern with isolated and tortuous microvessels, in which scanty microvessels do not connect with one another, is characteristic of poorly differentiated adenocarcinoma.

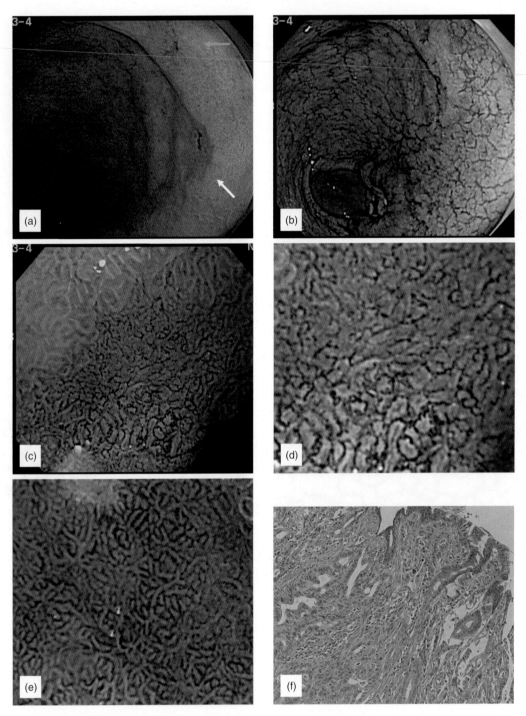

Figure 8.7 Type 0-IIc early gastric cancer: well-differentiated adenocarcinoma. (a) Conventional endoscopy and (b) chromoendoscopy show the presence of two reddish and erosive lesions on the posterior wall of gastric antrum. Magnifying endoscopy with NBI demonstrates the disappearance of fine mucosal structure and fine network microvasculature in the depressed lesion (white arrow in (a)), indicating that it is a well-differentiated adenocarcinoma (c, medium magnification; d, high magnification). (e) Magnifying endoscopy with NBI demonstrates the other depressed lesion (blue arrow in (a)) to have a tubular mucosal pattern and regular microvasculature, indicating that the lesion is noncancerous erosion. (f) Pathologic findings of early gastric cancer show well-differentiated adenocarcinoma (intestinal type), which is in accordance with the histologic prediction by magnifying endoscopy with NBI.

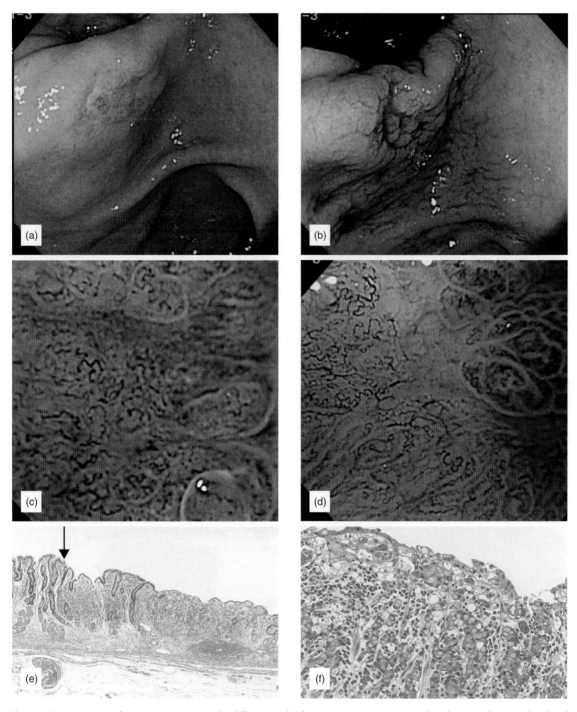

Figure 8.8 Type 0-IIc early gastric cancer: poorly differentiated adenocarcinoma. Conventional endoscopy shows a discolored depressed lesion with reddish granulation on the posterior wall of gastric angle (a), which chromoendoscopy with indigo carmine dye shows clearly (b), the morphology suggesting the possibility of poorly differentiated adenocarcinoma. (c, d) Magnifying endoscopy with NBI shows disappearance of fine mucosal structure and microvasculature with corkscrew pattern, indicating that the lesion is poorly differentiated adenocarcinoma. Upper right of (d) is equivalent to the slightly elevated area with granulation in the center of the lesion. This finding suggests that the area is not composed of cancerous tissue in all the layers, but is covered with regenerated epithelium. (e, f) Pathology of ESD specimen: (e) type 0-IIc to the right of arrow; (f) high magnification of H&E stained section shows poorly differentiated adenocarcinoma, which is in accordance with the histologic prediction by magnifying endoscopy with NBI.

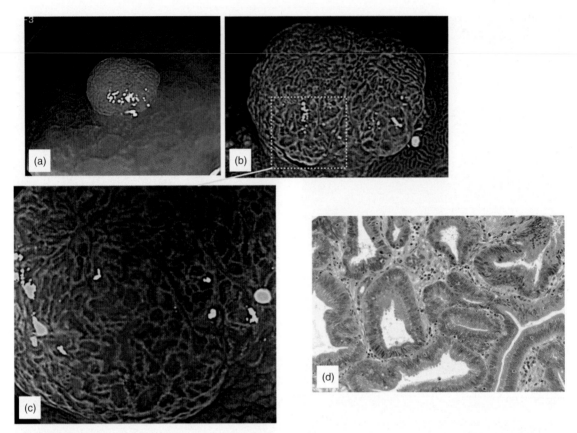

Figure 8.9 Type 0-IIa early gastric cancer: poorly differentiated adenocarcinoma. (a) Conventional endoscopy shows a discolored, small and white elevated lesion. (b, c) Microvasculature was not observed by magnifying endoscopy with NBI. Fine mucosal structure appears heterogeneous in shape, one of the specific findings in gastric cancer, suggesting that this lesion is cancer. (d) Pathology of ESD specimen shows well-differentiated adenocarcinoma.

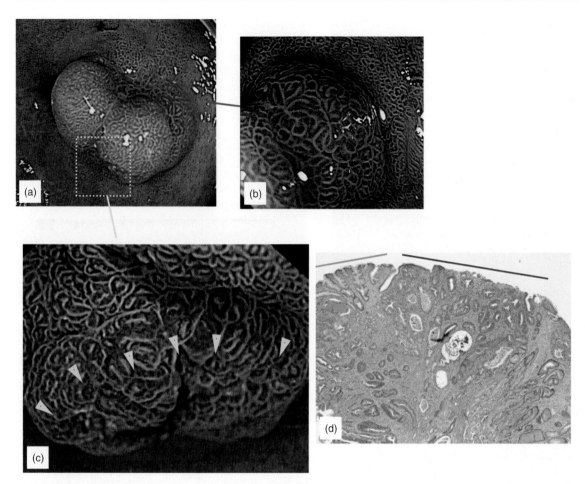

Figure 8.10 Cancer in hyperplastic polyps. (a) Conventional endoscopy shows an elevated lesion near to the pyloric ring. (b) Magnifying endoscopy with NBI shows large fine mucosal structure in the area within the blue square, which is compatible with hyperplastic polyp. (c) In contract, fine mucosal structure shows micrification in the area within the yellow square, one of the specific findings in gastric cancer. (d) Pathology of ESD specimen shows coexistence of cancerous glands (red line) and hyperplastic nonneoplastic glands (blue line).

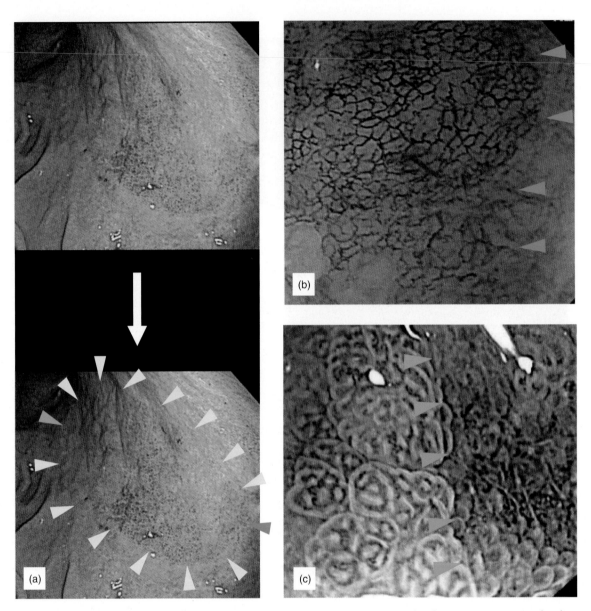

Figure 8.11 The existence or extent of gastric cancer is difficult to determine by conventional endoscopy. (a) Conventional endoscopy shows a reddish area on the posterior wall of the upper gastric corpus but it is still difficult to diagnosis as a cancerous lesion. However, magnifying endoscopy with NBI diagnoses it as an early gastric cancer, as delineated by arrowheads (type 0-IIc, well-differentiated adenocarcinoma). (b) Magnifying endoscopy with NBI shows irregular microvessels (margin delineated by green arrowheads), indicating that the lesion is well-differentiated adenocarcinoma. (c) Magnifying endoscopy with NBI shows a slight depression and irregular microvessels (margin delineated by blue arrowheads).

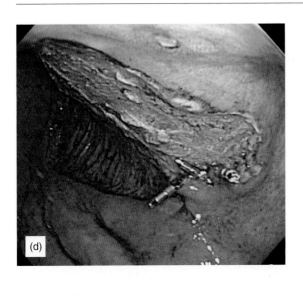

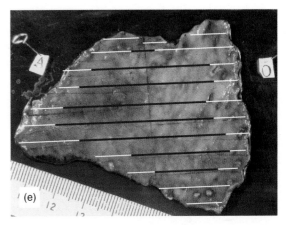

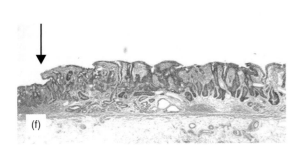

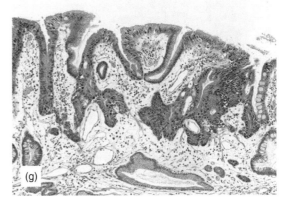

Figure 8.11 (Continued) (d) Endoscopic findings after ESD. (e) The resected specimen exhibits well-differentiated adenocarcinoma as shown by the red lines. A cancerous lesion is present within 5 mm from marking spots and this accords with the determination of extent by magnifying endoscopy with NBI, thus confirming that the modality is accurate for finding the extent of cancerous infiltration. (f) Pathology of ESD specimen shows a flat area (0-IIb) to the right of the arrow and a depressed area (0-IIc) to the left, in both of which well-differentiated adenocarcinoma is present. The finding is in accordance with the histologic prediction by magnifying endoscopy with NBI. (g) Type 0-IIb area is partially covered with non-neoplastic epithelium, which is the reason why the vertical margin is not clear by conventional endoscopy.

SECTION 3
Colon

9

Optical chromoendoscopy using NBI during screening colonoscopy: its usefulness and application

Yasushi Sano and Shigeaki Yoshida

Introduction

The detection and subsequent removal of neoplastic colorectal lesions, including adenomatous polyps and early cancers, have been reported to reduce the incidence of colorectal cancers, based on the concept of the adenoma–carcinoma sequence [1]. Therefore, the roles of screening colonoscopy and polypectomy are becoming more important because colorectal cancer is the third most common cause of cancer mortality, and the incidence of colorectal cancer in Japan is increasing [2]. Although efficacious colonoscopy is recommended, it has been reported that 10–30% of resected polyps are non-neoplastic lesions that did not need to be removed [3]. Therefore, the distinction of non-neoplastic lesions from neoplastic lesions can increase the efficiency of treatment by eliminating the time and cost of unnecessary polypectomy [4,5]. The narrowband imaging (NBI) system is based on modifying spectral features by narrowing the bandwidth of spectral transmittance with optical filters. Since 1999, we have been developing our own NBI system with support from a Grant for Scientific Research Expenses for Health and Welfare Programs, Japan. NBI modification provides a unique image emphasizing the capillary pattern (CP) and the surface structure [6–8]. In our pilot study, the NBI system was sufficient to differentiate non-neoplastic lesions from neoplastic lesions (optical chromoendoscopy), and had a special feature allowing otherwise invisible endoscopic findings to be visualized without a dye solution (high-contrast endoscopy) [8–11].

In this chapter, we describe the usefulness of NBI in screening colonoscopy and target optical chromoendoscopy, and discuss the utility of the detailed observation of the microvascular architecture for differential diagnosis during colonoscopy.

Improvement in visibility

Our pilot study found that, compared with normal observation, the NBI system is capable of clearer observation of the capillary vessels in the network on the surface layer of the mucosa [9]. Therefore, recognizing the lesion becomes easier since the permeable image of the vessels is interrupted. In the normal mucosa, a regular hexagonal or honeycomb-like pattern is found around the crypts of the glands. In contrast, these vessels become thicker in neoplastic lesions; as the abnormality worsens, endoscopy shows disruption of vessels, vessels with different diameters, and an increase in vessel density. Since the filter of NBI is adjusted to the absorption characteristics of hemoglobin, a brownish area can be found if the observing zone contains a large number of capillary vessels (Figure 9.1). Contrast enhancement of the lesion made disruption of the normal vessel network in colonic lesions obvious and improved visualization [11].

Improvement in observation of the surface structure (pit pattern) and the microcapillaries (capillary pattern)

Several studies have reported that observation using chromoendoscopy, and chromoendoscopy with magnifying function, is helpful in differentiating neoplasia from non-neoplasia. In our pilot study [9], the accuracy of endoscopic diagnosis was 79.1% for conventional colonoscopy and 93.4% for NBI colonoscopy. This was similar to that of chromoendoscopy with indigo carmine dye. Therefore, by combining NBI system with the magnifying function, it is possible to infer the pit pattern on the surface layer of the mucosa without any staining and therefore obtain as correct a diagnosis as with optical chromoendoscopy.

NBI modification provides a unique image that emphasizes the CP as well as the surface structure. Angiogenesis is critical in the transition from pre-malignant lesions in a hyperproliferative state to the malignant phenotype [12–14]. Therefore, a diagnosis based on angiogenic or vascular morphologic changes might be ideal for early detection or diagnosis of neoplasm. We have described the utility of detailed observation of microvascular architecture for differential diagnosis during NBI colonoscopy [10,15]. We have named the mucosal capillary meshwork arranged in a honeycomb pattern around the mucosal glands as "meshed capillary" (MC) and using NBI colonoscopy with magnification have classified the microvascular architecture into three types (CP types I, II, and III) [15]. These capillary vessels, which are observed clearly by NBI, are thought to be similar to capillary vessels of around 300 μm, according to the Monte Carlo simulation that we conducted [16]. The definition of each CP is summarized in Table 9.1 and described in detail in the following sections.

Normal colonic mucosa (CP type I)

Using NBI colonoscopy without magnification, not only thick veins and thick capillaries but also fine capillaries can be seen as a brown color. The vessel network of the mucosa is well visualized in much finer detail

on NBI colonoscopy compared with standard colonoscopy. However, the mucosal capillary meshwork (MC) arranged in a honeycomb pattern around the mucosal glands is invisible or faintly visible under magnifying observation using NBI colonoscopy (Figure 9.2a) because endoscopic resolution is insufficient to visualize the network. The vessel diameter was reported as 8.6 ± 1.8 to 12.4 ± 1.9 μm (range 6.4–20.9) [13,14].

Hyperplastic polyp (CP type I)

Most hyperplastic polyps can be seen as light-brown lesions without neovascular changes on NBI colonoscopy. Kudo's type II pit pattern can be seen by magnifying observation using NBI without any dye solution [17]. In many cases the mucosal capillary meshwork is invisible or faintly visible under magnifying observation using NBI colonoscopy, because endoscopic resolution is insufficient to visualize the network (Figure 9.2b). We have previously reported that intratumor microvessel density in small hyperplastic polyps is significantly higher than that in normal mucosa, but vessel diameter is not significantly increased in comparison to normal mucosa [18]. However, MC vessels are sometimes recognized in some

Table 9.1   Sano's endoscopic microvascular classification of colorectal lesions using NBI (Copyright Y. Sano and S. Yoshida).

	Schematic microvascular architecture	Capillary characteristics	Vessel diameter, μm (minimum to maximum)	Visibility using NBI
Normal mucosa		Mucosal capillary network (meshwork) arranged in a honeycomb pattern around the mucosal glands	8.6 ± 1.8 to 12.4 ± 1.9 (6.4–20.9)	MC vessel: invisible to faintly visible (CP type I)
Hyperplastic		Mucosal capillary network (meshwork) arranged in a honeycomb pattern around the mucosal glands	Usually less than 10	MC vessel: invisible to faintly visible (CP type I)
Adenoma		Vascular casts show that the microvasculature has a similar organization to the normal colon. However, capillaries are elongated and have increased diameters compared to normal	13.1 ± 3.3	MC vessel: clearly visible Slightly thicker capillary Capillary density: loose (CP type II)
Carcinoma		Vascular casts of colonic carcinoma are characterized by a disorganized structure and increased density of microvessels. The increased number and density of microvessels result in formation of nodular clusters of capillaries	18.3 ± 0.1 to 19.8 ± 7.6 (2.2–84.5)	MC vessel: clearly visible Uneven-sized thicker capillary with branching curtailed irregularity Capillary density: dense (CP type III)

hyperplastic polyps, such as large hyperplastic polyp [5,15] or hyperplastic polyp with serrated adenomatous change [5,15]. Nevertheless, when MC vessels are seen in hyperplastic polyps they are thin in caliber.

Adenomatous lesion (CP type II)

Adenomatous lesions, including the flat and depressed type, can be seen as dark-brown neovascular lesions (brownish area) on NBI colonoscopy without magnification and are easily detected when withdrawing the endoscope using NBI. Kudo's type IIIL or IV pit pattern demarcated by the appearance of MC vessels can be seen by magnifying observation using NBI without the application of dye solution [8,15]. MC vessels are clearly visible, because these capillaries are elongated and have increased diameters compared with normal ones (Figure 9.2c). Vessel diameter is reported as 13.1 ± 3.3 µm [13,14].

Cancerous lesion (CP type III)

The microvascular architecture of colonic carcinoma is characterized by disorganized structure and increased density of microvessels. Vessel diameter is reported as 18.3 ± 0.1 to 19.8 ± 7.6 (range 2.2–84.5) [13,14]. MC vessels are clearly visible and show uneven-sized thicker capillaries with branching, curtailed appearance, and irregularity (Figure 9.2d). When the lesion CP type III is identified during NBI colonoscopy, additional detailed observation using chromoendoscopy with indigo carmine or crystal violet dye is recommended [5].

The presence of MC vessels on magnifying endoscopy using NBI is useful for distinguishing between hyperplastic polyps and adenomatous polyps. Recently, we have developed the concept of detecting abnormal microcapillaries using NBI as a marker of neoplasia from the results of our prospective study. In this study, the overall diagnostic accuracy, sensitivity, and specificity using the presence of MC vessels for distinction between neoplastic and non-neoplastic lesions were 95.3%, 96.4%, and 92.3%, respectively (P <0.0001) [10]. We believe that this system speeds the assessment and simplifies the analysis of polyps as compared with real chromoendoscopy and helps the endoscopist to determine whether to remove a polyp. The combination of NBI as the initial optical chromoendoscopy and real chromoendoscopy when necessary for more advanced lesions may save time and cost in screening colonoscopy.

Histology of microvascular proliferation

We have evaluated microvascular proliferation with CD31 immunohistochemical staining in normal colonic mucosa, hyperplastic polyps, adenomas, and carcinomas (Figure 9.3). Many microcapillary vessels measuring less than 10 µm can be seen in the stroma at the surface of normal colonic mucosa and hyperplastic polyps. However, adenomatous and cancerous lesions with thicker capillary vessels (20–30 µm) can be seen surrounding glands just under the basal membrane at the surface. These findings suggest that MC vessels are histologically confirmed to be dilated, with increased microvasculature and vessel diameters in the superficial portion of adenomatous and cancerous lesions, on immunohistochemical staining with anti-human monoclonal CD31 antibody [19].

A bench study: comparison between endoscopic resolution and MC vessels

MC vessels in normal colonic mucosa and hyperplastic polyps are invisible or faintly visible under magnifying observation using NBI colonoscopy. To evaluate the correlation between endoscopic resolution and visibility of MC vessels, a squared plate (TOPPAN-TEST-CHART-NO1) was used in this bench study. As previously reported, the diameter of MC vessels ranges from 8 to 12 µm in normal colonic mucosa and hyperplastic polyps [12–14]. As shown in Figure 9.4(a), the approximately 8–12 mm bars on the squared plate adjusted to the same scale as the polyp are not clearly visible or distinguishable due to endoscopic resolution. In contrast, the diameter of MC vessels in adenomatous or cancerous lesion ranges from 13 to 20 µm [12–14]. These vessels are clearly visible on NBI colonoscopy with magnification (Figure 9.4c). In this bench study, the approximately 14–20 µm bars on the squared plate adjusted to the same scale as the polyp are clearly visible. Therefore, the presence of MC vessels on magnifying endoscopy using NBI is a useful indicator for distinguishing between hyperplastic polyps and adenomatous polyps.

Role and benefit of lesion detection and assessment of margins

The data described in this chapter establish a benefit for NBI in diagnosing a polyp as adenoma or non-adenoma, and describe the theoretical basis for this. Other relevant questions regarding the use and benefits of NBI light are in the initial detection of lesions and in the assessment of margins when attempting endoscopic removal. In our initial experiments, the use of high-resolution NBI colonoscopy had a benefit for the identification of flat lesions less than 10 mm in size. The detection rate of flat lesions using high-resolution NBI colonoscopy was approximately 20% higher than that using white light colonoscopy. While this and other studies have suggested a benefit in flat lesion detection, the preponderance of studies in the past decade have failed to demonstrate an increase in overall adenoma detection rate using NBI high resolution endoscopy as compared to white light high resolution endoscopy alone for average risk patients undergoing screening colonoscopy [20,21].

The observation of pit pattern using magnifying NBI colonoscopy is also useful for the assessment of resected margins after polypectomy or endoscopic mucosal resection. It may be necessary to perform subsequent management, such as hot biopsy or argon plasma coagulation, when neoplastic pit pattern (Kudo's IIIL or IV pits) is recognized at the margin of the resected tumor.

Future prospects

Diagnosis on the basis of mucosal pattern has been reported to be correlated with histologic diagnosis. Chromoendoscopy is often used, as it is a contrast staining method using a biocompatible dye such as indigo carmine. In mucosa with glands, the dye accumulates within crypt orifices. Although chromoendoscopy is effective in many applications, it is still only an optional diagnostic method because of its length, additional cost, and necessity of complete mucus removal. In this chapter, we have described the utility of detailed observation of the microvascular architecture for differential diagnosis during NBI colonoscopy. NBI modification provides a unique image that emphasizes the CP and the surface structure. Our initial data indicate that NBI may be as effective as, or more effective than, chromoendoscopy without having such problems [9].

Angiogenesis is critical to the transition from premalignant lesion in a hyperproliferative state to the malignant phenotype. Therefore, diagnosis based on angiogenic or vascular morphologic changes might be ideal for early detection or diagnosis of neoplasms. We have proposed the term "MC" for distinguishing between non-neoplastic and neoplastic lesions, and the capillary classification "CP" for the differential diagnosis of colorectal lesions. On the basis of previous investigations, the surface microvascular architecture in colorectal lesions can be divided into three patterns: (i) honeycomb-like capillaries in normal mucosa and hyperplastic polyps (8–12 μm); (ii) elongated meshwork capillaries of greater diameter in adenomatous lesions (~13 μm); and (iii) disorganized meshwork capillaries with increased density of microvessels in cancerous lesions (18–19 μm) [12–14]. These CPs can be easily recognized using NBI colonoscopy, and we believe that the combined use of NBI/optical chromoendoscopy and real chromoendoscopy decreases the time and cost of screening colonoscopy. The three-step strategy for the management of colorectal lesions using these procedures is shown in Figure 9.5. However, NBI colonoscopy may not be superior to chromoendoscopy for distinguishing between endoscopically treatable early invasive cancers and cancers requiring surgical management at this time. Attempts

to make this determination using magnification NBI analysis of microvessels will require further investigation. In the meantime, we should use the three different procedures outlined in Figure 9.5 without getting them confused. A number of colon lesions are presented in Figures 9.6–9.18 as examples of the appearance of different CPs under NBI at low and high magnification with chromoendoscopic and pathologic correlation.

In the near future, we hope that NBI procedures will become standard for screening and surveillance colonoscopy. To assess the feasibility and efficacy of using the NBI system, further studies are required for colorectal lesions and other lesions of the gastrointestinal tract.

 Video clips to accompany this book can be found in the online material at www.wiley.com/go/cohen/NBI

The following videos relate specifically to this chapter:

Video 48 Nice classification Type I hyper plastic polyps and WASP classification serrated polyps

Video 49 High confidence NICE Type II tubular adenomas and "valley signs"

Video 50 Colon polyps on NBI: detection and diagnosis. Optical diagnosis of a small adenoma

Video 51 Colon polyps on NBI: detection and diagnosis. Characterization of large sessile polyp and its margins

Video 52 Colon polyps on NBI: detection and diagnosis. The tip of the iceberg: detection of hidden extension of flat adenoma

Video 53 Familial polyposis: detection on NBI

Video 54 NBI characteristics of colon polyps: pit patterns and mesh capillary patterns

Video 55 Recurrent tubulovillous adenoma with scar

Video 56 Small sessile and pedunculated polyps

Video 59 Sessile depressed polyp

Video 61 Tubolovillous adenoma resection

Video 62 Pedunculated colon polyp with adenoma margin extending down stalk

Video 63 NBI optical diagnosis of diminutive adenoma

Video 64 Adenoma of the ileocecal valve

Video 65 Follow-up examination following resection of ileocecal valve polyp

Video 66 NICE 2 tubular adenoma optical diagnosis

Video 67 NICE 1 hyperplastic colon polyp

Video 68 NBI characterization of hyperplastic and adenomatous colon polyps

Video 69 Incomplete polypectomy and NBI margin assessment for colon adenoma

Video 70 NBI feature of advanced polyp and nonlifting sign

Video 71 Ileal transition zone mucosal examination

Video 75 High definition imaging WL and NBI to assess and fully resect giant near obstructing splenic flexure tubulovillous adenoma

References

1 Winawer SJ, Zauber AG, Ho MN *et al.* Prevention of colorectal cancer by colonoscopic polypectomy. The National Polyp Study Workgroup. *N Engl J Med* 1993;329:1977–81.

2 Saito H. Screening for colorectal cancer: current status in Japan. *Dis Colon Rectum* 2000;43:S78–S84.

3 Vatan MH, Stalsbert H. The prevalence of polyps of the large intestine in Oslo: an autopsy study. *Cancer* 1982;40:819–25.

4 Fu KI, Sano Y, Kato S *et al.* Chromoendoscopy using indigo carmine dye spraying with magnifying observation is the most reliable method for differential diagnosis between non-neoplastic and neoplastic colorectal lesions: a prospective study. *Endoscopy* 2004;36:1089–93.

5 Sano Y, Saito Y, Fu KI *et al.* Efficacy of magnifying chromoendoscopy for the differential diagnosis of colorectal lesions. *Dig Endosc* 2005;17:105–16.

6 Sano Y, Kobayashi M, Hamamoto Y *et al.* New diagnostic method based on color imaging using narrow band imaging (NBI) system for gastrointestinal tract. *Gastrointest Endosc* 2001;53:AB125.

7 Gono K, Obi T, Yamaguchi M *et al.* Appearance of enhanced tissue features in narrow-band endoscopic imaging. *J Biomed Opt* 2004;9:568–77.

8 Sano Y, Muto M, Tajiri H, Ohtsu A, Yoshida S. Optical/digital chromoendoscopy during colonoscopy using narrow band imaging system. *Dig Endosc* 2005;17:S60–S65.

9 Machida H, Sano Y, Hamamoto Y *et al.* Narrow band imaging for differential diagnosis of colorectal mucosal lesions: a pilot study. *Endoscopy* 2004;36:1094–8.

10 Sano Y, Horimatsu T, Fu KI *et al.* Magnified observation of micro-vascular architecture using narrow band imaging (NBI) for the differential diagnosis between non-

neoplastic and neoplastic colorectal lesion: a prospective study. *Gastrointest Endosc* 2006;63:AB102.

11 Tanaka S, Kaltenbach T, Chayama K, Soetikno R. High-magnification colonoscopy (with videos). *Gastrointest Endosc* 2006;64:604–13.

12 Konerding MA, Fait E, Gaumann A. 3D microvascular architecture of pre-cancerous lesions and invasive carcinomas of the colon. *Br J Cancer* 2001;84:1354–62.

13 Fait E, Malkusch W, Gnoth S-H *et al.* Microvascular patterns of the human large intestine: morphometric studies of vascular parameters in corrosion casts. *Scanning Microscopy* 1998;12:641–51.

14 Skinner SA, Frydman GM, O'Brien PE. Microvascular structure of benign and malignant tumors of the colon in humans. *Dig Dis Sci* 1995;40:373–84.

15 Sano Y, Horimatsu T, Fu KI *et al.* Magnified observation of microvascular architecture of colorectal lesions using narrow band imaging system. *Dig Endosc* 2006;18(Suppl 1):S44–S51.

16 Gono K, Yamazaki K, Doguchi N *et al.* Endoscopic observation of tissue by narrowband illumination. *Opt Rev* 2003;10:1–5.

17 Kudo S, Hirota S, Nakajima T *et al.* Colorectal tumours and pit pattern. *J Clin Pathol* 1994;47:880–5.

18 Sano Y, Maeda N, Kanzaki A *et al.* Angiogenesis in colon hyperplastic polyp. *Cancer Lett* 2005;218:223–8.

19 Muto M, Nakane M, Katada C *et al.* Squamous cell carcinoma in situ at oropharyngeal and hypopharyngeal mucosal sites. *Cancer* 2004;101:1375–81.

20 Nagorni A, Bjelakovic G, Petrovic B. Narrowband imaging versus conventional white light colonoscopy for the detection of colorectal polyps. *Cochrane Database Syst Rev* 2012;1:CD008361.

21 ASGE Technology Committee. Electronic chromoendoscopy. *Gastrointest Endosc* 2014; 81:249–261.

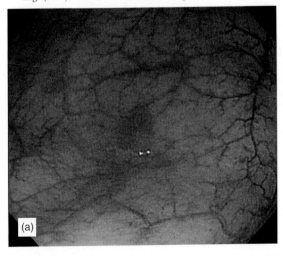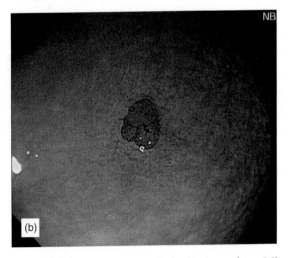

Figure 9.1 Brownish area with typical endoscopic features of flat adenomatous polyp on NBI. (a) Standard colonoscopy shows 0-IIa type lesion, 4 mm in size, in the rectum. (b) NBI without dye spraying. The lesion can be seen as a dark-brown area. (Copyright Y. Sano and S. Yoshida.)

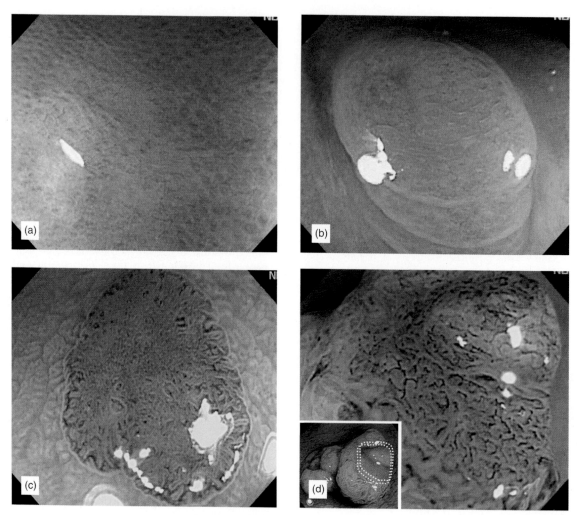

Figure 9.2 Magnifying endoscopic findings of macrocapillary vessels using NBI in normal colonic mucosa, hyperplastic polyps, adenomas, and carcinomas. (a) Normal colonic mucosa. In many cases the mucosal capillary meshwork, arranged in a honeycomb pattern around the mucosal glands, is invisible or faintly visible with magnifying observation using NBI colonoscopy, because endoscopic resolution is insufficient to visualize the network (MC –, CP type I). (b) Hyperplastic polyps. In many cases the mucosal capillary meshwork is invisible or only faintly visible with magnifying observation using NBI colonoscopy, because endoscopic resolution is insufficient to visualize the network (MC –, CP type I). (c) Adenomatous polyps. MC vessels are clearly visible, because these capillaries are elongated and have longer diameters than do normal capillaries. The honeycomb-like pattern of capillaries on the surface of the tumor is retained (MC +, CP type II). (d) Carcinoma in adenoma (magnifying view of the demarcated area in lower-left chromoendoscopic view). The microvascular architecture of colonic carcinoma is characterized by a disorganized structure and increased density of microvessels. MC vessels are clearly visible and show unevenly sized, thicker capillaries with branching curtailed irregularity (MC +, CP type III). (Copyright Y. Sano and S. Yoshida.)

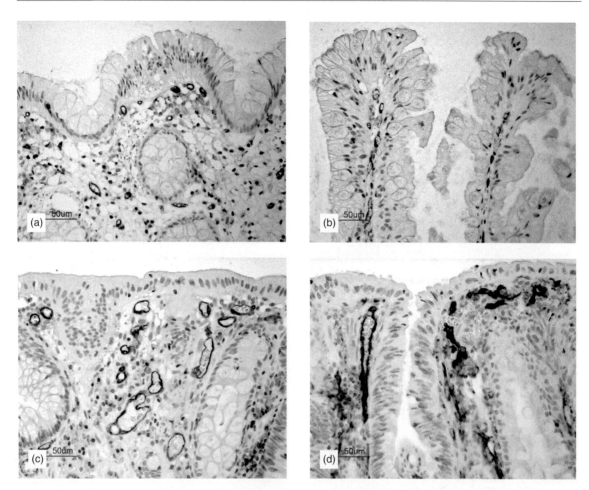

Figure 9.3 Histology of macrocapillary vessels in normal colonic mucosa, hyperplastic polyps, adenoma, and carcinoma. All specimens are stained for endothelial cells with an anti-CD31 antibody (clone JC/70A, DAKO, dilution 1 in 20). Original magnification ×100. (a) The superficial portion of normal colonic mucosa. Many microcapillary vessels measuring approximately 10 μm can be seen in the stromal tissue. (b) The superficial portion of hyperplastic polyp. Many microcapillary vessels measuring approximately 10 μm can be seen in the stromal tissue, as in normal mucosa. (c) The superficial portion of adenomatous polyp. Thicker capillary vessels can be seen surrounding the adenomatous glands. (d) The superficial portion of well-differentiated adenocarcinoma. Thicker capillary vessels can be seen surrounding the cancerous glands. (Copyright Y. Sano and S. Yoshida.)

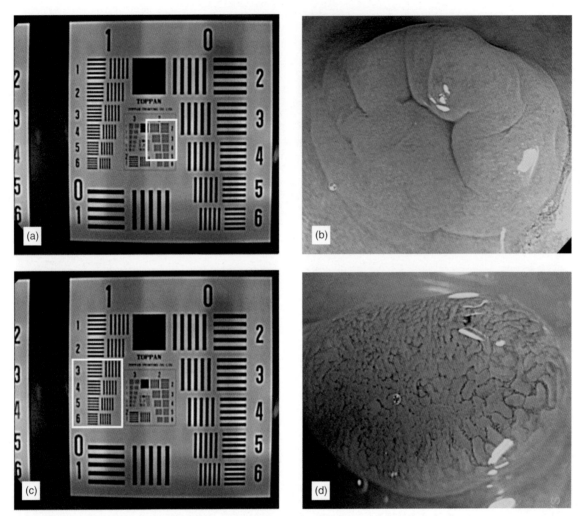

Figure 9.4 Comparison between endoscopic resolution and MC vessels. (a) Magnifying observation of squared plate (TOPPAN-TEST-CHART-NO1), 3 mm in size. The highlighted area relates to the approximately 8–12 μm bars, which are not clearly visible or distinguishable due to endoscopic resolution. (b) Magnifying observation of hyperplastic polyp, also 3 mm in size, MC −, CP type I. At this magnification, it is not possible to identify those MC vessels of 8–12 μm diameter shown in (a). (c) Magnifying observation of squared plate (TOPPAN-TEST-CHART-NO1), 3 mm in size. The highlighted area relates to the approximately 14–20 μm bars, which are clearly visible at this magnification. (d) Magnifying observation of adenomatous polyp, also 3 mm in size, MC +, CP type II. It is possible to identify those MC vessels of 14–20 μm diameter shown in (c). (Copyright Y. Sano and S. Yoshida.)

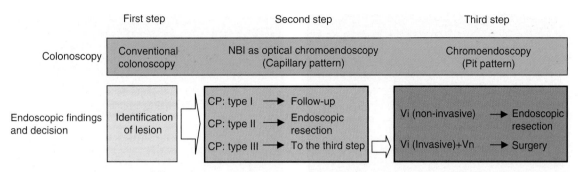

Figure 9.5 Three-step strategy for management of colorectal lesions using conventional colonoscopy, NBI colonoscopy, and chromoendoscopy. When a lesion is found with normal observation, it is then observed with NBI mode. If the result is CP type I, follow-up is recommended; for CP type II, resection is recommended; for CP type III, performing chromoendoscopy, observing the pit pattern carefully, and deciding the treatment policy are recommended. (Copyright Y. Sano and S. Yoshida.)

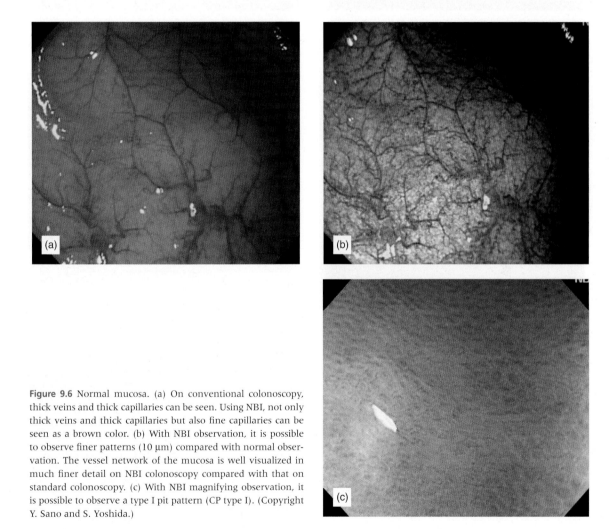

Figure 9.6 Normal mucosa. (a) On conventional colonoscopy, thick veins and thick capillaries can be seen. Using NBI, not only thick veins and thick capillaries but also fine capillaries can be seen as a brown color. (b) With NBI observation, it is possible to observe finer patterns (10 μm) compared with normal observation. The vessel network of the mucosa is well visualized in much finer detail on NBI colonoscopy compared with that on standard colonoscopy. (c) With NBI magnifying observation, it is possible to observe a type I pit pattern (CP type I). (Copyright Y. Sano and S. Yoshida.)

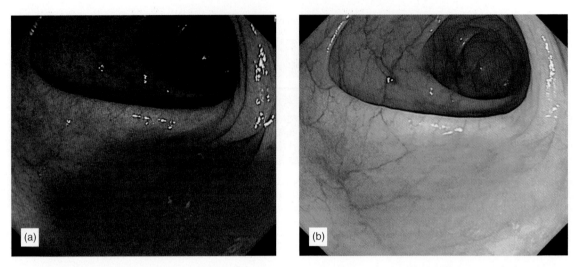

Figure 9.7 Intestinal fluids. (a) On NBI colonoscopy, intestinal fluids are recognized as a reddish color similar to blood. (b) This is a problem that may confuse the colonoscopist and if misinterpreted create a false cause of concern. (Copyright Y. Sano and S. Yoshida.)

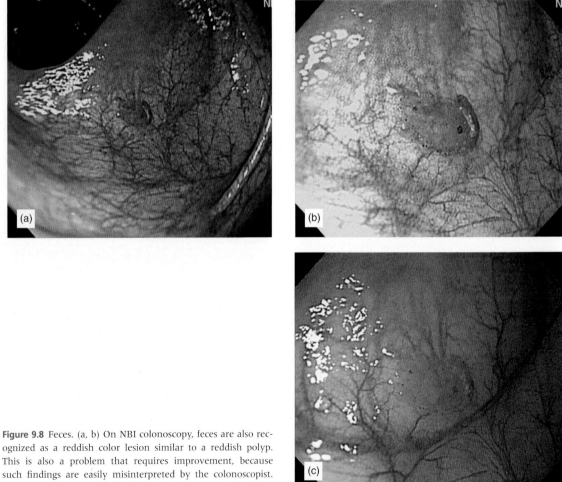

Figure 9.8 Feces. (a, b) On NBI colonoscopy, feces are also recognized as a reddish color lesion similar to a reddish polyp. This is also a problem that requires improvement, because such findings are easily misinterpreted by the colonoscopist. (c) Feces on the colonic wall. (Copyright Y. Sano and S. Yoshida.)

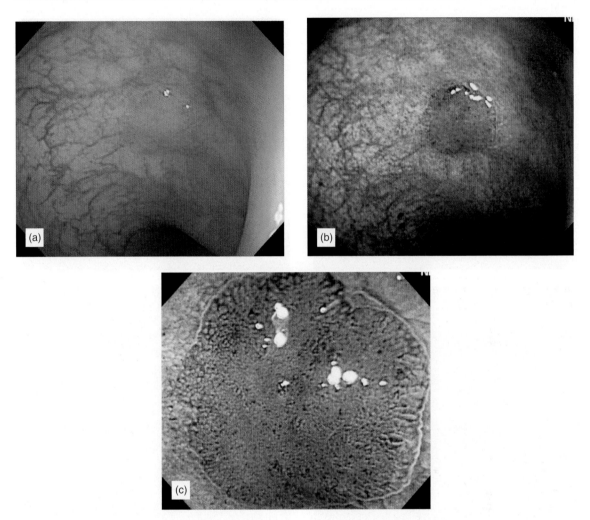

Figure 9.9 Tubular adenoma with moderate atypia, type IIa. (a) An 8-mm flat elevated lesion is recognized in the area where the visibility of the capillary vessels disappears in the sigmoid colon under conventional colonoscopic observation. (b) Capillary vessels of the background mucosa become clear under NBI observation, and with improved visibility the lesion is described as a round brown blob. (c) With NBI magnifying observation it is easy to observe IIIL + IIIs pit surrounded by MC (CP type II). (Copyright Y. Sano and S. Yoshida.)

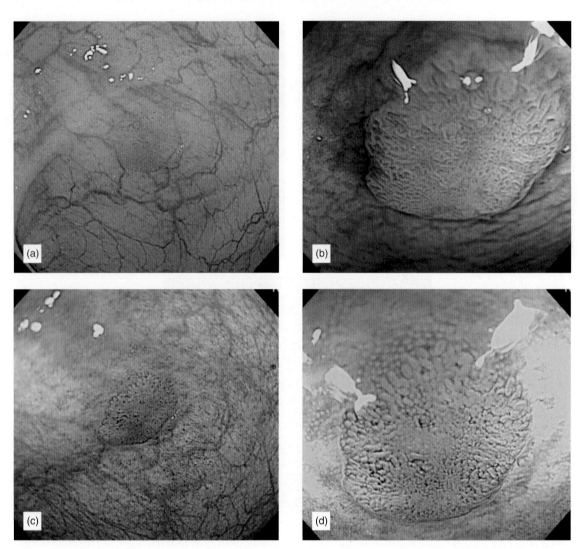

Figure 9.10 Tubular adenoma with moderate atypia, type IIa. (a) A 5-mm flat polyp is recognized in the area where the visibility of the blood vessels disappears in the sigmoid colon under normal observation. (b) With indigo carmine dye, IIIL and IIIs pit is recognized. (c) Capillary vessels of the background mucosa become clear under NBI observation, and with improved visibility the lesion is described as a round brown blob. (d) With NBI magnifying observation it is easy to observe IIIL + IIIs pit surrounded by MC (CP type II). (Copyright Y. Sano and S. Yoshida.)

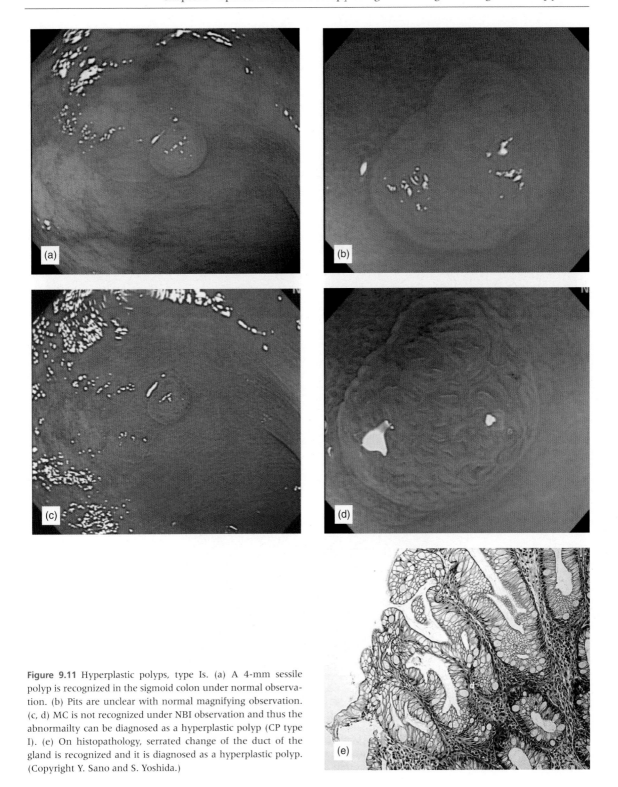

Figure 9.11 Hyperplastic polyps, type Is. (a) A 4-mm sessile polyp is recognized in the sigmoid colon under normal observation. (b) Pits are unclear with normal magnifying observation. (c, d) MC is not recognized under NBI observation and thus the abnormailty can be diagnosed as a hyperplastic polyp (CP type I). (e) On histopathology, serrated change of the duct of the gland is recognized and it is diagnosed as a hyperplastic polyp. (Copyright Y. Sano and S. Yoshida.)

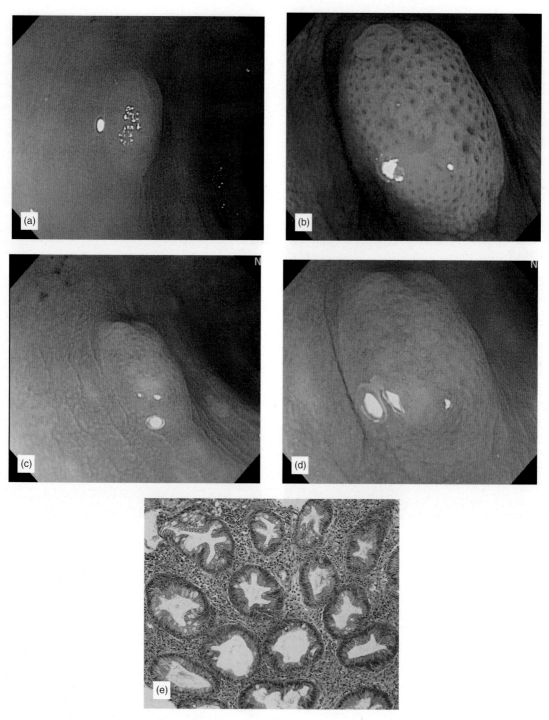

Figure 9.12 Hyperplastic polyp, type Is. (a) A faded color polyp in the sigmoid colon is recognized under normal observation. (b) Pit pattern is recognized as type II under magnifying observation with indigo carmine spread and thus diagnosed as a hyperplastic polyp. (c, d) MC is not recognized under NBI observation and thus the abnormailty can be diagnosed as a hyperplastic polyp (CP type I). (e) On histopathology, serrated change of the duct of the gland is recognized and it is diagnosed as a hyperplastic polyp. (Copyright Y. Sano and S. Yoshida.)

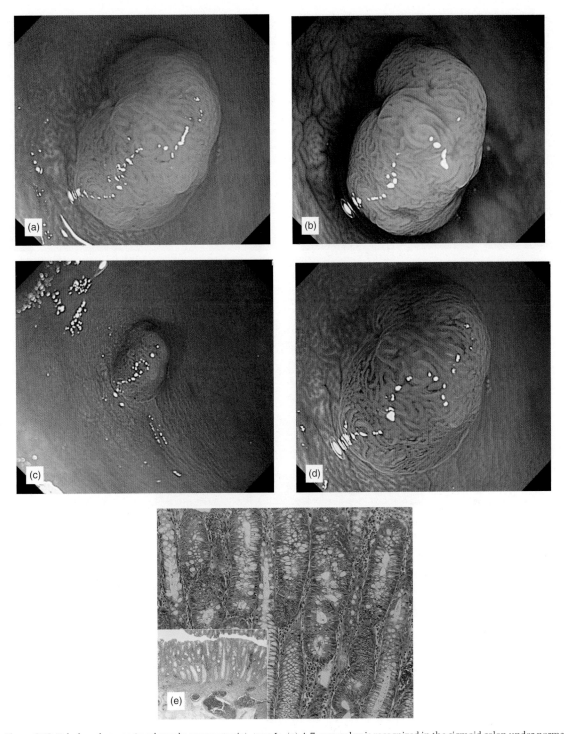

Figure 9.13 Tubular adenoma (moderately severe atypia), type Is. (a) A 7-mm polyp is recognized in the sigmoid colon under normal observation. (b) Type IIIL pit pattern is recognized under magnifying observation with indigo carmine spread and thus diagnosed as an adenomatous polyp. (c, d) Under NBI observation, type IIIL pit pattern is recognized by MC, which is surrounding the duct of the gland, and can thus be diagnosed as an adenomatous polyp (CP type II). (e) Abnormal cells are forming abnormal ducts of the gland and the nuclear and structural atypia are both moderately severe. (Copyright Y. Sano and S. Yoshida.)

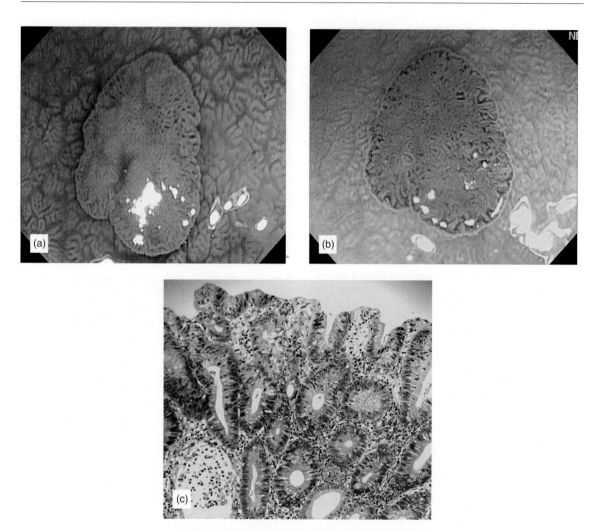

Figure 9.14 Tubular adenoma with moderate atypia, type IIa. (a) A 4-mm flat polyp is recognized in the rectosigmoid. Under magnifying observation, type IIIL pit pattern is recognized under magnifying observation with indigo carmine spread and thus diagnosed as an adenomatous polyp. (b) Under NBI magnifying observation, type IIIL pit pattern is clearly recognized by MC, which is surrounding the duct of the gland, and can thus be diagnosed as an adenomatous polyp (CP type II). (c) Abnormal cells are forming abnormal ducts of the gland and the nuclear and structural atypia are both moderately severe. The lesion is diagnosed as a tubular adenoma with moderate atypia. (Copyright Y. Sano and S. Yoshida.)

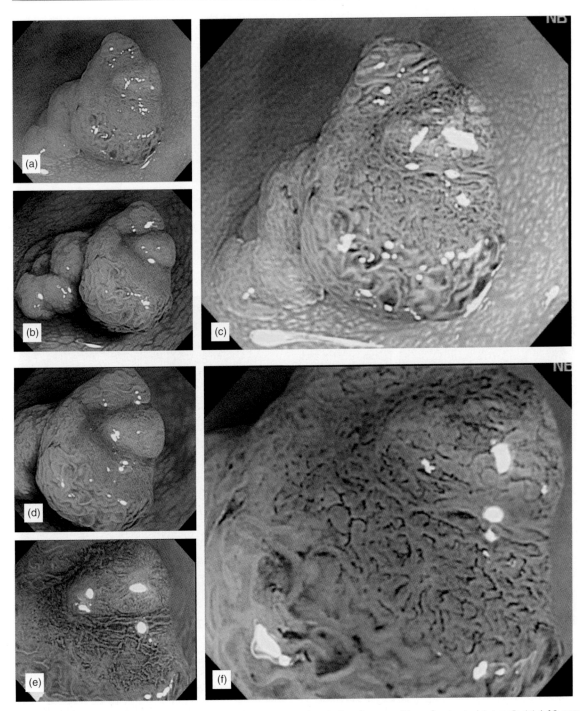

Figure 9.15 Cancer in adenoma (well-differentiated adenocarcinoma in tubular adenoma with moderate atypia), type Is. (a) A 10-mm sessile polyp is recognized in the sigmoid under normal observation. Depressed surface with a small elevation is also recognized on the right side of the polyp. (b) Depressed surface on the right side becomes clearer with indigo carmine spread under magnifying observation. (c) With NBI observation, irregular capillary vessels which irregularly surround the duct of the gland on the depressed surface on the right side can be recognized. (d) Indigo carmine dye with magnifying observation. Type IV pit pattern on the left side and slightly irregular type Vi pit are recognized on the depressed surface on the right side. (e) Crystal violet staining image. Low-grade irregular Vi pit is clearly recognized. The area of depressed surface is around 4 mm and it is not diagnosed as invasive pattern but cancer in mucosa. (f) With NBI observation, irregular capillary vessels which irregularly surround the duct of the gland on the depressed surface on the right side can be recognized. It is diagnosed as a cancer (CP type III). (continued)

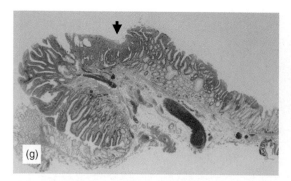

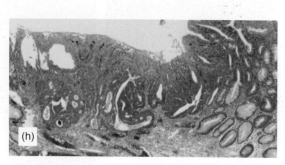

Figure 9.15 (Continued) (g) EMR resection specimen. Well-differentiated adenocarcinoma in tubular adenoma with moderate atypia. Cancer is recognized on the depressed surface on the right side (arrowhead). (h) Well-differentiated adenocarcinoma of the depressed surface. Muscularis mucosae is intact and the lesion is diagnosed as intramucosal cancer. (Copyright Y. Sano and S. Yoshida.)

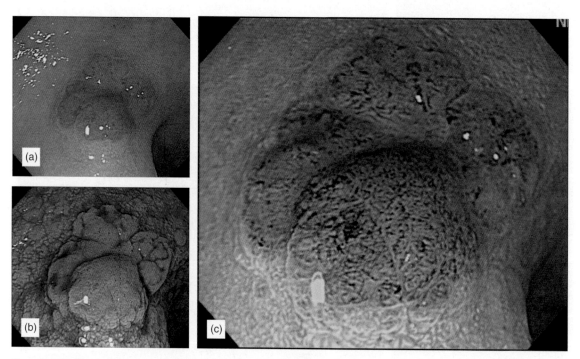

Figure 9.16 Cancer in adenoma (well-differentiated adenocarcinoma in tubular adenoma with moderate to severe atypia), type IIa (flat elevated cancer). (a) A 13-mm flat elevated lesion is recognized in the rectosigmoid under normal observation. A small elevation with red flare is recognized in front middle. (b) The small elevation becomes clearer with indigo carmine spread under magnifying observation. (c) With NBI observation, capillary vessels, which irregularly surround the duct of the gland in the area of small elevation, can be recognized.

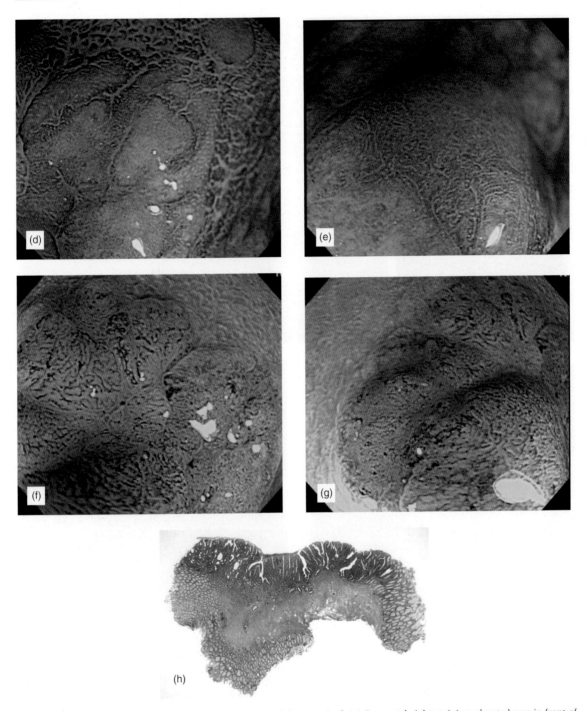

Figure 9.16 (Continued) (d) On crystal violet staining, a IIIL pit is recognized. (e) On crystal violet staining, elevated area in front of the lesion is observed as low-grade irregular VL pit. (f) With NBI magnifying observation, fine capillary vessels with thicker diameter which surround the duct of the gland are recognized on the flat elevated area on the right side (CP type II). (g) With NBI magnifying observation, blood vessels on the elevation in front of the lesion become thicker, presenting caliber variation and irregularly running and surrounding the duct of the gland (CP type III). (h) EMR resection specimen. Well-differentiated adenocarcinoma in tubular adenoma with moderate to severe atypia. Depth: intramucosal cancer. (Copyright Y. Sano and S. Yoshida.)

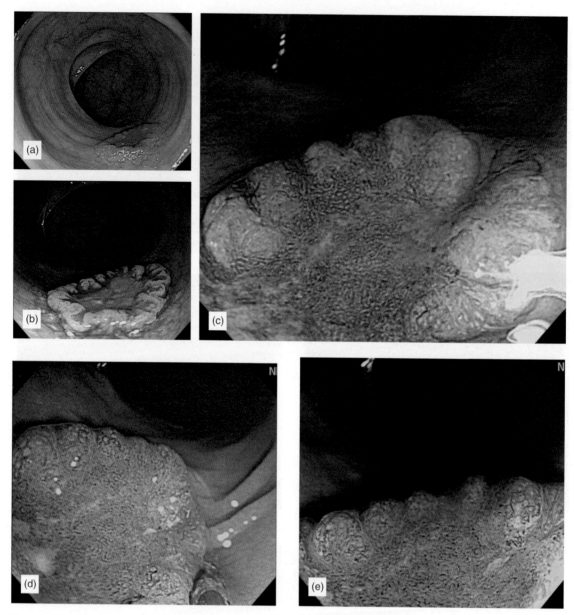

Figure 9.17 Moderately differentiated adenocarcinoma, type IIa + IIc, invasive cancer (sm1), T1. (a) A 23-mm depressed lesion with white spots is recognized under normal observation. Tightened fold can be found at margins. (b) Depressed surface becomes clearer with dye magnifying observation. Star-like irregularity is recognized on the margins of the depression. (c) Crystal violet staining image. Different-sized pits present in which the difference in size can be observed on the depressed surface of the lesion. The structure of the pit is not destroyed and it is diagnosed as a low-grade irregular type Vi pit. (d) With NBI magnifying observation, caliber variation and dense MC vessels are observed on the depressed surface (CP type III). (e) Region of type V pit (>3 mm) is recognized and it is diagnosed as submucosal cancer. (Copyright Y. Sano and S. Yoshida.)

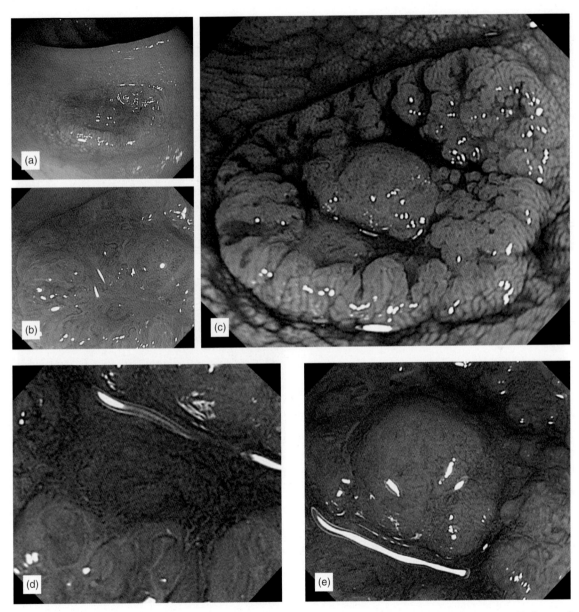

Figure 9.18 Moderately differentiated adenocarcinoma, type IIa + IIc, invasive cancer (sm1), T1. (a) A 17-mm IIa + IIc depressed lesion with white spots is recognized in the rectum under normal observation. A small elevation with red flare. (b) A small elevation that exhibits capillary vessels with thick bore becomes clearer. (c) With indigo carmine dye, star-like irregularity is recognized at margins of the depression. Pits of a different size are arranged on the depressed surface of the lesion located on the front left side. The structure of the pit is not destroyed and it is diagnosed as low-grade irregular type Vi pit. (d). Crystal violet staining under magnifying observation of the left lower part of the lesion. Unsteady high-grade irregular type Vi pit is observed as a whirlpool shape. (continued)

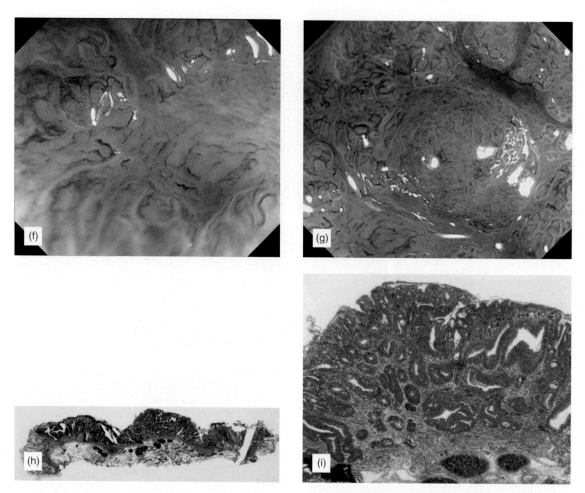

Figure 9.18 (Continued) (e) Crystal violet staining under magnifying observation of the middle part of the lesion. Low-grade irregular type Vi pit is observed. (f) NBI magnifying observation of the region shown in (d). Irregular disruption and meander is observed (CP type III). (g) NBI magnifying observation of the region shown in (e). Tumor blood vessels of different-sized bore that run irregularly are recognized. It is determined to be a blood vessel image of cancer (CP type III). (h, i) Moderately differentiated adenocarcinoma is recognized. Submucosal infiltration is found in the elevated area of the depressed area recognized by endoscopy (infiltration distance 375 μm). It was reported as ly0 and V0. (Copyright Y. Sano and S. Yoshida.)

10 Keys to effective performance of resect and discard NBI

Douglas K. Rex

Introduction

Resect and discard refers to a paradigm of polyp management in which diminutive (≤5 mm in size) and perhaps
small lesions (6–9 mm in size) are identified and then
have their pathology predicted or estimated using endoscopic criteria [1–3]. Those lesions that can be predicted
with high confidence can be discarded without submission to pathology and the subsequent surveillance
assigned based on the endoscopic prediction of pathology [1]. The target set of polyps in the United States is
the diminutive group [2]; in the UK the target group
is lesions of 9 mm or less [3]. One of the advantages
of resect and discard is the financial savings, with the
potential to recoup more than $1 billion per year esti-
mated for the United States [4]. An underpinning of the
resect and discard paradigm is the extremely low risk of
cancer in tiny polyps; for lesions of 5 mm or less in size,
this risk is less than 1 per 2000 lesions [5–13]. Certainly
any features that suggest cancer in a small or diminutive lesion is an absolute contraindication to discarding
the lesion without pathologic assessment. Such features
include surface ulceration, true depression, an amorphous or markedly irregular vessel pattern in a small
conventional adenoma, an atypical change in shape or
color or a suggestion of submucosal infiltration, or a suggestion of a hard or firm sensation with manipulation of
the lesion.

NICE classification

Several classification schemes for using NBI to differentiate conventional adenomas from serrated class lesions
have been proposed [14–16]. One validated classification
for this purpose is the narrowband imaging international
colorectal endoscopic (NICE) classification (Table 10.1)

[14]. The general and primary goal of current endoscopic
characterization using narrowband imaging (NBI) is to
classify diminutive lesions as being conventional adenomas or belonging to the serrated class. Secondarily, the
endoscopist should identify any features suggesting cancer, although such findings in diminutive lesions are rare.
With the conventional adenoma class of lesions, characterization with non-magnifying colonoscopes cannot
identify the presence of villous elements or determine
dysplasia grade [14]. This limitation is handled in the
overall management scheme by restricting the resect and
discard paradigm to lesions of 5 mm or less in size which
have a very low prevalence of both high-grade dysplasia
and villous elements [1]. The rationale for ignoring the
potential of high-grade dysplasia and villous elements
includes the realities that the pathologic definitions of
these findings are variable and not validated as clinically
significant and also subject to marked interobserver variation [17–22]. The high level of interobserver variation
reaches peak levels for diminutive lesions, related in part
to the very low prevalence of the findings [23].

Similarly, the NICE classification does not distinguish
between hyperplastic polyps (HPs) and sessile serrated
polyps (SSPs), the two major lesions within the serrated
class (traditional serrated adenoma is the third). Again,
the distinction between HP and SSP is managed in the
resect and discard paradigm by restricting the application of discard to lesions of 5 mm or less in size, for
which the prevalence of SSP is very small [24]. Particularly in the left colon, SSP elements are rare in serrated
lesions of 5 mm or less, and SSP with cytologic dysplasia is extremely rare in diminutive left colon serrated
lesions. Again, similar and analgous to the situation with
differentiation of villous elements and dysplasia grade
within conventional adenomas, pathologists showed
marked interobserver variation in differentiation of HPs
from SSPs [25,26]. Again, the pathologic criteria for the

Comprehensive Atlas of High-Resolution Endoscopy and Narrowband Imaging, Second Edition. Edited by Jonathan Cohen.
© 2017 John Wiley & Sons, Ltd. Published 2017 by John Wiley & Sons, Ltd.
Companion website: www.wiley.com/go/cohen/NBI

Table 10.1   The narrowband imaging international colorectal endoscopic (NICE) classification for differentiation of serrated class lesions (type 1) and conventional adenomas (type 2) and cancers with deep submucosal invasion (type 3).

	Type 1	Type 2	Type 3
Color	Same or lighter than background	Browner relative to background (verify color arises from vessels)	Brown to dark brown relative to background; sometimes patchy whiter areas
Vessels	None, or isolated lacy vessels may be present coursing across the lesion	Thick brown vessels surrounding white structures	Has area(s) with markedly distorted or missing vessels
Surface pattern	Dark spots surrounded by white	Oval, tubular, or branched white structures surrounded by brown vessels	Distortion or absence of pattern
Most likely pathology	Hyperplastic or sessile serrated polyp (adenoma)	Adenoma	Deep submucosal invasive cancer

distinction are not validated as being clinically significant. Outside the NICE classification, investigators have identified endoscopic features that distinguish SSPs from HPs [27,28]. First, SSPs are distinguished from HPs by general criteria such as large size, right colon location, and the presence of a mucus cap [28]. With regard to surface features, Hazewinkel *et al.* [27] found that, in white light, SSPs were characterized by indistinct edges and a "cloud-like" surface. In NBI, SSPs had the same features seen in white light as well as an irregular surface and dark spots on the crypts (Figure 10.1). When all or none of the four NBI features were present, the sensitivity, specificity, and accuracy of differentiating SSP from HP were 89%, 96%, and 93%, respectively.

The NICE classification includes elements for color, surface vessels, and surface pattern. The association of each element of the NICE classification with its respective polyp pathology has been validated in a study involving medical students, medical residents, and attending gastroenterologists [14]. In the resect and discard paradigm, a critical decision is whether the interpretation of a particular polyp can be made with high confidence. Polyps interpreted with high confidence can be subjected to discard, whereas polyps interpreted with low confidence should be submitted for formal pathologic assessment. In several trials, approximately 75–80% of diminutive polyps can be interpreted by experts with high confidence [29]. High confidence has been variably defined as more than a 90% probability of a correct estimate, arriving at a conclusion regarding the pathology prediction within 5 seconds, or having all the features of one type of lesion and none of the other type [2,29].

Figure 10.2 shows typical examples of diminutive NICE type 1 (serrated class) and Figure 10.3 shows high-confidence type 2 (conventional adenoma) lesions. Of the three criteria, the least reliable in my opinion is color.

While it is true that conventional adenomas (type 2) have a brown color, a dark color is commonly seen on the surface of type 1 lesions because the pits of a type 1 lesion can be either dark or white. It is critical for accurate interpretation that the endoscopist is able to differentiate pits from blood vessels, and to remember that both can be dark. In general, when pits are dark they tend to form the central aspect of structures for which the perimeter is white or light colored. Vessels, which are always dark in NBI and in conventional adenomas are often thick and have a browner hue (compared with the pits of type 1 lesions which trend toward a black color), typically appear to surround structures that are white.

High and low confidence

High confidence in type 2 is most appropriate when some or all of the white structures are tubular and/or variable in length (Figure 10.3). High confidence is also appropriate when these features are combined with a central valley that appears browner than the remaining polyp (Figure 10.4). This valley is not a true depression as implied by the 2c Paris classification [30]. The 2c depressions are typically larger, occupy more of the surface area of the lesion, and are characterized by a steep or sudden drop-off at the edge or transition from the elevated to depressed aspects. The central valley is sometimes called a "2a dip" or pseudo-depression and is not associated with the high prevalence of high-grade dysplasia and invasive cancer seen with true depressions. About 15% of conventional adenomas have such a central brown valley. Detailed inspection of the valley typically demonstrates that the more intense brown color is the result of a high concentration of relatively pinpoint brown vessels. Experienced examiners survey the entire surface of the polyp to determine the dominant pattern. For example, many high-confidence conventional adenomas will have portions of the polyp that meet the above criteria for tubular and variably shaped white structures, and another portion that has a concentration of relatively pinpoint vessels. The more pinpoint vessels may be difficult to differentiate from the pits of a type 1 lesion (which are also dark and very focal) without considering the context of the entire lesion.

The type 1 high-confidence lesion is characterized by a complete absence of vessels or by one or a few lacy vessels over the surface of the lesion (Figure 10.5). The pits of a type 1 lesion can be either white or dark (the color might reflect the angle at which light strikes the pit opening or the pit size) and should be relatively uniform in size. These vessels, when present on the surface of type 1 lesions, can be differentiated from the vessels of type 2 lesions because they are thinner and because they course past several pits, ending abruptly without surrounding pits. On the other hand, the vessels of type 2 lesions tend to brown and thick and appear to surround individual white structures without coursing across the lesion (Figure 10.6).

All of the features should be considered in predicting the pathology and in assigning the confidence level. Brown color in NBI can be the result of any red color in white light, including redness from congestion or bruising. If there are brown vessels but they are surrounding white structures of uniform size (Figure 10.7), caution should be exercised is assigning high-confidence type 2. A degree of variability in size of the white structures or a significant component of tubular white structures is needed to make a diagnosis of high-confidence type 2.

It is possible for both type 1 and type 2 features to be seen in the same lesion. This finding is uncommon and when present predicts an SSP with cytologic dysplasia (Figure 10.8). The area with type 2 features corresponds to the region of the polyp with cytologic dysplasia histologically. Such lesions are usually large and located in the proximal colon.

The fraction of lesions called with high confidence is of no importance to the principle of resect and discard, is likely to vary between examiners, and could change with experience for individual examiners. The 5-second rule implies that if the features are all consistent with type 1 or 2, then the diagnosis will be almost immediately evident. If the colonoscopist finds herself studying the lesion for longer than 5 seconds (certainly this is the case when many seconds are spent evaluating the lesion), then there is probably either a mix of type 1 and type 2 features or there is some other atypical aspect, and the lesion is best designated a low-confidence lesion.

Other considerations

Resect and discard is approaching status as an acceptable paradigm for diminutive polyp management in the United States. Recently, resect and discard has been endorsed by the American Society for Gastrointestinal Endoscopy [31] and the American Gastroenterological Association [32] as an effective strategy. Society endorsement provides a degree of medicolegal protection for the resect and discard practice. Table 10.2 lists a number of steps or events that would be necessary in most settings to initiate the resect and discard paradigm [33]. The medicolegal risk is extremely unlikely to be created by discard of lesions of 5 mm or less in size, since the risk of cancer in such lesions is negligible. The medicolegal risk arises when another larger lesion in the colon is missed and the patient presents with interval cancer. In this instance, the plaintiff's expert could allege that the discarded lesion contained cancer. A high-quality photograph of the *in vivo* lesion before resection is critical for establishing the appropriateness of the discard in a medicolegal proceeding. Second, the colonoscopist must be prepared to demonstrate that her adenoma detection rate (ADR) meets recommended thresholds [34]. Again, this step requires long-term storage of high-quality photographs demonstrating convincing conventional adenomas that can be counted by another expert in an ADR review [35]. Third, national, state, or local institutional rules that require submission of all resected tissue to be submitted for pathology must be revised. Given the extremely low risk of cancer in diminutive lesions, there is no rationale for continuing to require that these lesions be submitted to pathology, and several rationales exist for discarding the

Table 10.2 Remaining measures to make real-time determination of pathology a viable clinical practice for diminutive colorectal polyp management and target biopsy in Barrett's esophagus.

Development of credentialing protocols
Development of validated training tools
Documentation of endoscopic decision-making (image storage)
Medicolegal coverage
Documentation of adenoma detection rate[a]
Revision of institutional policies on requirements to submit tissue to pathology[a]
Reimbursement or other financial incentives for endoscopic determination of pathology

[a]Applies only to colorectal polyps.
Source: adapted from Rex [33].

lesions. For example, if an endoscopist were to estimate the pathology and destroy the lesions with an ablative tool such as the argon plasma coagulator, no objections would be raised. Such a strategy could be called "evaluate and destroy." Similarly, CT colonographers are told to not even report lesions of 5 mm or less in size [36]. Given these facts, the inappropriateness of requiring that tissue from lesions of 5 mm or less in size be submitted for histology is irrational, given that the lesions have already been removed in the resect and discard paradigm (unlike the practice in CT colonography) and can no longer harm the patient.

 Video clips to accompany this book can be found in the online material at www.wiley.com/go/cohen/NBI

The following videos relate specifically to this chapter:

Video 48 Nice classification Type I hyper plastic polyps and WASP classification serrated polyps

Video 49 High confidence NICE Type II tubular adenomas and "valley signs"

Video 50 Colon polyps on NBI: detection and diagnosis. Optical diagnosis of a small adenoma

Video 54 NBI characteristics of colon polyps: pit patterns and mesh capillary patterns

Video 56 Small sessile and pedunculated polyps

Video 59 Sessile depressed polyp

Video 66 NICE 2 tubular adenoma optical diagnosis

Video 67 NICE 1 hyperplastic colon polyp

Video 68 NBI characterization of hyperplastic and adenomatous colon polyps

References

1 Rex DK, Kahi C, O'Brien M *et al.* The American Society for Gastrointestinal Endoscopy PIVI (Preservation and Incorporation of Valuable Endoscopic Innovations) on real-time endoscopic assessment of the histology of diminutive colorectal polyps. *Gastrointest Endosc* 2011;73:419–22.

2 Rex DK. Narrow-band imaging without optical magnification for histologic analysis of colorectal polyps. *Gastroenterology* 2009;136:1174–81.

3 Ignjatovic A, East JE, Suzuki N, Vance M, Guenther T, Saunders BP. Optical diagnosis of small colorectal polyps at routine colonoscopy (Detect InSpect ChAracterise Resect and Discard; DISCARD trial): a prospective cohort study. *Lancet Oncol* 2009;10:1171–8.

4 Kessler WR, Imperiale TF, Klein RW, Wielage RC, Rex DK. A quantitative assessment of the risks and cost savings of forgoing histologic examination of diminutive polyps. *Endoscopy* 2011;43:683–91.

5 Chaput U, Alberto SF, Terris B *et al.* Risk factors for advanced adenomas amongst small and diminutive colo-

6 Gupta N, Bansal A, Rao D *et al.* Prevalence of advanced histological features in diminutive and small colon polyps. *Gastrointest Endosc* 2012;75:1022–30.

7. Shapiro R, Ben-Horin S, Bar-Meir S, Avidan B. The risk of advanced histology in small-sized colonic polyps: are non-invasive colonic imaging modalities good enough? *Int J Colorectal Dis* 2012;27:1071–5.

8 Tsai FC, Strum WB. Prevalence of advanced adenomas in small and diminutive colon polyps using direct measurement of size. *Dig Dis Sci* 2011;56:2384–8.

9 Unal H, Selcuk H, Gokcan H *et al.* Malignancy risk of small polyps and related factors. *Dig Dis Sci* 2007;52:2796–9.

10 Bretagne JF, Manfredi S, Piette C, Hamonic S, Durand G, Riou F. Yield of high-grade dysplasia based on polyp size detected at colonoscopy: a series of 2295 examinations following a positive fecal occult blood test in a population-based study. *Dis Colon Rectum* 2010;53:339–45.

11 Lieberman D, Moravec M, Holub J, Michaels L, Eisen G. Polyp size and advanced histology in patients undergoing colonoscopy screening: implications for CT colonography. *Gastroenterology* 2008;135:1100–5.

12 Lawrance IC, Sherrington C, Murray K. Poor correlation between clinical impression, the small colonic polyp and their neoplastic risk. *J Gastroenterol Hepatol* 2006;21:563–8.

13 Butterly LF, Chase MP, Pohl H, Fiarman GS. Prevalence of clinically important histology in small adenomas. *Clin Gastroenterol Hepatol* 2006;4:343–8.

14 Hewett DG, Kaltenbach T, Sano Y *et al.* Validation of a simple classification system for endoscopic diagnosis of small colorectal polyps using narrow-band imaging. *Gastroenterology* 2012;143:599–607.e1.

15 Rastogi A, Mathur S, Bansal A *et al.* Correlation of narrow band imaging (NBI) findings with colon polyp histology. *Gastroenterology* 2007;132:A92-A.

16 Sano Y, Ikematsu H, Fu KI *et al.* Meshed capillary vessels by use of narrow-band imaging for differential diagnosis of small colorectal polyps. *Gastrointest Endosc* 2009;69:278–83.

17 Costantini M, Sciallero S, Giannini A *et al.* Inter-observer agreement in the histologic diagnosis of colorectal polyps: the experience of the multicenter adenoma colorectal study (SMAC). *J Clin Epidemiol* 2003;56:209–14.

18 Yoon H, Antoine M, Robert B, Elisabeth L, Jacques D, Stanislas C. Inter-observer agreement on histological diagnosis of colorectal polyps: APACC study. *Gastroenterol Clin Biol* 2001;25:220–4.

19 Terry MB, Neugut AI, Bostick RM, Potter JD, Haile RW, Fenoglio-Preiser CM. Reliability in the classification of advanced colorectal adenomas. *Cancer Epidemiol Biomarkers Prev* 2002;11:660–3.

20 Brown LJ, Smeeton NC, Dixon MF. Assessment of dysplasia in colorectal adenomas: an observer variation and morphometric study. *J Clin Pathol* 1985;38:174–9.

21 Fenger C, Bak M, Kronborg O, Svanholm H. Observer reproducibility in grading dysplasia in colorectal adenomas: comparison between two different grading systems. *J Clin Pathol* 1990;43:320–4.

22 Jensen P, Krogsgaard MR, Christiansen J, Braendstrup O, Johansen A, Olsen J. Observer variability in the assessment of type and dysplasia of colorectal adenomas, analyzed using kappa-statistics. *Dis Colon Rectum* 1995;38:195–8.

23 Lasisi F, Mouchli A, Riddell R *et al.* Agreement in interpreting villous elements and dysplasia in adenomas less than one centimetre in size. *Dig Liver Dis* 2013;45:1049–55.

24 Abdeljawad K, Vemulapalli KC, Kahi CJ, Cummings OW, Snover DC, Rex DK. Sessile serrated polyp prevalence determined by a colonoscopist with a high lesion detection rate and an experienced pathologist. *Gastrointest Endosc* 2015;81:517–24.

25 Khalid O, Radaideh S, Cummings OW, O'Brien MJ, Goldblum JR, Rex DK. Reinterpretation of histology of proximal colon polyps called hyperplastic in 2001. *World J Gastroenterol* 2009;15:3767–70.

26 Tinmouth J, Henry P, Hsieh E *et al.* Sessile serrated polyps at screening colonoscopy: have they been under diagnosed? *Am J Gastroenterol* 2014;109:1698–704.

27 Hazewinkel Y, Lopez-Ceron M, East JE *et al.* Endoscopic features of sessile serrated adenomas: validation by international experts using high-resolution white-light endoscopy and narrow-band imaging. *Gastrointest Endosc* 2013;77:916–24.

28 Tadepalli US, Feihel D, Miller KM *et al.* A morphologic analysis of sessile serrated polyps observed during routine colonoscopy (with video). *Gastrointest Endosc* 2011;74:1360–8.

29 McGill SK, Evangelou E, Ioannidis JP, Soetikno RM, Kaltenbach T. Narrow band imaging to differentiate neoplastic and non-neoplastic colorectal polyps in real time: a meta-analysis of diagnostic operating characteristics. *Gut* 2013;62:1704–13.

30 Paris endoscopic classification of superficial neoplastic lesions: esophagus, stomach, and colon: November 30 to December 1, 2002. *Gastrointest Endosc* 2003;58(6 Suppl):S3–S43.

31 Abu Dayyeh BK, Thosani N, Konda V *et al.* ASGE Technology Committee systematic review and meta-analysis assessing the ASGE PIVI thresholds for adopting real-time endoscopic assessment of the histology of diminutive colorectal polyps. *Gastrointest Endosc* 2015;81:502e1–e16.

32 Lieberman D, Brill J, Canto M *et al.* Management of diminutive colon polyps based on endoluminal imaging. *Clin Gastroenterol Hepatol* 2015;13:1860–6.

33 Rex DK. Prediction of colorectal polyp pathologic lesions with image-enhanced endoscopy: what will it take to make it matter? *Gastrointest Endosc* 2014;80:1088–93.

34 Rex DK, Schoenfeld PS, Cohen J *et al.* Quality indicators for colonoscopy. *Gastrointest Endosc* 2015;81:31–53.

35 Rex DK, Hardacker K, MacPhail M, Rahmani F, Vemulapalli KC, Kahi CJ. Determining the adenoma detection rate and adenomas per colonoscopy by photography alone: proof-of-concept study. *Endoscopy* 2015;47:245–50.

36 Zalis ME, Barish MA, Choi JR *et al.* CT colonography reporting and data system: a consensus proposal. *Radiology* 2005;236:3–9.

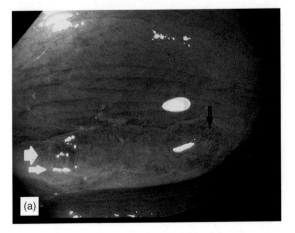
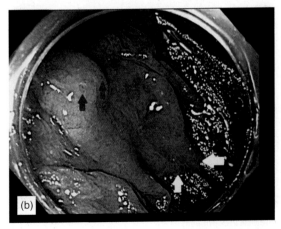

Figure 10.1 Narrowband imaging photographs of sessile serrated polyps. Features that suggest sessile serrated polyp over hyperplastic polyp include indistinct edges (yellow arrows), large dark pits (orange arrows), and an irregular surface (black rectangles). (continued)

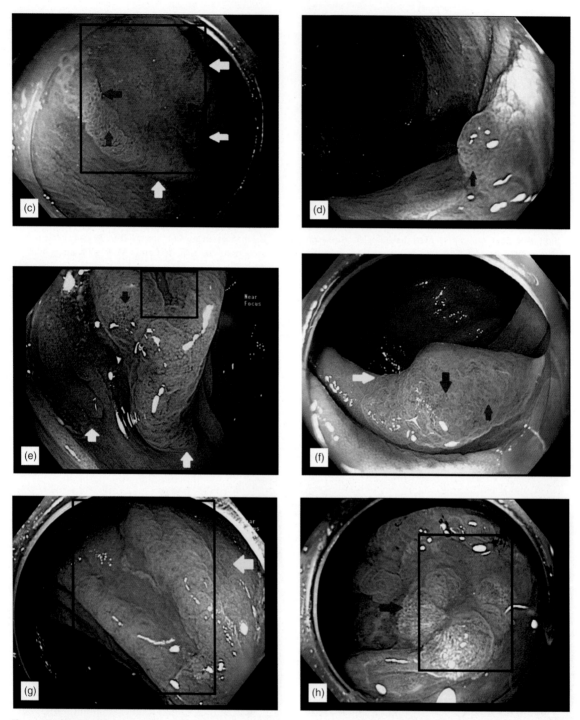

Figure 10.1 (Continued)

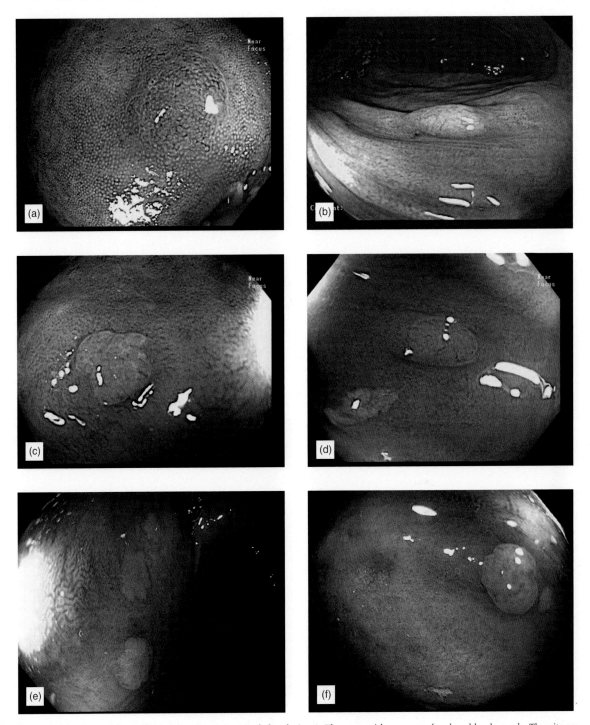

Figure 10.2 High-confidence diminutive type 1 (serrated class lesions). There are either no or a few lacy blood vessels. The pits are relatively uniform in size.

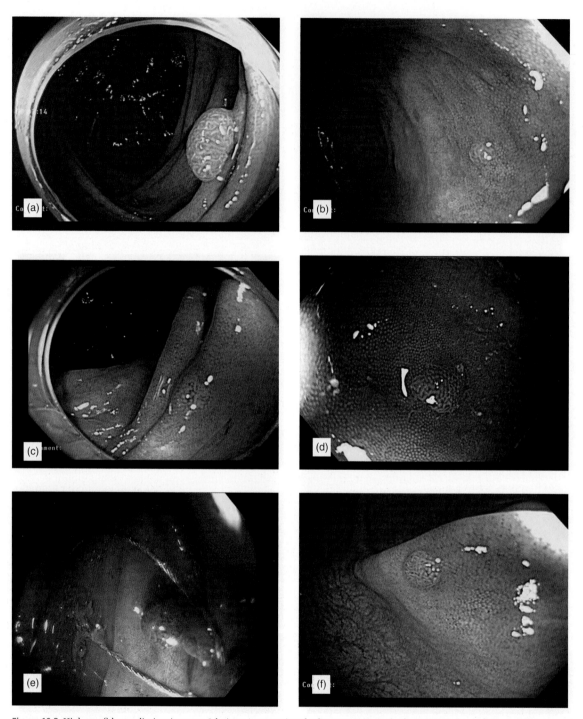

Figure 10.3 High-confidence diminutive type 2 lesions (conventional adenomas). Note the brown vessels, and the variably shaped white structures including tubular shaped structures.

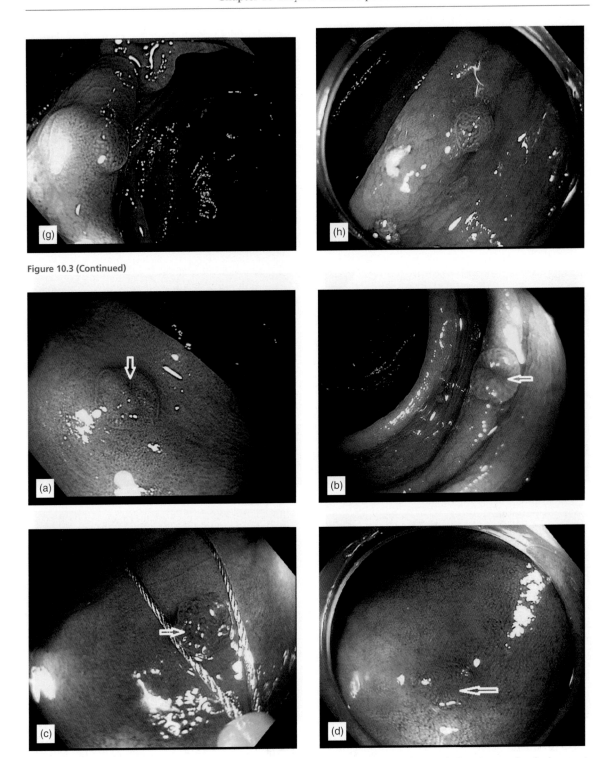

Figure 10.3 (Continued)

Figure 10.4 The arrows point to the darker brown colored valley seen in about 15% of type 2 lesions (conventional adenomas). These areas are specific but not sensitive for type 2.

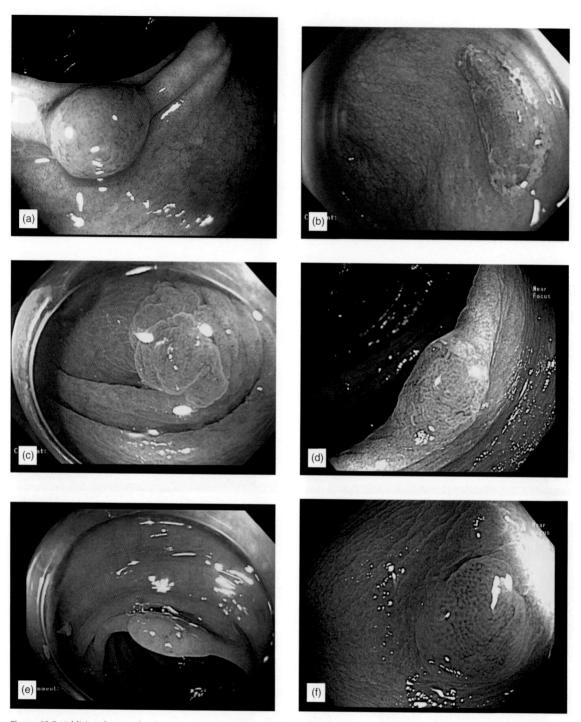

Figure 10.5 Additional examples demonstrating features of type 1 lesions. There are no vessels or only a few lacy vessels. The pits may be light or dark but are of uniform size.

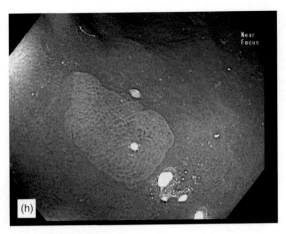

Figure 10.5 (Continued)

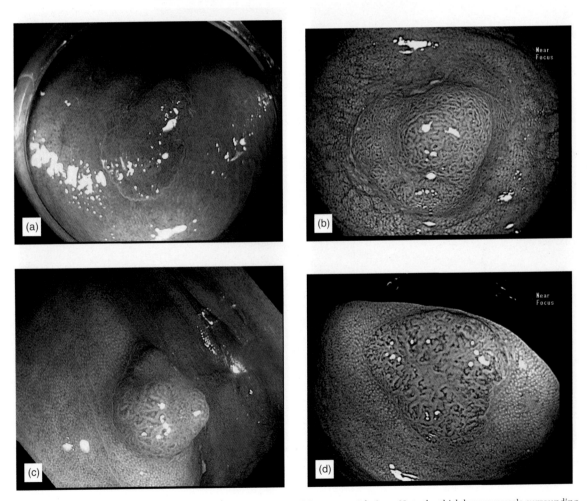

Figure 10.6 Additional polyps demonstrating features of high-confidence type 2 lesions. Note the thick brown vessels surrounding white structures of variable shape including tubular shapes. (continued)

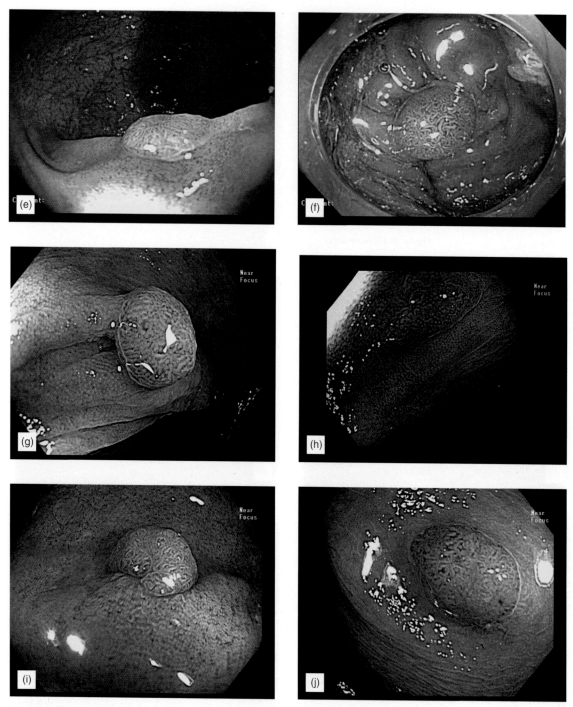

Figure 10.6 (Continued)

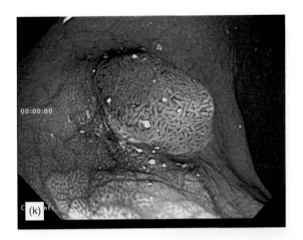

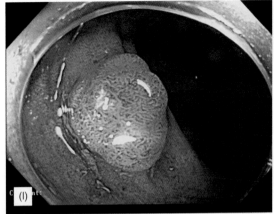

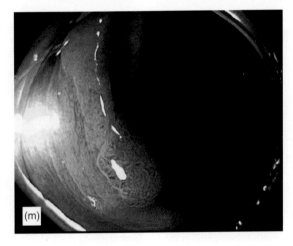

Figure 10.6 (Continued)

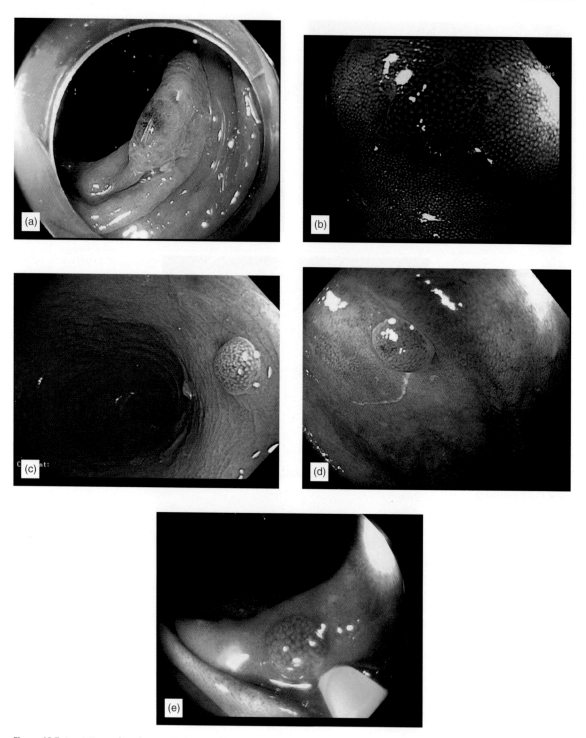

Figure 10.7 (a–e) Examples of type 1 lesions easily mistaken for type 2: (a) dark area of congestion but there are no vessels and the pits are uniform small white dots; (b–d) dark vessels surrounding pits, but the pits are of relatively uniform size.

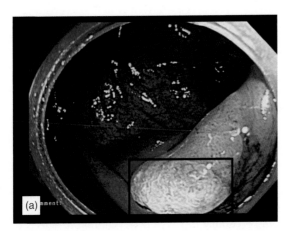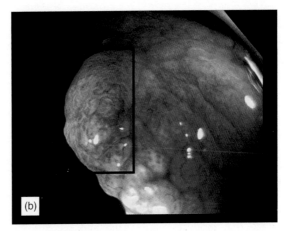

Figure 10.8 Sessile serrated polyps with cytologic dysplasia. The area in the black rectangle demonstrates type 2 features and is the dysplastic portion of the lesion. The remainder of the lesion is typical sessile serrated polyp histologically and shows type 1 features endoscopically.

11 The significance of NBI observation for inflammatory bowel diseases

Takayuki Matsumoto, Tetsuji Kudo, Mitsuo Iida, and James East

Introduction

Narrowband imaging (NBI) is characterized by a light source that produces narrowband and spectroscopically characteristic light. NBI enhances specific depth and color tone. In the NBI system, the narrowband filter wavelength matches the absorption peak of hemoglobin, and vascular architecture and surface structure as outlined by vessels in the gastrointestinal mucosa are enhanced. As a result, NBI is potentially useful for the detection of neoplasms and the diagnosis of tumor depth in the gastrointestinal tract; however, the application of NBI where background inflammation already exists is potentially more challenging.

Comparisons of images of colonic ulcers among conventional colonoscopy, NBI, and chromoendoscopy with indigo carmine are illustrated in Figure 11.1. In NBI, vascular-like structures are observed clearly and crypt openings in the reddish mucosa around the ulcer are enhanced. On the other hand, the elevated or depressed areas become more obvious by chromoendoscopy, even though the vascular pattern is obscure.

Ulcerative colitis

Determination of endoscopic severity

In active ulcerative colitis (UC), conventional colonoscopy shows disappearance of mucosal vascular pattern (MVP), fine or coarse granular mucosa, mucous exudates, and mucosal defects. In quiescent UC, distorted MVP, inflammatory polyps, and scarred ulcers are observed. On some occasions, the conventional colonoscopic findings completely normalize. Because NBI is a procedure that highlights the vasculature, MVP is the best target for NBI observation in UC to determine the severity.

In addition, the histologic severity may be assessed, and subsequent response to therapy may be predicted when NBI is coupled with magnifying endoscopy. According to Fujiya et al. [1], minute defects of epithelium, mucous exudates, and villous- or coral reef-like mucosa are characteristic magnifying colonoscopic findings in histologically active UC. Among these findings, coral reef-like mucosa, which is presumed to conform to invisible network pattern without crypt openings in our classification, seems to be the most significant finding and indicates histologically active disease. Villous mucosa, which may be better seen with NBI, is considered to indicate long-standing inflammation.

Active UC

Small yellowish spots (Figures 11.2 and 11.3) and mucous exudates (Figures 11.4 and 11.5) seen under conventional colonoscopy are observed as localized white spots under NBI. On the other hand, actively inflamed mucosa, which is marked by disappearance of MVP, fine granular mucosa, and spontaneous bleeding on conventional colonoscopy, is depicted as brownish mucosa under NBI observation. NBI in active UC occasionally depicts vessels in the deep layer, which cannot be observed by conventional colonoscopy (Figures 11.4 and 11.5). These vessels in the deep layer, which appear commonly in NBI under normal conditions as linear green structures, are generally obscure in active UC (Figures 11.4–11.6). When observation with appropriate distance from the mucosa is applied, NBI can detect patchy and skipped involvement that is found in approximately 30% of patients with active UC (Figure 11.7).

With NBI observation, circular pits of crypt openings and mucosal surface patterns, which conform to either coral reef-like appearance (Figures 11.4 and 11.5) or villous appearance (Figure 11.6), can be easily observed in active UC. However, there is a need for the assessment of round pits under both white light and NBI, because crypt openings cannot be distinguished from yellowish spots by the procedure alone. While conventional colonoscopy is superior to NBI for the determination of small yellowish spots (Figures 11.2 and 11.3), crypt openings are better emphasized by NBI (Figures 11.4–11.6).

Quiescent UC and mucosal healing

As has been described, NBI is useful for the assessment of MVP. This is especially the case for quiescent UC. Under NBI observation, MVP comprises two distinctive patterns: (i) a deep vasculature appearing green in color and (ii) superficial vasculature that is brown in color.

When UC has completely healed, conventional colonoscopy depicts MVP as seen in normal subjects. In this situation, both green vessels in the deep layer and brownish vessels in the more superficial layer are observed clearly by NBI (Figures 11.8 and 11.9). By simultaneous application of magnifying observation, the small and regular hexagonal vascular network in the superficial layer can be depicted more clearly. However, MVP in the superficial layer may become obscure under NBI observation in the mucosa with slightly distorted MVP (Figure 11.10).

On the other hand, the pattern of MVP is divided into two types when quiescent UC with pale mucosa is observed by NBI colonoscopy. In one pattern, the superficial brown vessels are enhanced (Figures 11.11 and 11.12) and in the other pattern the brownish vessels become obscure with obvious crypt openings (Figures 11.13–11.15). When compared with histologic findings, the obscure brown vessel pattern tended to represent more severe inflammatory infiltrates, and more frequent goblet cell depletion and basal plasmacytosis. It remains unclear whether detailed observation of the mucosal structure using magnification following healing in UC can predict relapse. Mucosal pattern observation with chromoendoscopy seems to be predictive as does intestinal permeability with confocal laser endomicroscopy. Early observations with NBI suggest that microvessel pattern is abnormal even in normal-appearing mucosa with white light [2] but prospective data are currently lacking. European Crohn's and Colitis Organization (ECCO) guidelines in 2013 highlight the potential role of advanced endoscopic techniques with magnification to enhance assessment of mucosal healing [3].

Diagnosis of dysplasia

Because patients with UC are at high risk for the development of colorectal cancer, endoscopic surveillance is a recommended strategy for the disease. In recent years, international guidelines have endorsed targeted biopsy with chromoendoscopy as useful for the detection of neoplastic lesions during surveillance colonoscopy [3,4]. As has been demonstrated previously, chromoendoscopy can help identify minimally protruding or depressed lesions, with magnifying colonoscopy helping to identify pit pattern specific to neoplastic lesions [5].

NBI colonoscopy is a procedure to enhance vessels and the corresponding pit pattern, rather than to emphasis subtle height differences (topography) of the mucosa. Because of the difficulty of identifying hypervascular dysplastic lesions on an inflamed background, NBI has not improved detection of dysplasia in colitis compared with white light, nor is it superior to chromoendoscopy for wide-field detection in colitis; meta-analysis demonstrated a 6% per patient detection rate in favor of chromoendoscopy (95% CI, −1 to 14%) (Figure 11.16) [4]. However, comparisons used the LUCERA SPECTRUM EXERA II systems; data for the brighter LUCERA ELITE EXERA III system is awaited.

Thus, the major value of NBI colonoscopy for surveillance colonoscopy in UC is to confirm in a suspected raised or depressed lesion the presence of a pit pattern specific to neoplasia. One potential application is in combination with autofluorescence imaging (AFI). AFI is a widefield "red flag" technique, but produces many false positives in colitis. The addition of NBI with magnification (termed "endoscopic trimodal imaging") to characterize AFI-identified lesions may improve diagnostic performance [6].

Figure 11.17 shows dysplasia in a patient with UC, which was found by NBI. Although the lesion was not discernible by conventional colonoscopy, a diminutive localized lesion with IIIL pit pattern was detected by NBI observation. Biopsy specimen obtained from the lesion contained high-grade dysplasia. In order to improve the diagnostic value of NBI in this field, it seems that further investigation will be necessary to elucidate more precisely the pit patterns of dysplasia in UC. It seems that these may differ from the classical Kudo pit pattern, e.g., honeycomb and tortuous patterns [7].

Crohn's disease

In addition to major intestinal manifestations, such as cobblestone appearance of the intestine and longitudinal ulcers, patients with Crohn's disease manifest small aphthoid ulcers within the gastrointestinal tract. In cases of Crohn's disease, we could not confirm any practical significance of NBI for the observation of major disease involvement; much of this is readily apparent under white light examination. In contrast, NBI observation was useful for the identification of aphthoid ulcer and lymphoid hyperplasia, which coexisted frequently in patients with Crohn's disease. As indicated in Figures 11.18 and 11.19, a small elevation with central depression, which was not depicted by conventional colonoscopy, became evident by means of NBI colonoscopy. This is an early feature of Crohn's disease and NBI might be helpful in detecting Crohn's disease at earlier stages [8].

Conclusion

As described in this chapter, NBI observation may provide important information for the assessment of pathophysiology in patients with chronic inflammatory bowel disease. This seems to be especially the case for the evaluation of MVP in UC, which has not been systematically and objectively scored by conventional colonoscopy. In addition, NBI seems to contribute to the diagnosis of dysplasia in these patients, but not to detection.

 Video clips to accompany this book can be found in the online material at www.wiley.com/go/cohen/NBI

The following videos relate specifically to this chapter:
Video 71 Ileal transition zone mucosal examination
Video 72 Crohn's colitis
Video 73 Flat polyp with low-grade dysplasia on chromoendoscopy surveillance examination in chronic ulcerative colitis
Video 74 Scarring on chromoendoscopy 1 year following resection of flat adenomatous polyp in chronic ulcerative colitis
Video 76 Normal ileum with stool mimicking a lesion
Video 77 Ulcerative colitis surveillance in a patient with primary sclerosing cholangitis

Video 78 Pseudopolyp features on NBI
Video 79 Large inflammatory polyp vs. DALM in UC

References

1 Fujiya M, Saitoh Y, Nomura M *et al.* Minute findings by magnifying colonoscopy are useful for the evaluation of ulcerative colitis. *Gastrointest Endosc* 2002;56:535–42.

2 Danese S, Fiorino G, Angelucci E *et al.* Narrow-band imaging endoscopy to assess mucosal angiogenesis in inflammatory bowel disease: a pilot study. *World J Gastroenterol* 2010;16:2396–400.

3 Annese V, Daperno M, Rutter MD *et al.* European evidence based consensus for endoscopy in inflammatory bowel disease. *J Crohns Colitis* 2013;7:982–1018.

4 Laine L, Kaltenbach T, Barkun *et al.* SCENIC international consensus statement on surveillance and management of dysplasia in inflammatory bowel disease. *Gastroenterology* 2015;148:639–51.

5 Kudo S, Tamura S, Nakajima T *et al.* Diagnosis of colorectal tumorous lesions by magnifying colonoscopy. *Gastrointest Endosc* 1996;44:8–14.

6 van den Broek FJ, Fockens P, van Eeden S *et al.* Endoscopic tri-modal imaging for surveillance in ulcerative colitis: randomised comparison of high-resolution endoscopy and autofluorescence imaging for neoplasia detection and evaluation of narrow-band imaging for classification of lesions. *Gut* 2008;57:1083–9.

7 Matsumoto T, Kudo T, Jo Y *et al.* Magnifying colonoscopy with narrow band imaging system for the diagnosis of dysplasia in ulcerative colitis: a pilot study. *Gastrointest Endosc* 2007;66:957–65.

8 Sanders DS. Mucosal integrity and barrier function in the pathogenesis of early lesions in Crohn's disease. *J Clin Pathol* 2005;58:568–72.

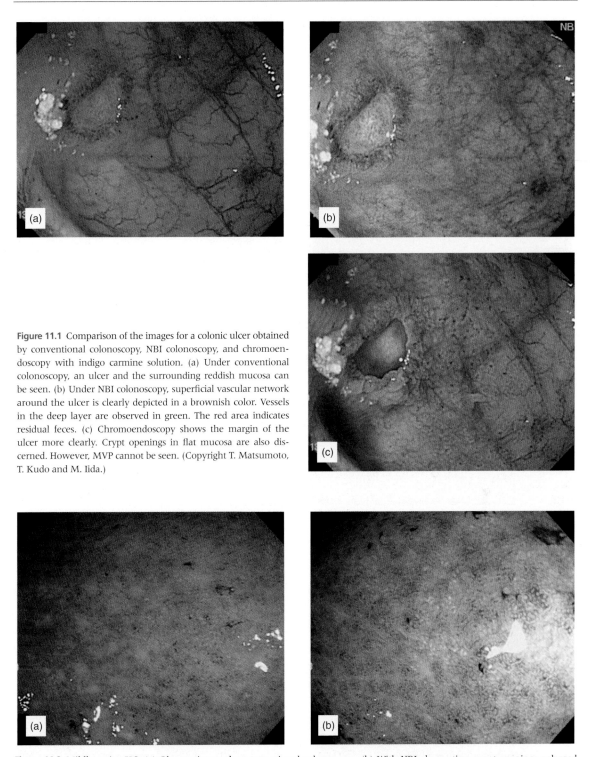

Figure 11.1 Comparison of the images for a colonic ulcer obtained by conventional colonoscopy, NBI colonoscopy, and chromoendoscopy with indigo carmine solution. (a) Under conventional colonoscopy, an ulcer and the surrounding reddish mucosa can be seen. (b) Under NBI colonoscopy, superficial vascular network around the ulcer is clearly depicted in a brownish color. Vessels in the deep layer are observed in green. The red area indicates residual feces. (c) Chromoendoscopy shows the margin of the ulcer more clearly. Crypt openings in flat mucosa are also discerned. However, MVP cannot be seen. (Copyright T. Matsumoto, T. Kudo and M. Iida.)

Figure 11.2 Mildly active UC. (a) Observation under conventional colonoscopy. (b) With NBI observation, crypt openings enlarged to villous-like structure is clearly observed. Deep green-colored vessels can be seen. (Copyright T. Matsumoto, T. Kudo and M. Iida.)

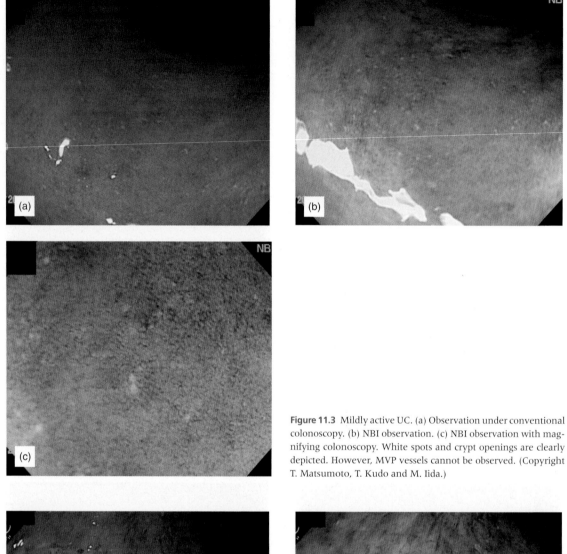

Figure 11.3 Mildly active UC. (a) Observation under conventional colonoscopy. (b) NBI observation. (c) NBI observation with magnifying colonoscopy. White spots and crypt openings are clearly depicted. However, MVP vessels cannot be observed. (Copyright T. Matsumoto, T. Kudo and M. Iida.)

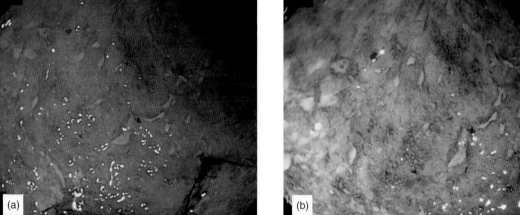

Figure 11.4 Moderately active UC. (a) Observation under conventional colonoscopy. (b) On NBI observation, mucous exudates are depicted as whitish area. Coral reef-like mucosa is evident. (Copyright T. Matsumoto, T. Kudo and M. Iida.)

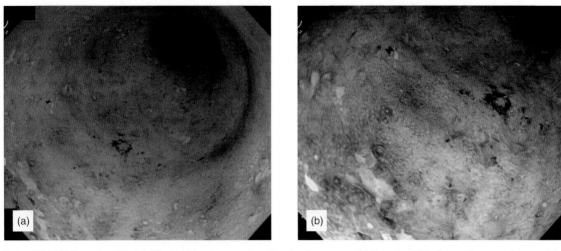

Figure 11.5 Mildly active UC. (a) Observation under conventional colonoscopy. (b) Even on NBI observation, vessels cannot be observed. There is coral reef-like mucosa. (Copyright T. Matsumoto, T. Kudo and M. Iida.)

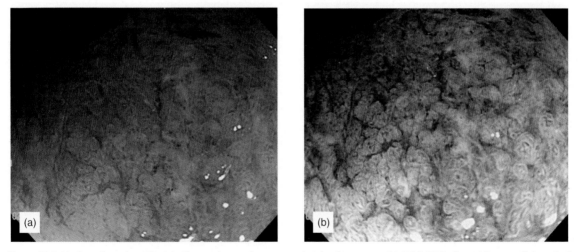

Figure 11.6 Moderately active UC. (a) Observation under conventional colonoscopy. (b) With NBI observation, small intestinal villous structure becomes clear. (Copyright T. Matsumoto, T. Kudo and M. Iida.)

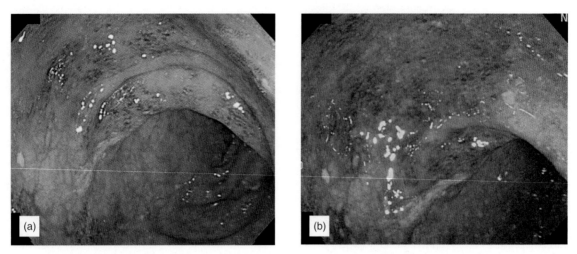

Figure 11.7 Skipped involvement. (a) Observation under conventional colonoscopy. (b) With NBI observation, a discontinuous lesion can be observed as a brownish area. (Copyright T. Matsumoto, T. Kudo and M. Iida.)

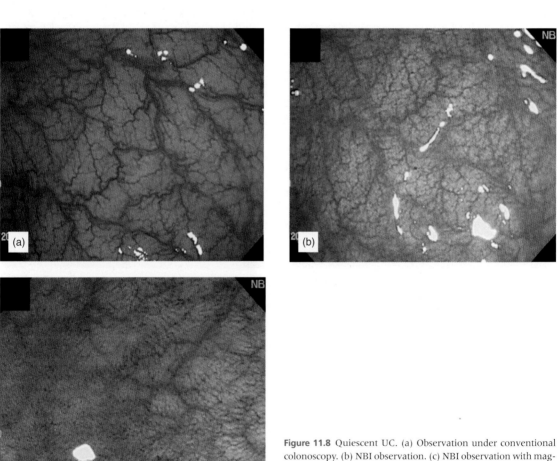

Figure 11.8 Quiescent UC. (a) Observation under conventional colonoscopy. (b) NBI observation. (c) NBI observation with magnifying colonoscopy. With NBI, it is possible to clarify deep green vessels and brownish superficial vessels. Magnifying observation shows vessels and crypt openings clearly. (Copyright T. Matsumoto, T. Kudo and M. Iida.)

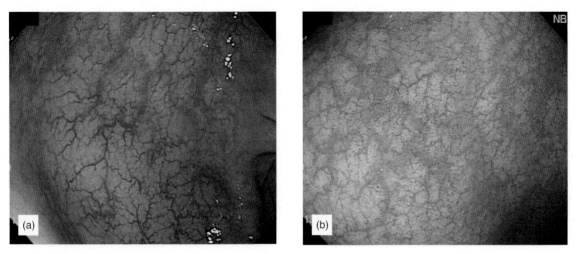

Figure 11.9 Quiescent UC. (a) Observation under conventional colonoscopy. (b) NBI observation shows clear MVP. (Copyright T. Matsumoto, T. Kudo and M. Iida.)

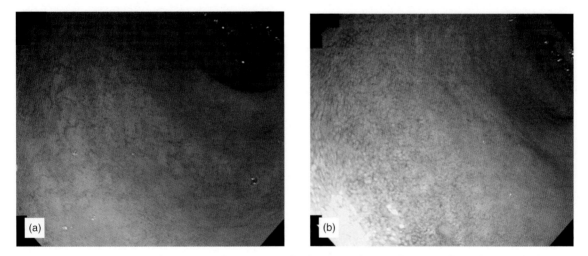

Figure 11.10 Quiescent UC. (a) Observation under conventional colonoscopy. (b) NBI observation shows deep vessels. However, superficial vessels are not discerned. (Copyright T. Matsumoto, T. Kudo and M. Iida.)

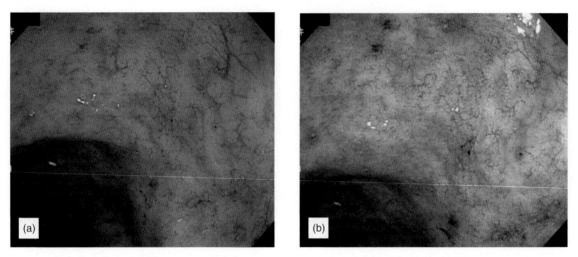

Figure 11.11 Quiescent UC. (a) Observation under conventional colonoscopy. (b) With NBI observation, deep vessels and tortuous superficial vessels can be seen. (Copyright T. Matsumoto, T. Kudo and M. Iida.)

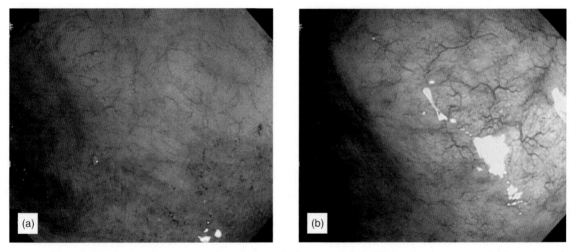

Figure 11.12 Quiescent UC. (a) Observation under conventional colonoscopy. (b) With NBI observation, superficial vessels can be clearly observed. (Copyright T. Matsumoto, T. Kudo and M. Iida.)

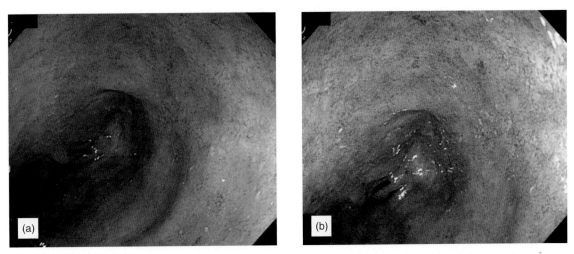

Figure 11.13 Quiescent UC. (a) Observation under conventional colonoscopy. (b) NBI observation. Although deep vessels can be seen, superficial vessels are obscure. (Copyright T. Matsumoto, T. Kudo and M. Iida.)

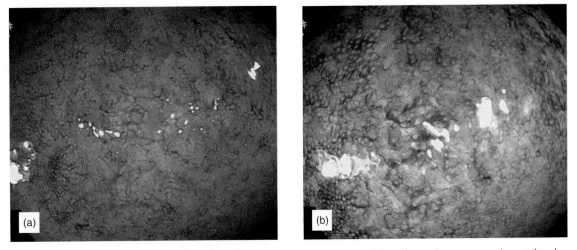

Figure 11.14 Quiescent UC. (a) Observation under conventional colonoscopy. (b) With NBI observation, crypt openings, rather than superficial vessels, are clear. (Copyright T. Matsumoto, T. Kudo and M. Iida.)

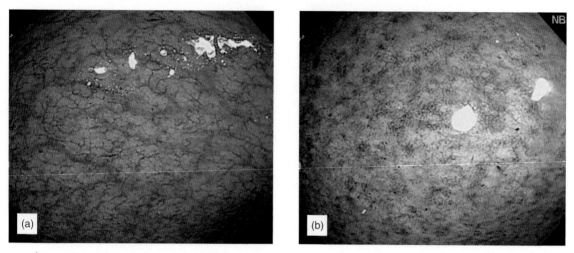

Figure 11.15 Quiescent UC. (a) Observation under conventional colonoscopy. (b) NBI observation. Although deep vessels can be seen, superficial vessels are obscure. (Copyright T. Matsumoto, T. Kudo and M. Iida.)

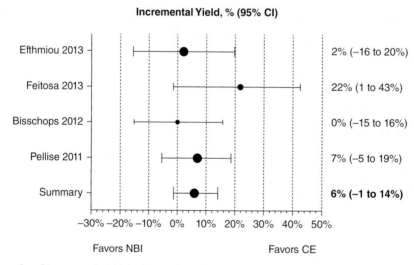

Figure 11.16 Forest plot of incremental yield in the number of patients with endoscopically visible dysplasia during surveillance colonoscopy comparing chromoendoscopy to narrowband imaging. CI, confidence interval; CE, chromoendoscopy; NBI, narrowband imaging. (Reproduced from Laine *et al.*, *Gastrointest Endosc* 2015;81:489–501.e26, with permission from Elsevier.)

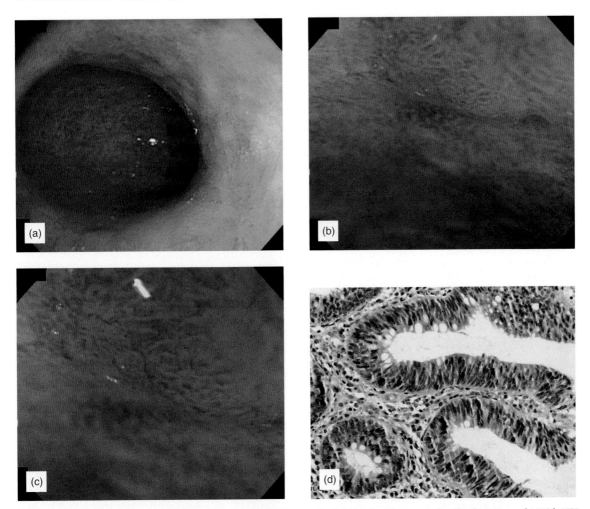

Figure 11.17 A case of high-grade dysplasia in UC. (a) No lesion can be discerned under conventional colonoscopy. (b) With NBI observation, there is an area of IIIL pit pattern, which is distinct from the surrounding mucosa. (c) Magnifying observation shows the area to be composed of IIIL and IIIs pit patterns. (d) Histology of the biopsy specimen shows high-grade dysplasia. (Copyright T. Matsumoto, T. Kudo and M. Iida.)

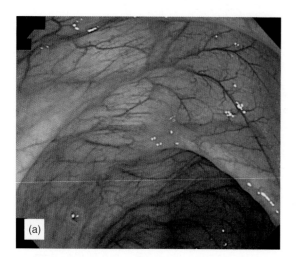

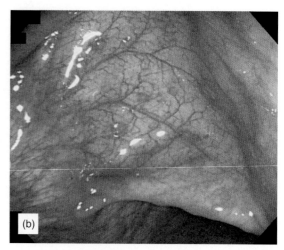

Figure 11.18 Colonoscopic findings in a case of Crohn's disease of ileitis type. (a) Observation under conventional colonoscopy. (b) With NBI observation, lymphoid hyperplasia becomes evident. (Copyright T. Matsumoto, T. Kudo and M. Iida.)

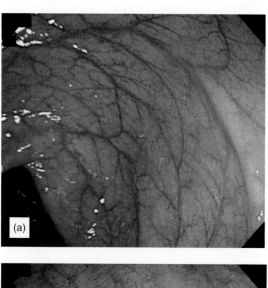

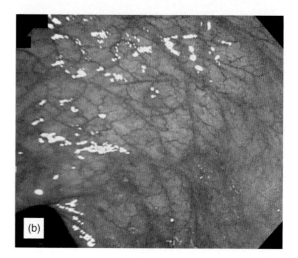

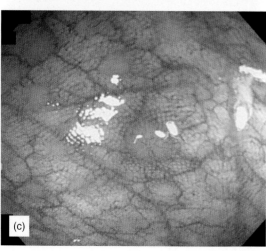

Figure 11.19 Colonoscopic findings in a case of Crohn's disease of aphthous type. (a) Observation under conventional colonoscopy. (b) NBI observation. (c) Close-up view under NBI. Lymphoid hyperplasia is seen clearly. (Copyright T. Matsumoto, T. Kudo and M. Iida.)

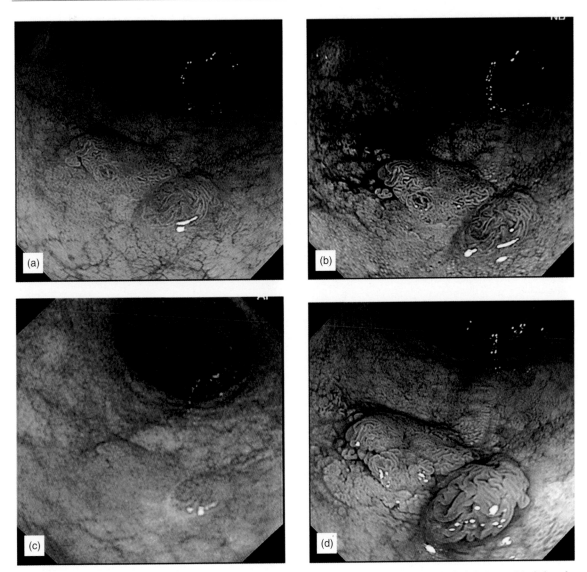

Figure 11.20 A 10-mm sessile polypoid area (Paris 0-Is) with abnormal pit pattern was seen during high-definition white light colonoscopy for surveillance of long-standing UC. (a) Assessment with NBI (Olympus, Tokyo) was used to clarify the pit pattern (Kudo type IV). (b) Assessment with autofluorescence imaging (Olympus, Tokyo) helps differentiate the neoplastic tissue (pink/purple) from the surrounding normal mucosa (green) (endoscopic trimodal imaging). (c) Chromoendoscopy (dye-spray) with indigo carmine 0.2% is used to clarify the lesion margin. (d) Biopsy confirmed low-grade dysplasia.

New Horizons for High-Resolution Endoscopy and Narrowband Imaging

12 NBI and high-resolution endoscopy in the bile duct and pancreas

Takao Itoi

Introduction

Peroral fiberoptic cholangiopancreatoscopy emerged as a diagnostic endoscopy technique to inspect indeterminate pancreaticobiliary lesions in the late 1970s [1,2]. Since then, it has been developed as a technique of close examination with tissue sampling under direct endoscopic visualization. However, cholangiopancreatoscopy at the time was limited because it had an ultra-slim endoscope with optical fibers and image quality was not optimal. In the early 2000s, peroral video cholangiopancreatoscopy was developed, providing comparatively more precise white-light imaging (WLI) than possible with fiberoptic cholangiopancreatoscopy, Furthermore, narrowband imaging (NBI) emerged as a new endoscopic system based on narrowing the bandwidth of spectral transmittance of red/green/blue (RGB) optical filters [3]. NBI with magnifying endoscopy facilitates the imaging of certain features such as mucosal structures and mucosal microvessels in gastrointestinal diseases [4–6]. In terms of pancreaticobiliary diseases, we have reported the first study of the usefulness of NBI although this did not incorporate any magnification [7,8]. In this chapter, we describe the use of NBI and high-resolution video cholangiopancreatoscopy in the bile duct and pancreas.

Role of video cholangiopancreatoscopy

Video cholangioscopy

Video cholangioscopy has two important roles in the diagnosis of biliary diseases as follows:

1 Endoscopic inspection and pathologic sampling in primary biliary strictures and polypoid lesions in which the cholangiogram shows indeterminate biliary stricture or filling defects.
2 Endoscopic evaluation and pathologic sampling in superficial tumor spreading lesions, as is often seen in intraductal papillary neoplasms of the bile duct or common type bile duct cancers showing papillary growth. Endoscopic inspection using cholangioscopy is often performed to help differentiate between benign and malignant strictures. These strictures usually have intrinsic origins (e.g., bile duct cancers) and extrinsic origins (e.g., lymphadenopathy). With regard to the growth pattern of bile duct cancer, it is divided into three categories, namely papillary, nodular, and flat. Of these growth patterns, most bile duct cancers show a nodular growth pattern. Our results have revealed that most papillary and partially nodular type bile duct cancers show lateral mucosal cancer spreading [9]. In contrast, most flat-type bile duct cancers showed intramural invasion cancer spreading (e.g., lymph permeation, venous permeation, and perineural invasion) instead of mucosal spreading [9]. Therefore, papillary or nodular growth type bile duct cancers appear most suitable for diagnosis using cholangioscopy.

Video pancreatoscopy

Video pancreatoscopy has more limited application than video cholangioscopy because the diameter of the normal pancreatic duct is small (<2 mm). Thus, it seems to be suitable for when there is a dilated pancreatic duct, as seen in intraductal papillary mucinous neoplasms (IPMNs). Particularly, main pancreatic duct IPMNs often show superficial tumor spread lesions in the dilated pancreatic duct. Thus, pancreatoscopy can be important for deciding the surgical margin for curative operation.

System of video cholangiopancreatoscopy and NBI

Currently, mother–baby video cholangiopancreatoscopy scopes (CHF-B260, outer diameter 3.4 mm, accessory channel diameter 1.2 mm; CHF-BP260, outer diameter

Comprehensive Atlas of High-Resolution Endoscopy and Narrowband Imaging, Second Edition. Edited by Jonathan Cohen.
© 2017 John Wiley & Sons, Ltd. Published 2017 by John Wiley & Sons, Ltd.
Companion website: www.wiley.com/go/cohen/NBI

2.6 mm, accessory channel diameter 0.5 mm; Olympus Medical Systems, Tokyo, Japan), which have two-way tip deflection, are commercially available in limited regions of the world. In contrast, ultra-slim upper gastrointestinal or nasal endoscopes (e.g., GIF-N260, Olympus) for direct cholangiopancreatoscopy, which have four-way tip deflection and an approximately 2.0-mm working channel, are widely used throughout the world. Although mother–baby video cholangiopancreatoscopy needs two skilled endoscopists for better observation and accurate biopsy with 1-mm forceps, direct video cholangiopancreatoscopy can be performed by only one skilled endoscopist. The NBI system can be used for both of these types of video cholangiopancreatoscopy (CV-260SL/CV-290 processor, CVL-260SL/CVL-290SL light source, Olympus).

Since the contents of the bile duct and pancreatic duct tend to be turbid because of mucus, blood, and biliary sludge, clear visualization of targeted lesions immediately after insertion is possible in only a few cases. Therefore, traditionally, irrigation of the bile duct and pancreatic duct with saline is usually conducted before observation. However, this often entails a lengthy procedure to reach satisfactory images. Recently, several investigators revealed that CO_2 insufflation is another option during video cholangiopancreatoscopy [10].

Diagnostic ability of video cholangiopancreatoscopy

Typical video cholangiopancreatoscopy findings

The mucosal appearance of a bile duct lesion as observed by cholangiopancreatoscopy under WLI can be characterized as follows.

Malignant findings

1 Irregular, dilated, and tortuous vessels (tumorigenic vessels) (Figure 12.1).
2 Friability.
3 Irregular papillogranular surface (Figure 12.2).
4 Leaf-like projection (Figure 12.3).
5 Fish-egg-like projection (Figure 12.4).
6 A nodular elevated surface-like submucosal tumor (Figure 12.5).

Benign findings

1 Fine network of thin vessels and flat surface without definite neovascularization (Figure 12.6).
2 Slightly homogeneous papillogranular surface or scale-like appearance without a primary mass, suggesting hyperplasia (Figure 12.7).
3 Irregular surface with or without pseudodiverticula, suggesting inflammation.

4 White surface with convergence of folds, suggesting cicatricial formation (Figure 12.8).

Mucosal cancerous extension findings

1 Irregular fine granular patterns and fish-egg-like appearance of the surface surrounding the primary tumor (Figure 12.9) [7,8,11–21].

To date, several retrospective and prospective studies have been published that used video and fiberoptic cholangioscopy for the diagnosis of indeterminate biliary strictures and filling defects [11,13–19] (Table 12.1). In terms of video cholangioscopy, no study examined visual diagnostic ability alone because the final diagnosis (diagnostic accuracy, 93–98%) was calculated based on the histologic diagnosis by cholangioscopy-guided or fluoroscopic-guided biopsy. Interestingly, with regard to fiberoptic cholangioscopy, visual diagnosis was superior to target biopsy in two studies [16,17]. In contrast, in terms of pancreatoscopy, although there is no study on the visual diagnostic ability of video pancreatoscopy, one retrospective study has shown that sensitivity, specificity, and diagnostic accuracy in distinguishing benign from malignant lesions in IPMNs were 100%, 71%, and 88%, respectively [22]. Since the evidence for visual diagnosis by video choangiopancreatoscopy is extremely low, prospective evaluation is necessary in the near future.

Differential diagnosis

Video cholangiopancreatoscopy can distinguish benign from malignant relatively well based on the criteria described here. However, in terms of primary sclerosing cholangitis (PSC) and IgG4-related sclerosing cholangitis, a definite diagnosis is not easy to make because the cholangioscopic findings in these diseases are similar to those in bile duct cancers [23]. With regard to PSC, the typical cholangioscopic findings are bile duct strictures without neovascular change, scar formation, and relatively large pseudodiverticula. Although it appears to be easy to distinguish PSC and cancers, care should be taken in the case of possible bile duct cancer derived from PSC (Figure 12.10). On the other hand, cholangioscopic findings in IgG4-related sclerosing cholangitis often show a bile duct stricture with thick and tortuous vessels resembling cancerous strictures, resulting in misdiagnosis (Figure 12.11a,b) [23]. Thus, clinical information, for example serum IgG4, pancreatography by endoscopic retrograde cholangiopancreatography (ERCP) or magnetic resonance cholangiopancreatography (MRCP) (Figure 12.12), is mandatory for making a definite diagnosis. In the case of strongly suspected IgG4-related sclerosing cholangitis, steroid administration may be one of the options because after a trial of steroids, the stricture with thick and tortuous vessels can show dramatic changes compared to before treatment (Figure 12.11c,d). Cholangioscopic findings in IgG4-related sclerosing cholangitis include, although rarely, scar formation, a bumpy surface, and pseudodiverticula (Figure 12.13).

NBI can enhance the imaging of these lesions. However, since there is no magnifying function yet possible in cholangiopancreatoscopy, more detailed observation and interpretation, as has been shown in luminal gastrointestinal diseases, is limited. Another serious limitation of NBI cholangioscopy, apart from pancreatic juice, is that bile is recognized as a reddish color fluid similar to blood. At times, it precludes more detailed endoscopic bile duct imaging, and frequently time-consuming irrigation is necessary to clean the bile duct. In contrast, video cholangiopancreatoscopy under CO_2 insufflation can provide better imaging than with saline irrigation in the absence of bile or thick mucin. However, it is important to note that saline irrigation may allow a better-quality image in patients with severe stenosis or protruded papillary lesions [10].

Conclusions

Peroral video cholangiopancreatoscopy has high potential for diagnosis of pancreaticobiliary lesions. Furthermore, NBI in combination with WLI can enhance the characteristics of these lesions.

Acknowledgment

Thanks are due to Dr Edward Barroga for reviewing and editing this chapter.

 Video clips to accompany this book can be found in the online material at www.wiley.com/go/cohen/NBI

The following videos relate specifically to this chapter:
Video 1 NBI examination of the oropharynx
Video 2 Benign lesion, hyperplasia
Video 3 Neoplastic lesion, low-grade intraepithelial neoplasia
Video 4 Diagnosis of superficial squamous cell carcinoma
Video 44 Bleeding vessels in nodular cholangiocarcinoma
Video 45 Nodular cholangiocarcinoma with abnormal tumor vessels
Video 46 Benign bile duct stricture
Video 47 Hyperplastic mucosa in benign bile duct stricture

References

1 Rösch W, Koch H, Demling L. Peroral cholangioscopy. *Endoscopy* 1976;8:172–5.

2 Nakajima M, Akasaka Y, Fukumoto K *et al.* Peroral cholangiopancreatoscopy (PCPS) under duodenoscopic guidance. *Am J Gastroenterol* 1978;66:241–7.

3 Gono K, Yamazaki K, Doguchi N *et al.* Endoscopic observation of tissue by narrowband illumination. *Opt Rev* 2003;10:211–15.

4 Yoshida T, Inoue H, Usui S *et al.* Narrow-band imaging system with magnifying endoscopy for superficial esophageal lesions. *Gastrointest Endosc* 2004;59:288–95.

5 Machida T, Sano Y, Hamamoto Y *et al.* Narrow-band imaging in the diagnosis of colorectal mucosal lesions: a pilot study. *Endoscopy* 2004;36:1094–8.

6 Nakayoshi T, Tajiri H, Matsuda K *et al.* Magnifying endoscopy combined with narrow band imaging system for early gastric cancer: correlation of vascular pattern with histopathology. *Endoscopy* 2004;36:1080–4.

7 Itoi T, Sofuni A, Itokawa F *et al.* Peroral cholangioscopic diagnosis of biliary tract diseases using narrow-band imaging. *Gastrointest Endosc* 2007;66:730–6.

8 Itoi T, Sofuni A, Itokawa F *et al.* Initial experience of peroral pancreatoscopy combined with narrow-band imaging in diagnosis of intraductal papillary mucinous neoplasms of the pancreas (with video). *Gastrointest Endosc* 2007;66:793–7.

9 Itoi T, Sofuni A, Itokawa F *et al.* What's new on the cholangioscopy? Is narrow-band imaging cholangioscopy next generation? *Dig Endosc* 2007;19:S87–S94.

10 Doi S, Yasuda I, Nakashima M *et al.* Carbon dioxide insufflation versus conventional saline irrigation for the peroral video cholangioscopy. *Endoscopy* 2011;43:1070–5.

11 Itoi T, Osanai M, Igarashi Y *et al.* Diagnostic peroral video cholangioscopy is an accurate diagnostic tool for patients with bile-duct lesions. *Clin Gastroenterol Hepatol* 2010;8:934–8.

12 Itoi T, Neuhaus H, Chen YK. Diagnostic value of imaging-enhanced video cholangiopancreatoscopy. *Gastrointest Endosc Clin North Am* 2009;19:557–66.

13 Osanai M, Itoi T, Igarashi Y *et al.* Peroral video cholangioscopy to evaluate indeterminate bile duct lesions and preoperative mucosal cancerous extension: a prospective multicenter study. *Endoscopy* 2013;45:635–42.

14 Fukuda Y, Tsuyuguchi T, Sakai Y *et al.* Diagnostic utility of peroral cholangioscopy for various bile duct lesions. *Gastrointest Endosc* 2005;62:374–82.

15 Shah RJ, Langer DA, Antillon MR *et al.* Cholangioscopy and cholangioscopic forceps biopsy in patients with indeterminate pancreaticobiliary pathology. *Clin Gastroenterol Hepatol* 2006;4:219–25.

16 Chen YK, Parsi MA, Binmoeller KF *et al.* Single-operator cholangioscopy in patients requiring evaluation of bile duct disease or therapy of biliary stones (with videos). *Gastrointest Endosc* 2011;74:805–14.

17 Ramchandani M, Reddy DN, Gupta R *et al.* Role of single-operator peroral cholangioscopy in the diagnosis

of indeterminate biliary lesions: a single-center, prospective study. *Gastrointest Endosc* 2011;74:511–19.

18 Draganov PV, Chauhan S, Wagh MS *et al.* Diagnostic accuracy of conventional and cholangioscopy-guided sampling of indeterminate biliary lesions at the time of ERCP: a prospective, long-term follow-up study. *Gastrointest Endosc* 2012;75:347–53.

19 Nisikawa T, Tsuyuguchi T, Sakai Y *et al.* Comparison of the diagnostic accuracy of peroral video cholangioscopic visual findings and cholangioscopy-forceps biopsy findings for indeterminate biliary lesion: a prospective study. *Gastrointest Endosc* 2013;77:219–26.

20 Kawakami H, Kuwatani M, Etoh K *et al.* Endoscopic retrograde cholangiography versus peroral cholangioscopy

to evaluate intraepithelial tumor spread in biliary cancer. *Endoscopy* 2009;41:959–64.

21 Nishikawa T, Tsuyuguchi T, Sakai Y *et al.* Preoperative assessment of longitudinal extension of cholangiocarcinoma with peroral video-cholangioscopy: a prospective study. *Dig Endosc* 2014;26:450–7.

22 Hara T, Yamaguchi T, Ishihara T *et al.* Diagnosis and patient management of intraductal papillary-mucinous tumor of the pancreas by using peroral pancreatoscopy and intraductal ultrasonography. *Gastroenterology* 2002;122:34–43.

23 Itoi T, Kamisawa T, Igarashi Y *et al.* The role of peroral video cholangioscopy in patients with IgG4-related sclerosing cholangitis. *J Gastroenterol* 2013;48:504–14.

Table 12.1 Diagnostic ability of mother–baby cholangioscopy in combination with forceps biopsy for the diagnosis of indeterminate biliary strictures and filling defects.

Study (year)	N	Study	Center	Scope	Sensitivity (%)	Specificity (%)	PPV (%)	NPV (%)	Accuracy (%)
Fukuda *et al.* (2007) [14]	97[a]	R	Single	Fiber	100	87	88	100	94
Shah *et al.* (2007) [15]	62[a]	R	Single	Fiber	86	96	89	96	NA
Itoi *et al.* (2010) [11]	144[a]	R	Single	Video	99	96	99	96	98
Chen *et al.* (2011) [16]	226/140[b]	P	Multi	Fiber	77/49[b]	82/98[b]	NA	NA	80/75[b]
Ramchandani *et al.* (2011) [17]	36/33[b]	P	Single	Fiber	95/82	79/82[b]	NA	NA	89/82[b]
Draganov *et al.* (2012) [18]	26[a]	P	Single	Fiber	77	NA	NA	NA	85
Nishikawa *et al.* (2013) [19]	33[a]	P	Single	Video	100	92	96	100	97
Osanai *et al.* (2013) [13]	87[a]	P	Multi	Video	94	92	NA	NA	93

R, retrospective study; P, prospective study; PPV, positive predictive value; NPV, negative predictive value.
[a] Visual diagnosis plus histologic diagnosis by forceps biopsy.
[b] Impression diagnosis/histologic diagnosis by forceps biopsy.

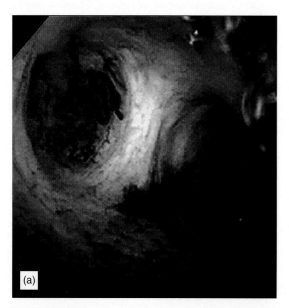 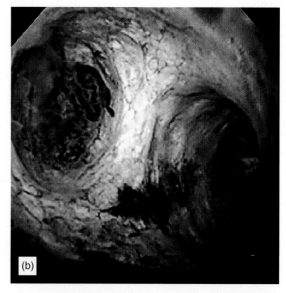

Figure 12.1 Cholangiocaricnoma. (a) WLI: irregular, dilated and tortuous vessels (tumorigenic vessels). (b) NBI: these findings are enhanced by NBI.

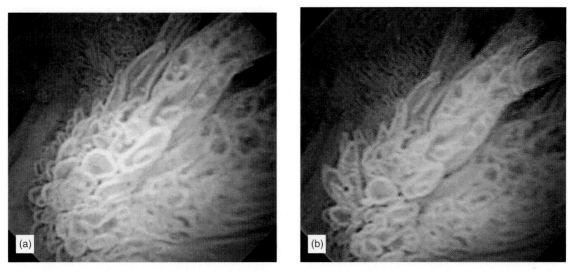

Figure 12.2 Cholangiocaricnoma. (a) WLI: irregular papillogranular projection. (b) NBI: these findings are enhanced by NBI.

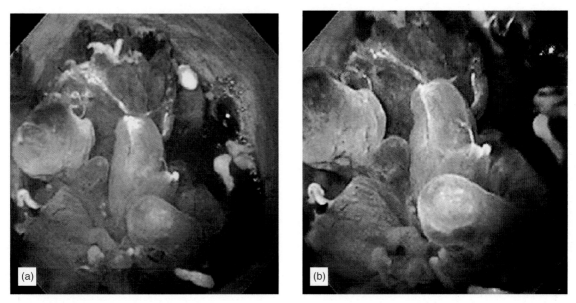

Figure 12.3 Intraductal papillary neoplasms of the bile duct. (a) WLI: leaf-like projection. (b) NBI: these findings are enhanced by NBI.

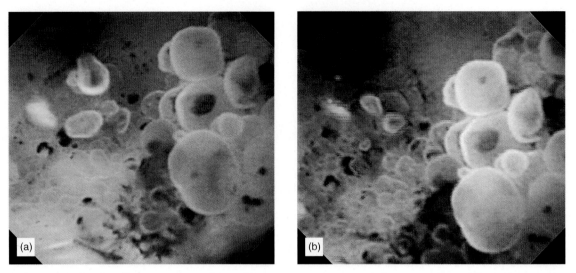

Figure 12.4 Intraductal papillary mucinous neoplasms of the pancreas (main pancreatic duct type). (a) WLI: fish-egg-like projection. (b) NBI: these findings are enhanced by NBI.

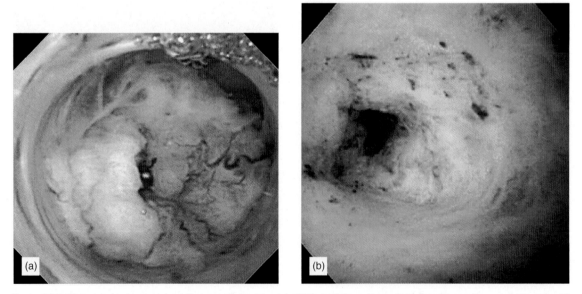

Figure 12.5 Cholangiocarcinomas (nodular growth type). (a) WLI: nodular elevated surface-like submucosal tumor with tumorigenic vessels. (b) WLI: nodular elevated surface-like submucosal tumor with friability mucosa.

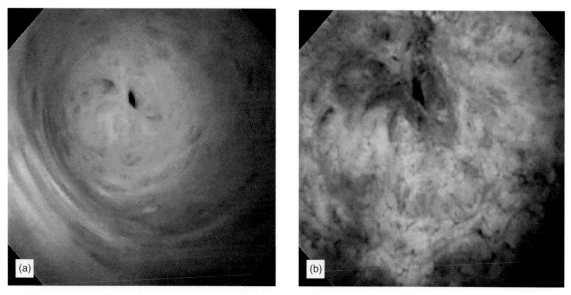

Figure 12.6 Benign biliary stricture. (a) WLI: fine network of thin vessels and flat surface without definite neovascularization. (b) NBI: these findings are enhanced by NBI.

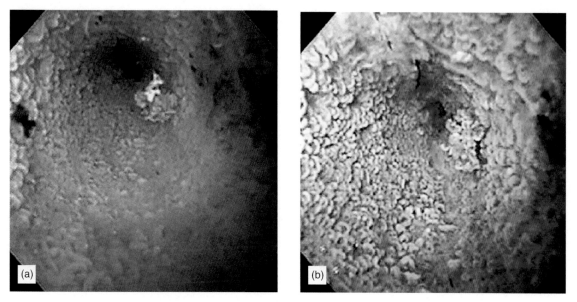

Figure 12.7 Normal mucosa with hyperplasia. (a) WLI: flat surface with mucosal hyperplasia. (b) NBI: these findings are enhanced by NBI.

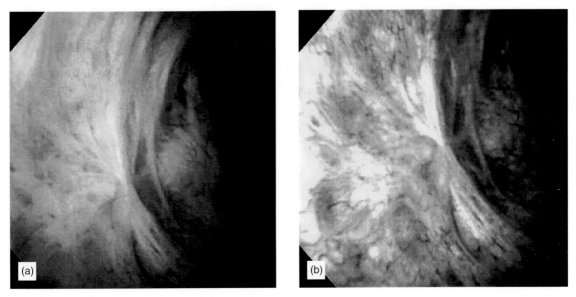

Figure 12.8 Normal mucosa with scarring. (a) WLI: white surface with convergence of folds, suggesting cicatricial formation. (b) NBI: these findings are enhanced by NBI.

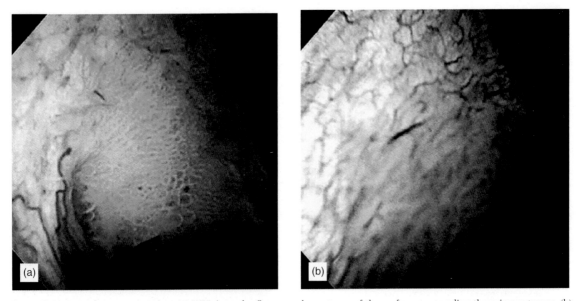

Figure 12.9 Mucosal cancer extension. (a) WLI: irregular fine granular patterns of the surface surrounding the primary tumor. (b) NBI: these findings are enhanced by NBI.

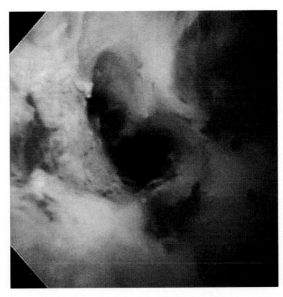

Figure 12.10 Cholangiocarcinoma derived from PSC. WLI: irregular and fragile mucosa based on PSC.

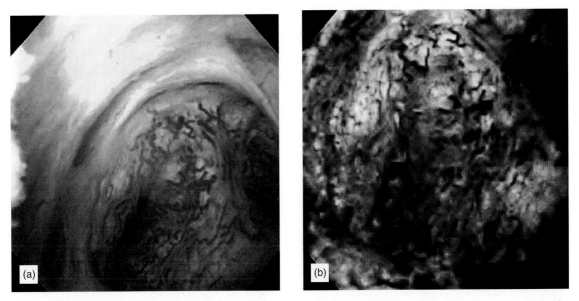

Figure 12.11 IgG4-related sclerosing cholangitis (a, b, before steroid treatment; c, d, after steroid treatment). (a) WLI: irregular, dilated and tortuous vessels like tumorigenic vessels. (b) NBI: these findings are enhanced by NBI (same site as (a)). (continued)

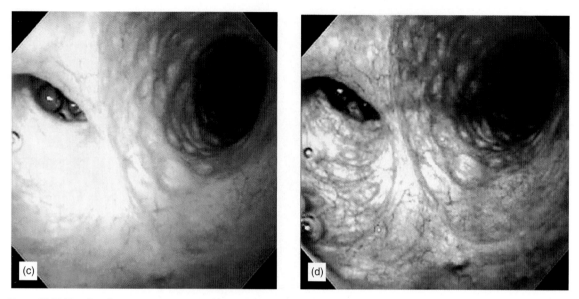

Figure 12.11 (Continued) (c) WLI: tumorigenic-like vessels have disappeared. (d) NBI: these findings are enhanced by NBI (same site as (c)).

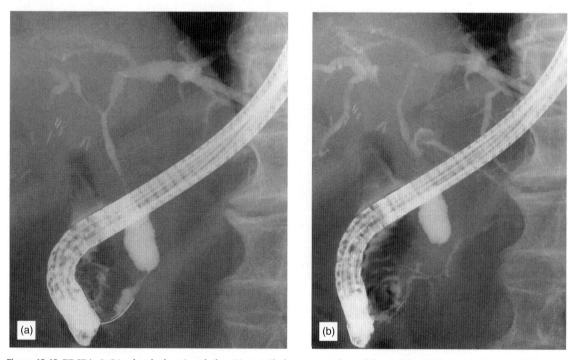

Figure 12.12 ERCP in IgG4-related sclerosing cholangitis. (a) Cholangiogram shows hilar and distal bile duct strictures. (b) Pancreatogram shows diffuse pancreatic duct stricture.

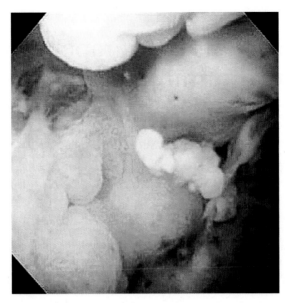

Figure 12.13 IgG4-related sclerosing cholangitis. WLI shows a bumpy surface.

Applications in therapeutic endoscopy: impact on timing and completeness of mucosal ablation and resections

Michael J. Bartel, Lijia Jiang, and Michael B. Wallace

Introduction

Advances in imaging as well as advances in mucosal resection and ablation techniques have resulted in substantial changes over the last decade in how gastroenterologists approach diagnosis and treatment especially of Barrett's esophagus and advanced colorectal neoplasia. Treatment options have shifted from surgical resection as the only treatment option to surgical-sparing therapies with lower mortality rates, making mucosal resection and ablation the treatment of choice of early neoplasia in Barrett's esophagus and lateral spreading polyps in the colorectum. Dedicated surveillance following ablation or resection is necessary due to the risk for recurrence [1–4].

Advances in imaging and resection techniques

Advanced endoscopic imaging encompasses a multitude of optical enhancing techniques utilizing either topical dyes (indigo carmine, methylene blue) or equipment-based enhanced techniques, such as narrowband imaging (NBI, Olympus), Fujinon intelligent chromoendoscopy (FICE, Fujifilm), i-scan (Pentax), and confocal laser endomicroscopy, with the goal of improving the detection, characterization and recognition of borders and surface topography of pathologic lesions in the esophagus and colon in real time [5]. At present, advanced imaging predicts diminutive colorectal polyp histology reliably in experienced hands, which may make certain biopsies obsolete [6,7]. Further, advanced imaging

predicts the presence of invasive cancer, but with large variability, making biopsies in this setting inevitable. In this context, the main question is the depth of invasion, which reflects the risk of lymphangitic cancer spread. This question cannot be answered yet with sufficient accuracy by advanced imaging in both colorectal and esophageal neoplasia [8]. Whether volumetric laser endomicroscopy will fill this gap for Barrett's esophagus is unclear.

The development of mucosal resection and ablation went hand in hand with advances in imaging. Radiofrequency ablation (RFA) is now the preferred ablation technique for Barrett's esophagus given its low complication rate compared with photodynamic therapy [1]. Mucosal resection of suspicious lesions, particularly raised nodules in Barrett's esophagus, allows precise staging of early cancers, as well as other features which may predict the completeness of endoscopic resection. Thus the paradigm of targeted endoscopic resection, followed by ablation of the remaining Barrett's, has emerged as the preferred treatment. Endoscopic mucosal resection (EMR) encompasses submucosal injection with lifting of the mucosa and subsequent snare resection, often also referred to as the "inject-and-cut" technique (Figure 13.1). Alternatively, cap-assisted band-ligation can be performed in the esophagus with or without injection to separate the mucosa from the submucosa.

Another endoscopic resection technique mainly performed in East Asian countries is endoscopic submucosal dissection (ESD) [1,9,10]. Both EMR and ESD allow histologic assessment of neoplasia and its depth of invasion (T staging) with subsequent conclusion on the likelihood of lymph node metastasis.

Comprehensive Atlas of High-Resolution Endoscopy and Narrowband Imaging, Second Edition. Edited by Jonathan Cohen.
© 2017 John Wiley & Sons, Ltd. Published 2017 by John Wiley & Sons, Ltd.
Companion website: www.wiley.com/go/cohen/NBI

Barrett's esophagus

Nondysplastic Barrett's esophagus harbors a risk of 0.1–0.3% per year for the development of esophageal adenocarcinoma, whereas high-grade dysplasia progresses at a rate of 6–19% per year [1,11]. A recent study by Phoa *et al.* [12] demonstrated that endoscopic ablation prevents progression of low-grade dysplasia to high-grade dysplasia and adenocarcinoma in 25% of patients. Based on this data, current guidelines recommend surveillance or endoscopic ablation for patients with low-grade dysplasia and ablation alone for high-grade dysplasia [11].

Regarding the risk to benefit ratio, RFA is the preferred option for endoscopic esophageal ablation. RFA yields high complete eradication of dysplasia and intestinal metaplasia (90.5% and 77.4%) compared with sham treatment (22.7% and 2.3%) at 12 months [13]. Complete remission of all dysplasia (95%) and intestinal metaplasia (93%) at 2 years was demonstrated in another study, including patients with low-grade and high-grade dysplasia [14]. In another study by Phoa *et al.* [15], 90% of patients had complete remission of neoplasia and intestinal metaplasia at 5 years, with all recurrent neoplasia being managed endoscopically. Haidry *et al.* [16] calculated that a mean of 2.5 RFA applications was required to eradicate high-grade dysplasia in 86% and all dysplasia in 81% at 12-month follow-up. A prior EMR did not provide any benefit for RFA treatment in terms of dysplasia eradication, but provided precise disease staging. Surveillance of Barrett's esophagus following dysplasia eradication is important, as 4% showed recurrent dysplasia after a median follow-up of 19 months [16]. In another study, Gupta *et al.* [17] detected recurrence of intestinal metaplasia in 33% at 24 months after complete remission of intestinal metaplasia, of which 22% harbored dysplasia. The importance of advanced imaging technologies for Barrett's esophagus surveillance was outlined by Qumseya *et al.* [18]. Based on a meta-analysis, advanced imaging technology increased the diagnostic yield for detection of dysplasia or cancer by 34% compared with white light endoscopy (Figures 13.2 and 13.3). As Barrett's esophagus can recur up to 10 years after ablation, long-term endoscopic surveillance is required, although optimal time intervals are yet to be determined. The acquisition of an adequate biopsy specimen, which includes targeted biopsies as well as four-quadrant biopsies every 1–2 cm, is crucial for optimal histology assessment. In this context, advanced imaging is able to predict dysplasia in Barrett's esophagus, as delineated in a recent meta-analysis. Based on irregular mucosal pit patterns and irregular microvasculature, NBI predicted high-grade dysplasia

with a pooled sensitivity and specificity of 96% and 94%, but specialized intestinal metaplasia with a specificity of only 65% [19]. Moreover, these results must be seen in the context of a moderate interobserver agreement between expert and nonexpert endoscopists [20]. Confocal laser endomicroscopy imaging has been shown to increase the detection of dysplasia in comparison to white light imaging but has not been shown to be superior to NBI [21,22]. Similarly, for detection of residual or recurrent neoplasia in Barrett's esophagus, confocal imaging was not superior to the combination of high-definition white light plus NBI in a randomized controlled trial [23]. Currently, confocal laser endomicroscopy cannot be recommended as part of the routine protocol for screening or surveillance of Barrett's esophagus.

Another limitation of advanced imaging is its virtually inability to visualize buried Barrett's esophagus (subsquamous intestinal metaplasia), which was shown to be present in up to 98.2% of patients with underlying dysplastic Barrett's esophagus, making ablation and resection margins inaccurate [24]. Interestingly, buried Barrett's esophagus appears to have less neoplastic potency than macroscopically visible Barrett's, although this was not addressed in long-term outcome studies [25]. In contrast, advanced imaging was shown to be of utility in determining the endoscopic resection borders of endoscopically treatable early gastric cancer and colorectal neoplasia, reaching an accuracy of up to 100% in early gastric cancer [26,27].

Colorectal neoplasia

Approximately 5% of all colorectal neoplastic lesions are classified as advanced colorectal neoplasia. EMR permits the removal of nearly all large (≥20 mm) noninvasive lesions as well as early cancers limited to the superficial submucosa, resulting in avoidance of surgery in more than 90% of such cases [28,29]. In this context, advanced endoscopic imaging can predict the presence of invasive malignancy, which makes any endoscopic resection obsolete. Macroscopic polyp appearance (Paris classification), colonic mucosal pit pattern (Kudo classification), the narrowband imaging international colorectal endoscopic (NICE) classification, and Sano classification are the most frequently utilized classification systems assessing the likelihood of malignancy of colorectal neoplasia [30–32].

Amendable polyps are resected in Europe and North America mainly utilizing EMR. Depending on expertise, polyp site, polyp size, and polyp assessment, curative resection can be performed in nearly all lesions [33]. The endoscopic polyp assessment is of particular importance in this context, as the presence of Kudo V pattern, especially when nonstructured (Vn) and in the setting of a Paris IIc and III polyp variant, is highly suspicious for invasive carcinoma that is not amendable for resection [34,35]. Another important predictor for resectability is the lifting sign following submucosal injection [36]. Its absence can indicate submucosal invasion in treatment-naive polyps. However, following attempted polypectomy, a desmoid reaction can mimic submucosal invasion by absence of the lifting sign. In this case, EMR can be attempted in the absence of Kudo V with Paris IIc or III polyp variant [37,38].

Similar to any surgical oncologic operation, the achievement of a negative resection margin is a principal goal of polypectomy. To achieve negative resection margins, the preferred resection modality is an en bloc versus a piecemeal resection, given its advantage of superior assessment of resection margins and lower rate of neoplasia recurrence. Most endoscopists assess the polypectomy site with advanced imaging to document complete resection. Imaging can be used both prior to resection and following resection to delineate margins and confirm normal pit patterns at the resection edge. The clinical impact of this growing practice, particularly for large polyps, is not yet fully determined. High-magnification chromoendoscopy has been shown to predict incomplete resection after EMR in 93% and 95%, for involvement of lateral and deep margins, respectively; however, no study has demonstrated its impact on residual or recurrent neoplasia during polyp surveillance [39,40]. Woodward *et al.* [38] demonstrated that polyp size, absence of lifting sign and, especially, piecemeal resection of advanced neoplasia are risk factors for residual neoplasia, which was detected in 12% on follow-up colonoscopy at 3–6 months after index procedure. Other studies have identified the presence of intra-procedural bleeding and advanced polyp histology to be associated with higher risk of neoplasia recurrence [41]. Generally, recurrence rates of up to 55% following colorectal EMR have been reported, although the vast majority of recurrences can be easily and successfully treated by further resection or ablation [4]. An important consideration for the timing of surveillance colonoscopy is the occurrence of "late recurrences" following piecemeal resection. Despite the absence of neoplasia at the resection site during the first surveillance colonoscopy, recurrent neoplasia was demonstrated in 4–16% of cases after 6 months [4,42].

Moreover, inconspicuous polypectomy scars harbored neoplasia in 7% based on biopsies [42]. In this context, incomplete polypectomy, besides missed polyps, is believed to account for a significant number of interval colorectal cancers (Figures 13.4 and 13.5) [43,44]. Pohl *et al.* [44] demonstrated incomplete resection of 23.3%

of polyps measuring 15–20 mm and 31% of sessile serrated adenoma/polyps (SSA/P). This is of particular importance as SSA/P harbor high-grade dysplasia in up to 9.5% [45].

Adjuvant techniques to diminish colorectal neoplasia recurrence are limited. In some studies, argon plasma coagulation has been shown to decrease the risk of residual neoplasia following a piecemeal resection, both when utilized during the index resection and when used as an ablative technique for neoplasia recurrence [46,47]. Salvage EMR following previous unsuccessful resection attempts, which induce scar tissue at the polypectomy site, can be performed successfully in experienced hands, yielding an en-bloc resection rate of 53.5% and residual neoplasia of only 27% at follow-up [37].

Advanced imaging including NBI and confocal microscopy have been shown to be valuable at detecting recurrent and residual neoplasia after colorectal EMR. With a negative predictive value of nearly 100%, these technologies have the potential to reduce the need for surveillance biopsy and overtreatment of non-neoplastic scar tissue [40].

ESD, which is primarily used in East Asian countries, yields particular high R0 rates (88%) and en-bloc resection rates (91.6%), with the downside of higher perforation rates (4%) and substantially longer procedure times. A recent systematic review calculated a pooled risk of recurrence of only 0.07% following colorectal ESD [48]. An important observation is also a lower recurrence rate for colorectal neoplasia following ESD of 2% compared with EMR of 14% [49]. The lower recurrence rate following ESD is based on its technical strength, yielding high rates of en bloc resection and wider resection margins. Assessment of the polypectomy site with advanced imaging for incomplete resection is used widely by gastroenterologists who undertake resection of these large colon polyps. Although a formal study in this context has not been performed, it is unlikely that these differences in recurrence rates are related to variation in the use of advanced imaging to assess margins before or after resection.

Surveillance colonoscopy remains the backbone of colorectal cancer prevention following colorectal EMR and ESD. Current standard of care is a follow-up interval of 3–6 months after resection, with a low recurrence rate at the polypectomy site if residual neoplasia is absent at the first follow-up [2,4]. However, in light of "late recurrences," which range from 4 to 16%, a 3-month follow-up appears to be too early [4,42]. Moreover, experts recommend visualization of previous EMR sites with white light as well as with advanced endoscopic imaging techniques. However, at present, not enough studies are available which address the impact of advanced imaging for post-polypectomy surveillance [2].

Video clips to accompany this book can be found in the online material at www.wiley.com/go/cohen/NBI

The following videos relate specifically to this chapter:

Video 14 Band EMR of focal high-grade dysplasia in Barrett's

Video 15 Radiofrequency ablation of Barrett's tongues

Video 16 Barrett's cap EMR of high-grade dysplasia

Video 17 Barrett's HGD cap EMR: bleeding management

Video 18 Advanced obstructing esophageal adenocarcinoma

Video 36 NBI detection of poorly differentiated superficial gastric cancer not seen on white light

Video 37 Endoscopic submucosal dissection of superficial gastric cancer

Video 51 Colon polyps on NBI: detection and diagnosis. Characterization of large sessile polyp and its margins

Video 52 Colon polyps on NBI: detection and diagnosis. The tip of the iceberg: detection of hidden extension of flat adenoma

Video 58 Management of large sessile polyp

Video 60 Saline injection, polypectomy and tattooing

Video 61 Tubolovillous adenoma resection

Video 62 Pedunculated colon polyp with adenoma margin extending down stalk

Video 63 NBI optical diagnosis of diminutive adenoma

Video 64 Adenoma of the ileocecal valve

Video 65 Follow-up examination following resection of ileocecal valve polyp

Video 69 Incomplete polypectomy and NBI margin assessment for colon adenoma

Video 70 NBI feature of advanced polyp and nonlifting sign

Video 75 High definition imaging WL and NBI to assess and fully resect giant near obstructing splenic flexure tubulovillous adenoma

References

1 Spechler SJ, Souza RF. Barrett's esophagus. *N Engl J Med* 2014;371:836–45.

2 Lieberman DA, Rex DK, Winawer SJ *et al*. Guidelines for colonoscopy surveillance after screening and polypectomy: a consensus update by the US Multi-Society Task Force on Colorectal Cancer. *Gastroenterology* 2012;143:844–57.

3 Ahlenstiel G, Hourigan LF, Brown G *et al*. Actual endoscopic versus predicted surgical mortality for treatment of advanced mucosal neoplasia of the colon. *Gastrointest Endosc* 2014;80:668–76.

4 Khashab M, Eid E, Rusche M, Rex DK. Incidence and predictors of "late" recurrences after endoscopic piecemeal resection of large sessile adenomas. *Gastrointest Endosc* 2009;70:344–9.

5 Bartel MJ, Picco MF, Wallace MB. Chromocolonoscopy. *Gastroenterol Clin North Am* 2015;25:243–60.

6 Abu Dayyeh BK, Thosani N, Konda V *et al*. ASGE Technology Committee systematic review and meta-analysis assessing the ASGE PIVI thresholds for adopting real-time endoscopic assessment of the histology of diminutive colorectal polyps. *Gastrointest Endosc* 2015;81:502e1–e16.

7 Kaminski MF, Hassan C, Bisschops R *et al*. Advanced imaging for detection and differentiation of colorectal neoplasia: European Society of Gastrointestinal Endoscopy (ESGE) Guideline. *Endoscopy* 2014;46:435–49.

8 Kudo S, Rubio CA, Teixeira CR, Kashida H, Kogure E. Pit pattern in colorectal neoplasia: endoscopic magnifying view. *Endoscopy* 2001;33:367–73.

9 Kaltenbach T, Soetikno R. Endoscopic resection of large colon polyps. *Gastrointest Endosc Clin North Am* 2013;23:137–52.

10 Repici A, Pellicano R, Strangio G *et al*. Endoscopic mucosal resection for early colorectal neoplasia: pathologic basis, procedures, and outcomes. *Dis Colon Rectum* 2009;52:1502–15.

11 Bennett C, Vakil N, Bergman J *et al*. Consensus statements for management of Barrett's dysplasia and early-stage esophageal adenocarcinoma, based on a Delphi process. *Gastroenterology* 2012;143:336–46.

12 Phoa KN, van Vilsteren FG, Weusten BL *et al*. Radiofrequency ablation vs endoscopic surveillance for patients with Barrett esophagus and low-grade dysplasia: a randomized clinical trial. *JAMA* 2014;311:1209–17.

13 Shaheen NJ, Sharma P, Overholt BF *et al*. Radiofrequency ablation in Barrett's esophagus with dysplasia. *N Engl J Med* 2009;360:2277–88.

14 Shaheen NJ, Overholt BF, Sampliner RE *et al*. Durability of radiofrequency ablation in Barrett's esophagus with dysplasia. *Gastroenterology* 2011;141:460–8.

15 Phoa KN, Pouw RE, van Vilsteren FG *et al*. Remission of Barrett's esophagus with early neoplasia 5 years after radiofrequency ablation with endoscopic resection: a Netherlands cohort study. *Gastroenterology* 2013;145:96–104.

16 Haidry RJ, Dunn JM, Butt MA *et al*. Radiofrequency ablation and endoscopic mucosal resection for dysplastic Barrett's esophagus and early esophageal adenocarcinoma: outcomes of the UK National Halo RFA Registry. *Gastroenterology* 2013;145:87–95.

17 Gupta M, Iyer PG, Lutzke L *et al*. Recurrence of esophageal intestinal metaplasia after endoscopic mucosal resection and radiofrequency ablation of Barrett's esophagus: results from a US Multicenter Consortium. *Gastroenterology* 2013;145:79–86.e71.

18 Qumseya BJ, Wang H, Badie N *et al*. Advanced imaging technologies increase detection of dysplasia and

neoplasia in patients with Barrett's esophagus: a meta-analysis and systematic review. *Clin Gastroenterol Hepatol* 2013;11:1562–70.e2.

19 Mannath J, Subramanian V, Hawkey CJ, Ragunath K. Narrow band imaging for characterization of high grade dysplasia and specialized intestinal metaplasia in Barrett's esophagus: a meta-analysis. *Endoscopy* 2010;42:351–9.

20 Silva FB, Dinis-Ribeiro M, Vieth M *et al.* Endoscopic assessment and grading of Barrett's esophagus using magnification endoscopy and narrow-band imaging: accuracy and interobserver agreement of different classification systems (with videos). *Gastrointest Endosc* 2011;73:7–14.

21 Sharma P, Meining AR, Coron E *et al.* Real-time increased detection of neoplastic tissue in Barrett's esophagus with probe-based confocal laser endomicroscopy: final results of an international multicenter, prospective, randomized, controlled trial. *Gastrointest Endosc* 2011;74:465–72.

22 Canto MI, Anandasabapathy S, Brugge W *et al.* In vivo endomicroscopy improves detection of Barrett's esophagus-related neoplasia: a multicenter international randomized controlled trial (with video). *Gastrointest Endosc* 2014;79:211–21.

23 Wallace MB, Crook JE, Saunders M *et al.* Multicenter, randomized, controlled trial of confocal laser endomicroscopy assessment of residual metaplasia after mucosal ablation or resection of GI neoplasia in Barrett's esophagus. *Gastrointest Endosc* 2012;76:539–47.e1.

24 Anders M, Lucks Y, El-Masry MA *et al.* Subsquamous extension of intestinal metaplasia is detected in 98% of cases of neoplastic Barrett's esophagus. *Clin Gastroenterol Hepatol* 2014;12:405–10.

25 Hornick JL, Mino-Kenudson M, Lauwers GY *et al.* Buried Barrett's epithelium following photodynamic therapy shows reduced crypt proliferation and absence of DNA content abnormalities. *Am J Gastroenterol* 2008;103:38–47.

26 Nonaka K, Namoto M, Kitada H *et al.* Usefulness of the DL in ME with NBI for determining the expanded area of early-stage differentiated gastric carcinoma. *World J Gastrointest Endosc* 2012;4:362–7.

27 Nagahama T, Yao K, Maki S *et al.* Usefulness of magnifying endoscopy with narrow-band imaging for determining the horizontal extent of early gastric cancer when there is an unclear margin by chromoendoscopy (with video). *Gastrointest Endosc* 2011;74:1259–67.

28 Hassan C, Pickhardt PJ, Kim DH *et al.* Systematic review: distribution of advanced neoplasia according to polyp size at screening colonoscopy. *Aliment Pharmacol Ther* 2010;31:210–17.

29 Swan MP, Bourke MJ, Alexander S, Moss A, Williams SJ. Large refractory colonic polyps: is it time to change our practice? A prospective study of the clinical and economic impact of a tertiary referral colonic mucosal resection and polypectomy service (with videos). *Gastrointest Endosc* 2009;70:1128–36.

30 Sano Y, Ikematsu H, Fu KI *et al.* Meshed capillary vessels by use of narrow-band imaging for differential diagnosis of small colorectal polyps. *Gastrointest Endosc* 2009;69:278–83.

31 Tanaka S, Sano Y. Aim to unify the narrow band imaging (NBI) magnifying classification for colorectal tumors: current status in Japan from a summary of the consensus symposium in the 79th Annual Meeting of the Japan Gastroenterological Endoscopy Society. *Dig Endosc* 2011;23(Suppl 1):131–9.

32 Kudo S, Tamura S, Nakajima T *et al.* Diagnosis of colorectal tumorous lesions by magnifying endoscopy. *Gastrointest Endosc* 1996;44:8–14.

33 Kaltenbach T, Friedland S, Maheshwari A *et al.* Short- and long-term outcomes of standardized EMR of non-polypoid (flat and depressed) colorectal lesions ≥1 cm (with video). *Gastrointest Endosc* 2007;65:857–65.

34 The Paris endoscopic classification of superficial neoplastic lesions: esophagus, stomach, and colon: November 30 to December 1, 2002. *Gastrointest Endosc* 2003;58:S3–43.

35 Soetikno RM, Kaltenbach T, Rouse RV *et al.* Prevalence of nonpolypoid (flat and depressed) colorectal neoplasms in asymptomatic and symptomatic adults. *JAMA* 2008;299:1027–35.

36 Kato H, Haga S, Endo S *et al.* Lifting of lesions during endoscopic mucosal resection (EMR) of early colorectal cancer: implications for the assessment of resectability. *Endoscopy* 2001;33:568–73.

37 Buchner AM, Guarner-Argente C, Ginsberg GG. Outcomes of EMR of defiant colorectal lesions directed to an endoscopy referral center. *Gastrointest Endosc* 2012;76:255–63.

38 Woodward TA, Heckman MG, Cleveland P *et al.* Predictors of complete endoscopic mucosal resection of flat and depressed gastrointestinal neoplasia of the colon. *Am J Gastroenterol* 2012;107:650–4.

39 Hurlstone DP, Cross SS, Brown S, Sanders DS, Lobo AJ. A prospective evaluation of high-magnification chromoscopic colonoscopy in predicting completeness of EMR. *Gastrointest Endosc* 2004;59:642–50.

40 Shahid MW, Buchner AM, Coron E *et al.* Diagnostic accuracy of probe-based confocal laser endomicroscopy in detecting residual colorectal neoplasia after EMR: a prospective study. *Gastrointest Endosc* 2012;75:525–33.

41 Burgess NG, Metz AJ, Williams SJ *et al.* Risk factors for intraprocedural and clinically significant delayed bleeding after wide-field endoscopic mucosal resection of large colonic lesions. *Clin Gastroenterol Hepatol* 2014;12:651–61.e1–3.

42 Knabe M, Pohl J, Gerges C *et al.* Standardized long-term follow-up after endoscopic resection of large,

nonpedunculated colorectal lesions: a prospective two-center study. *Am J Gastroenterol* 2014;109:183–9.

43 Pohl H, Robertson DJ. Colorectal cancers detected after colonoscopy frequently result from missed lesions. *Clin Gastroenterol Hepatol* 2010;8:858–64.

44 Pohl H, Srivastava A, Bensen SP *et al.* Incomplete polyp resection during colonoscopy: results of the complete adenoma resection (CARE) study. *Gastroenterology* 2013;144:74–80.e1.

45 Bouwens MW, van Herwaarden YJ, Winkens B *et al.* Endoscopic characterization of sessile serrated adenomas/polyps with and without dysplasia. *Endoscopy* 2014;46:225–35.

46 Regula J, Wronska E, Polkowski M *et al.* Argon plasma coagulation after piecemeal polypectomy of sessile

colorectal adenomas: long-term follow-up study. *Endoscopy* 2003;35:212–18.

47 Brooker JC, Saunders BP, Shah SG *et al.* Treatment with argon plasma coagulation reduces recurrence after piecemeal resection of large sessile colonic polyps: a randomized trial and recommendations. *Gastrointest Endosc* 2002;55:371–5.

48 Repici A, Hassan C, De Paula Pessoa D *et al.* Efficacy and safety of endoscopic submucosal dissection for colorectal neoplasia: a systematic review. *Endoscopy* 2012;44:137–50.

49 Saito Y, Fukuzawa M, Matsuda T *et al.* Clinical outcome of endoscopic submucosal dissection versus endoscopic mucosal resection of large colorectal tumors as determined by curative resection. *Surg Endosc* 2010;24:343–52.

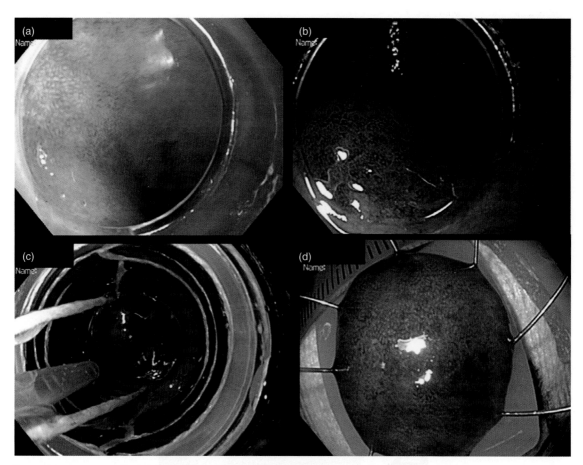

Figure 13.1 Barrett's esophagus with nodule seen by white light and NBI. EMR of nodule and preparation of specimen for histology confirmed only low-grade dysplasia.

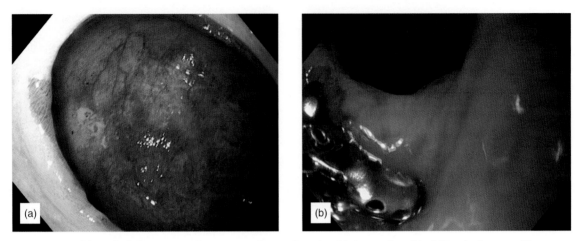

Figure 13.2 Possible residual short tongue of Barrett's esophagus after prior ablation confirmed by NBI and subsequent biopsy.

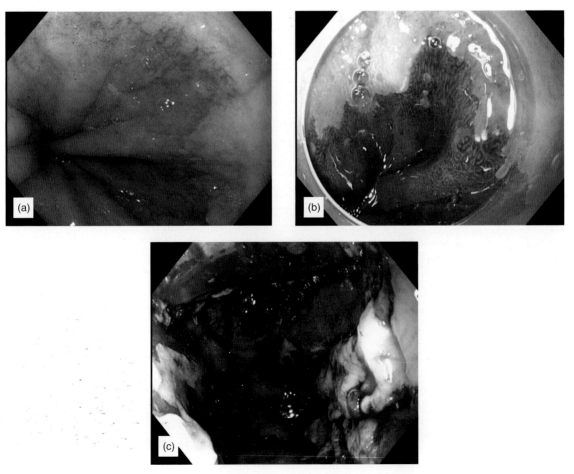

Figure 13.3 Residual tongue of Barrett's esophagus by white light and NBI, ablation by focal RFA.

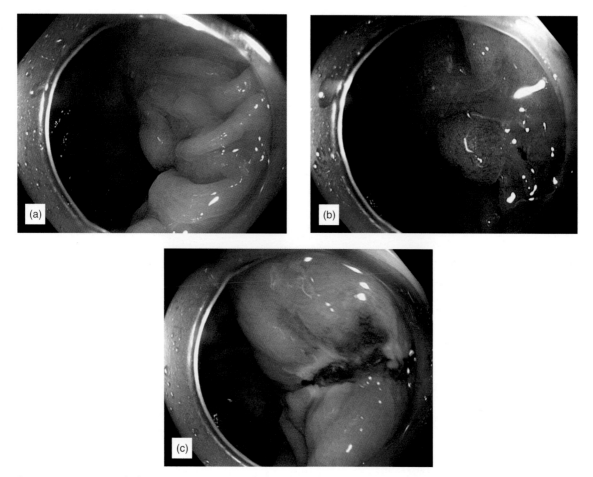

Figure 13.4 Recurrence of adenoma at prior EMR site, detected by white light, NBI and re-resection by repeat EMR.

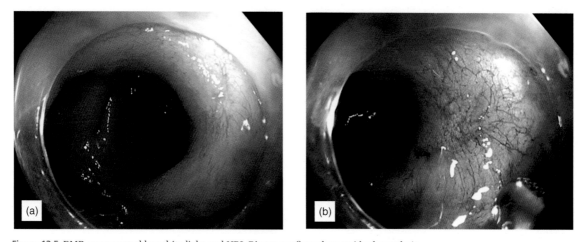

Figure 13.5 EMR scar assessed by white light and NBI. Biopsy confirmed no residual neoplasia.

PART 3

Atlas of Images and Histopathologic Correlates

14 Pharynx and esophagus atlas

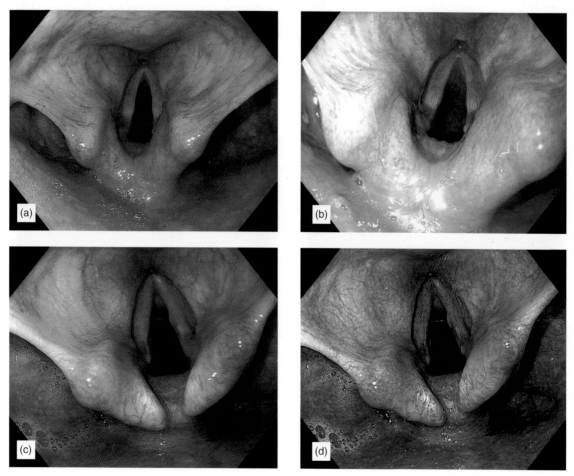

Figure 14.1 (a, b) Normal cords, WL and H190 NBI. (c, d) Inflamed red aryepiglottic folds in a patient undergoing evaluation for possible laryngeal reflux. (Jonathan Cohen, NYU Langone School of Medicine.)

Comprehensive Atlas of High-Resolution Endoscopy and Narrowband Imaging, Second Edition. Edited by Jonathan Cohen.
© 2017 John Wiley & Sons, Ltd. Published 2017 by John Wiley & Sons, Ltd.
Companion website: www.wiley.com/go/cohen/NBI

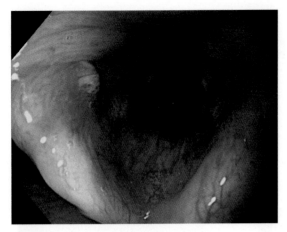

Figure 14.2 Small nodule on arytenoid and cyst on vocal cord WL H180. (Jacques Deviere, Erasmus University Hospital.)

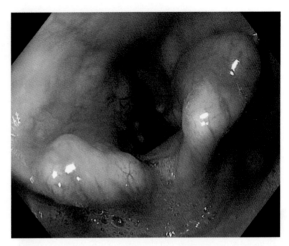

Figure 14.3 Distorted cords WL HRE H180 low magnification view. (Jonathan Cohen, NYU Langone School of Medicine.)

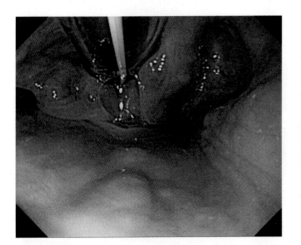

Figure 14.4 WL H190 image of esophageal intubation alongside endotracheal tube placed for airway protection. (Jonathan Cohen, NYU Langone School of Medicine.)

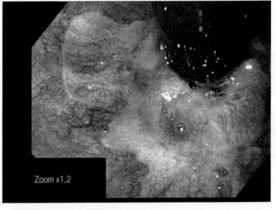

Figure 14.5 Turnaround view highlights normal stratified squamous mucosa of the distal esophagus well delineated on NBI H180 magnification view. (Jean-François Rey, Institute Arnault Tzanck.)

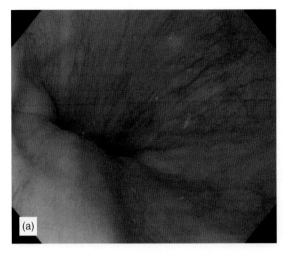
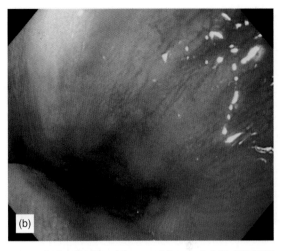

Figure 14.6 (a) Palisade vessels in normal esophageal mucosa, important to the localization of the top of the gastric folds WL H180. (b) NBI view of palisade vessels in normal distal esophageal mucosa. (Guido Costamagna, Catholic University of the Sacred Heart).

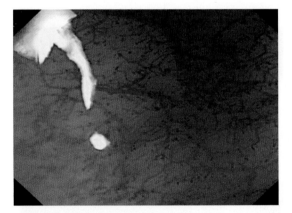

Figure 14.7 Type I intraepithelial papillary capillary loops (IPCLs) seen under NBI low-magnification view of normal esophageal mucosa. These appear here as characteristic brown dots in a "pin-hair" pattern. (Copyright H. Inoue, Northern Yokohama Hospital.)

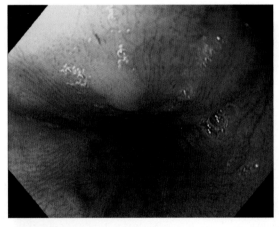

Figure 14.8 Normal esophagus in NBI H180 view with normal IPCL pattern to the left of the image and no visible IPCL pattern to the right. (Jacques Deviere, Erasmus University Hospital.)

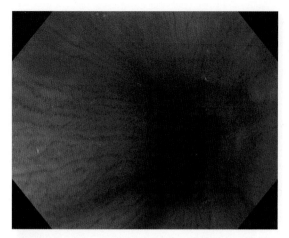

Figure 14.9 Normal esophageal stratified squamous epithelium, IPCL Type 1 pattern seen as brown dots, NBI H180 1.5 × magnification (Jonathan Cohen, NYU Langone School of Medicine.)

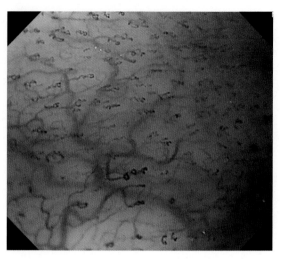

Figure 14.10 Normal brown IPCL pattern with deeper green branching vessels below. (Copyright M. Muto, Kyoto University Hospital Cancer Center.)

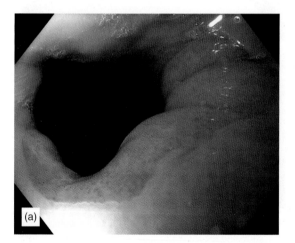

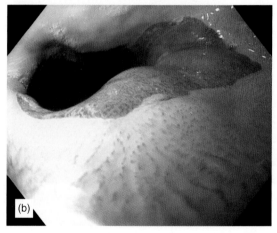

Figure 14.11 (a, b) H190 near-focus WL and NBI images of normal gastroesophageal junction. Compared with earlier EXERA 180 models, squamous IPCLs can now ae more clearly delineated on NBI but require near-focus magnification and often NBI mode to be appreciated. (Jonathan Cohen, NYU Langone School of Medicine.)

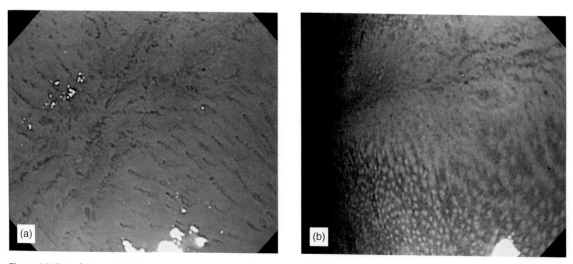

Figure 14.12 (a, b) Type II IPCL in gastroesophageal reflux disease (GERD). Enlarged but regularly arranged IPCLs are observed. (Copyright H. Inoue, Northern Yokohama Hospital.)

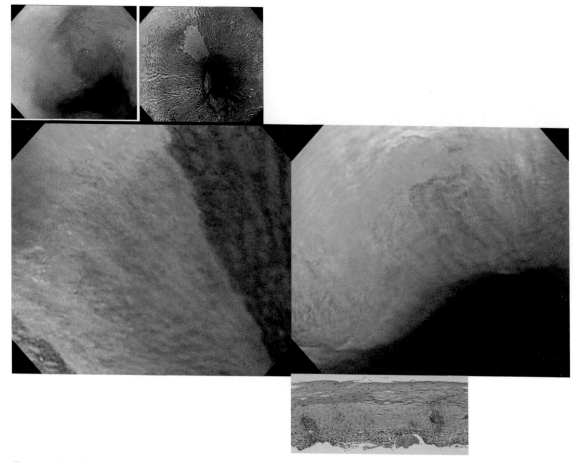

Figure 14.13 IPCL type III pattern present in chronic esophagitis. IPCL type III reflects Lugol-void area with no IPCL proliferation. The magnification view of the capillary pattern shows that this is a benign lesion despite the nonstaining with iodine similar to squamous cell carcinoma (SCC). (Copyright H. Inoue, Northern Yokohama Hospital.)

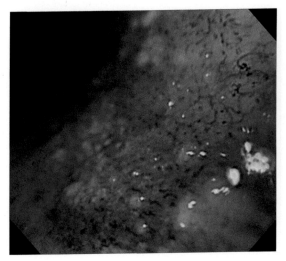

Figure 14.14 Type IV IPCL seen on magnification NBI. IPCL type IV reflects an area with IPCL proliferation. (Copyright H. Inoue, Northern Yokohama Hospital.)

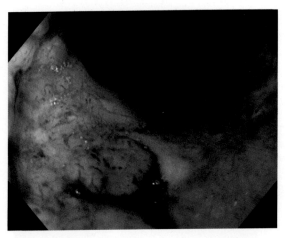

Figure 14.15 Irregular vessels in SCC, close-up with WL H180 HRE and NBI without zoom. (University Medical Center Hamburg Eppendorf.)

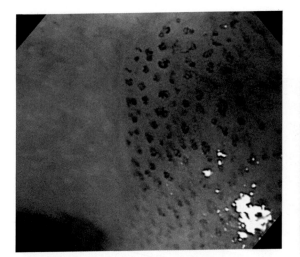

Figure 14.16 Type V1 IPCL seen on magnification NBI in a superficial SCC. IPCL type V1 reflects an area with marked IPCL proliferation and meandering. Note the combination of irregular high-density and thicker vessels with a sharp demarcation in this flat cancer. (Copyright H. Inoue, Northern Yokohama Hospital.)

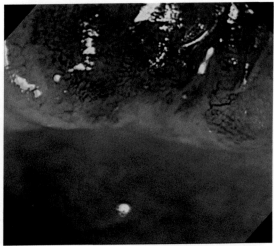

Figure 14.17 NBI magnification view of invasive SCC as manifest by neovessel IPCL (Type VN). (Copyright H. Inoue, Northern Yokohama Hospital.)

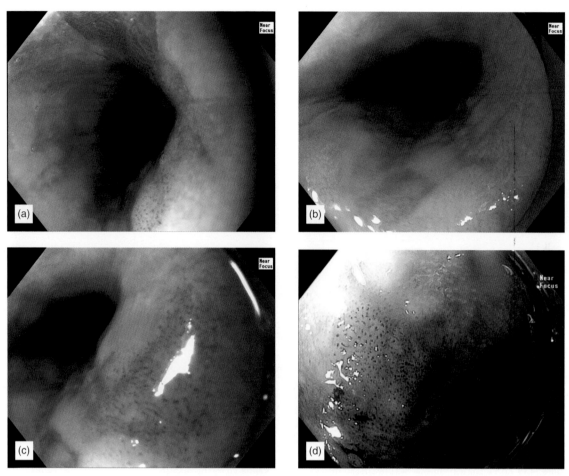

Figure 14.18 Proximal esophageal squamous cell esophageal cancer Type 0 IIc adjacent to inlet patch NBI view (a) with sharp demarcation and clearly abnormal type V IPCLs visible on WL (b) better seen on NBI H190 near focus view (c); best view of magnification with clear cap (d). (Jonathan Cohen, NYU Langone School of Medicine.)

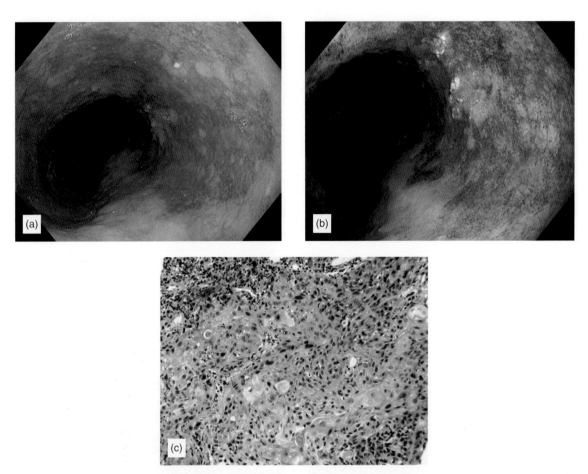

Figure 14.19 (a) Esophageal mucosal SCC, WL H180 HRE low-magnification view. This appears on WL as a flat reddened area and might be mistaken for an inlet patch of ectopic gastric mucosa without better examination of the mucosal surface and vascular pattern with NBI and magnification. (b) Esophageal mucosal NBI low-magnification view of esophageal SCC. Magnification required to really assess the vascular pattern. Dense dark vessels and irregular surface are evident, as well as demarcation from normal tissue. (c) Histologic image demonstrating SCC. (Mayo Clinic, Jacksonville.)

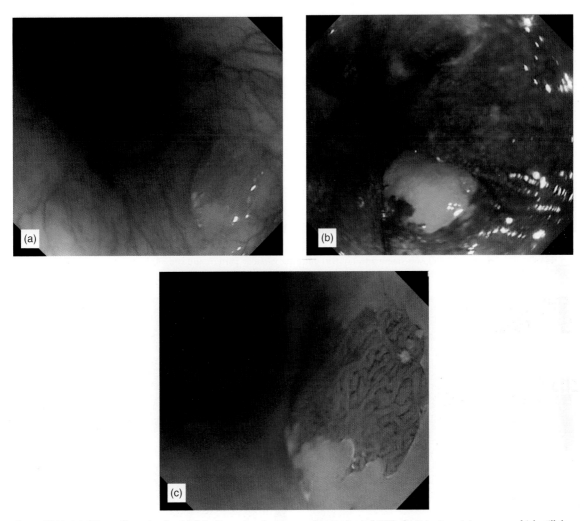

Figure 14.20 (a) This small proximal reddish lesion may raise concern for esophageal SCC. (b) Ectopic gastric mucosa which still does not stain by iodine solution, similar to SCC. (c) Magnification NBI image shows regular gastric mucosal pattern with no abnormal brown IPCLs that would be present in an SCC. (Copyright M. Muto, Kyoto University Hospital Cancer Center).

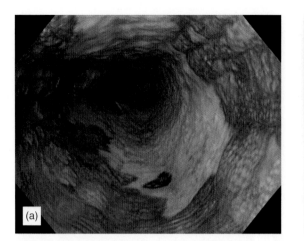

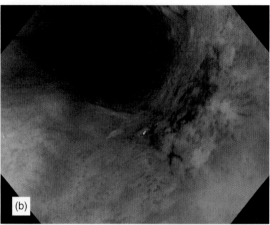

Figure 14.21 (a) Flat SCC, Lugol non-staining under H180 WL. The margin of the lesion is distinguished easily. (b) HRE NBI H180 image corresponding to the area of Lugol non-staining in (a). NBI adds the vascular pattern and still allows margins to be distinguished. (University Medical Center Hamburg Eppendorf.)

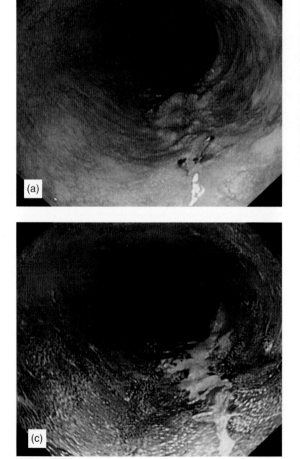

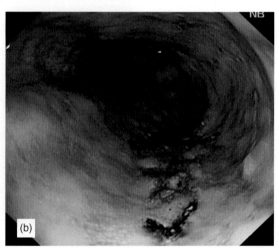

Figure 14.22 (a) WL magnified view of squamous cell esophageal carcinoma. Histology revealed an invasive well-differentiated SCC. (b) NBI H180 image of this lesion prior to Lugol staining delineates margins well. (c) Lugol stain shows similar outline of tumor extent to the NBI image. (University of Amsterdam.)

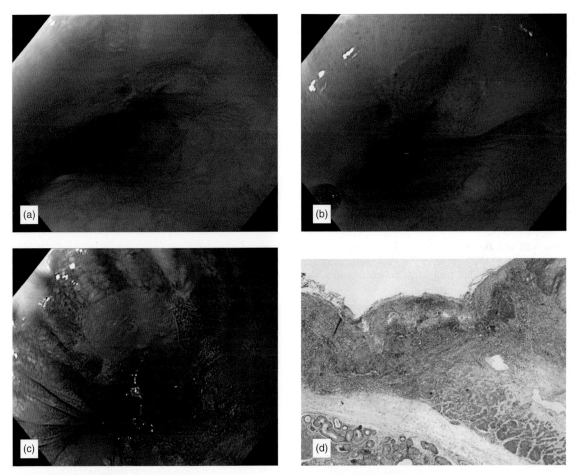

Figure 14.23 (a) SCC on WL HRE H180 view detected as slightly depressed, erythroplastic area. (b, c) Slightly depressed SCC: (b) red–brown on NBI (because of hypervascularization). Note the sharp demarcation and the irregular IPCL pattern. (c) Lugol image provides similar information to the NBI view. (d) SCC invades the mucosa and superficial submucosa. (Thierry Ponchon, Edouard Herriot Hospital.)

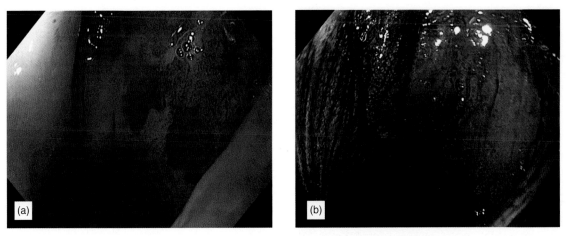

Figure 14.24 Lower limit of a superficial SCC: (a) good delineation of the extent of the lesion with NBI H180; (b) Lugol staining provides the same information as NBI in this case. (Thierry Ponchon, Edouard Herriot Hospital.)

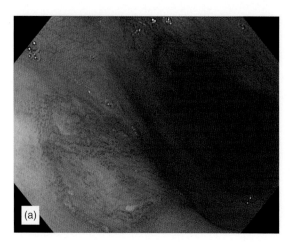

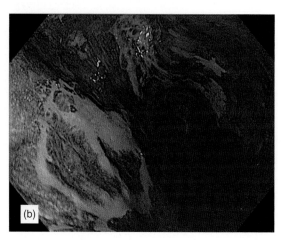

Figure 14.25 (a) NBI H180 image reveals two lesions of superficial SCC. The abnormal IPCL pattern is evident on the proximal lesion. (b) The same two lesions of superficial SCC: Lugol (same pattern as with NBI). When iodine is used, nonstaining area should be watched for transition into pink color indicative of carcinoma. (Thierry Ponchon, Edouard Herriot Hospital.)

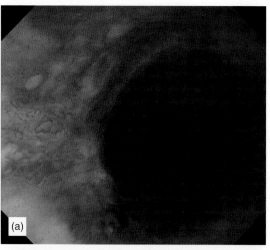

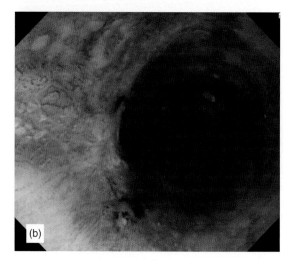

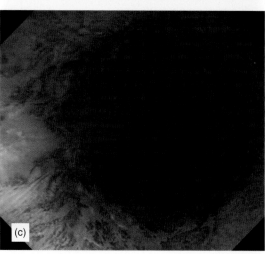

Figure 14.26 (a) WL view of a superficial SCC of the esophagus notable for nonspecific discoloration and bumpy surface appearance. (b) NBI nicely delineates the margin of this SCC occupying a wide proportion of the circumference of the esophagus. (c) In this case, Lugol staining provides similar information to NBI view in terms of margin. (Copyright M. Muto, Kyoto University Hospital Cancer Center.)

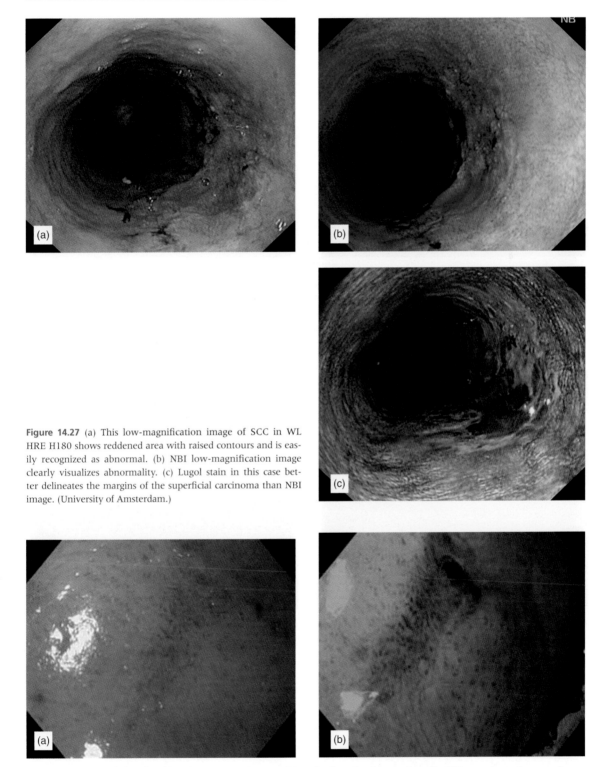

Figure 14.27 (a) This low-magnification image of SCC in WL HRE H180 shows reddened area with raised contours and is easily recognized as abnormal. (b) NBI low-magnification image clearly visualizes abnormality. (c) Lugol stain in this case better delineates the margins of the superficial carcinoma than NBI image. (University of Amsterdam.)

Figure 14.28 (a) Small discolored lesion seen on WL H180 and found to be a (3 × 7 mm) triangular SCC on endoscopic mucosal resection (EMR) specimen. (b) Better delineation of extent of this lesion is possible with NBI, low-magnification view. (Thierry Ponchon, Edouard Herriot Hospital.)

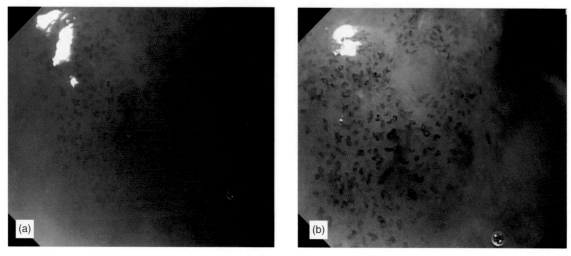

Figure 14.29 Hypopharynx, left pyriform sinus, SCC. (a) Lesion appears on WL HRE only as a small red blush, much better appreciated with NBI. (b) Note the sharp demarcation and the abnormal Type V IPCL pattern within the lesion. (Copyright M. Muto, Kyoto University Hospital Cancer Center.)

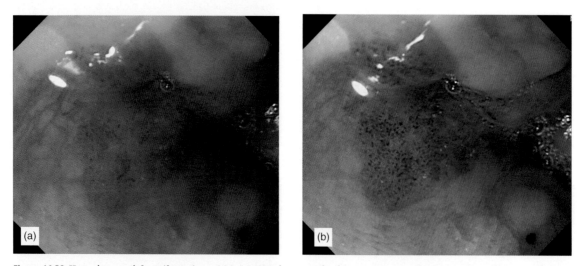

Figure 14.30 Hypopharynx, left pyriform sinus, SCC. (a) HRE does reveal a demarcation. Examination to detect lesions in the pharynx is best performed initially under NBI light. (b) The lesion demonstrates a sharp border and dense irregular brown IPCL vessels seen on NBI. (Copyright M. Muto, Kyoto University Hospital Cancer Center.)

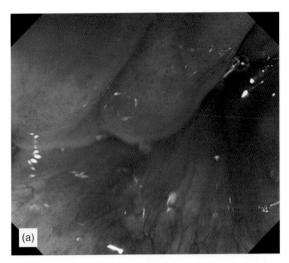

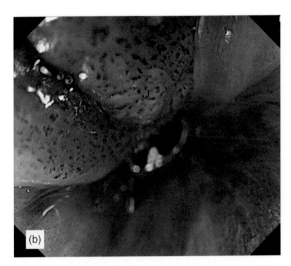

Figure 14.31 (a) Line of discoloration on magnification WL image in right pyriform sinus in patient with multifocal pharyngeal carcinoma. (b) NBI magnification view shows irregular IPCL pattern as well as a demarcation line indicative of carcinoma. (Copyright M. Muto, Kyoto University Hospital Cancer Center.)

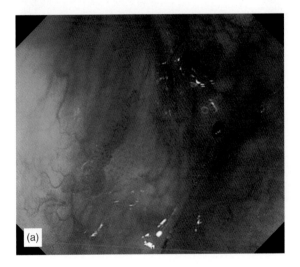

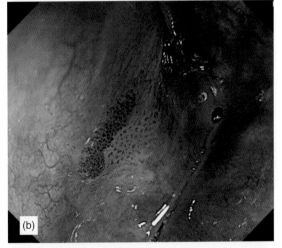

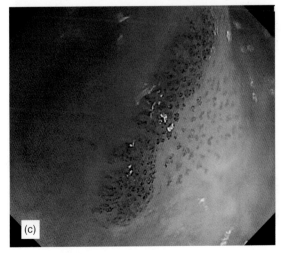

Figure 14.32 (a) Low-magnification WL image shows sharp red line in this patient after chemoradiotherapy for SCC of the esophagus. (b) NBI view demonstrates a demarcation line with thick irregular brown vessels suspicious for residual carcinoma. (c) Magnified NBI view shows type V IPCL brown background colour and sharp demarcation in this residual carcinoma post treatment. (Copyright M. Muto, Kyoto University Hospital Cancer Center.)

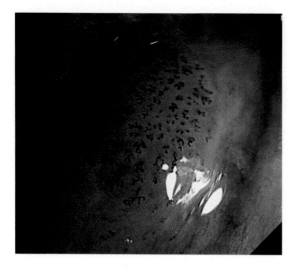

Figure 14.33 Magnified view of this hyperplastic lesion under NBI light to accentuate irregular IPCL pattern. Note the lack of clear demarcation of the prominent IPCLs. Unlike (c) there is no brown background color. (Copyright M. Muto, Kyoto University Hospital Cancer Center.)

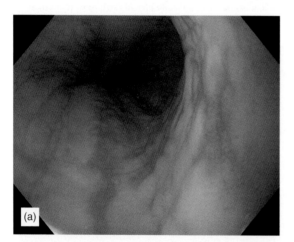

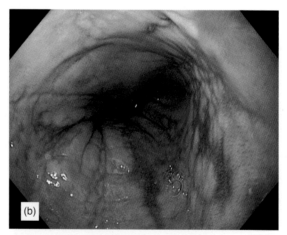

Figure 14.34 (a) High-resolution WL H180 image demonstrates the furrows of mucosal erosion found in early erosive esophagitis. (b) The subtle erythematous furrows of early erosive esophagitis are clearly demonstrated with NBI. (Mayo Clinic, Jacksonville.)

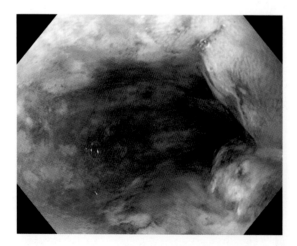

Figure 14.35 Los Angeles Grade 4 gastroesophageal reflux-induced esophagitis WL H180. (James DiSario, University of Utah Health Sciences Center.)

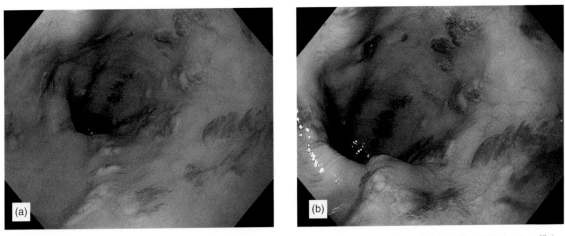

Figure 14.36 (a) High-resolution image demonstrating the white curd-like exudate of Candida esophagitis. WL H180 view is sufficient to make this diagnosis. (b) Candida lesions appear pink on this NBI image given the yellow WL appearance of these lesions. More often, Candida appears white on NBI in stark contrast to the blue–gray background. (Mayo Clinic, Jacksonville.)

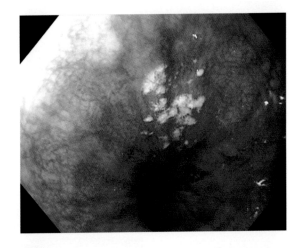

Figure 14.37 Patient with dysmotility of the esophagus found to have these more common white punctate lesions of Candida esophagitis NBI H180 low magnification view. (University Medical Center Hamburg Eppendorf.)

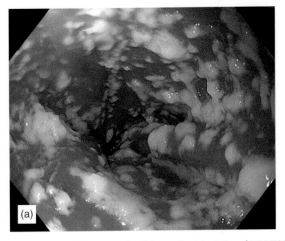
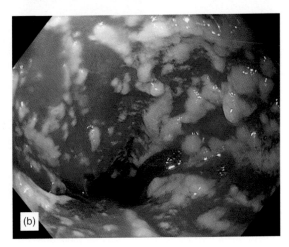

Figure 14.38 (a, b) Severe Candida esophagitis, WL and NBI H190. (Jonathan Cohen, NYU Langone School of Medicine.)

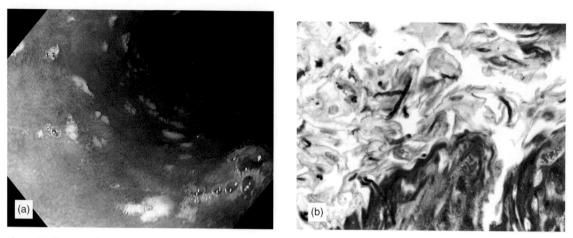

Figure 14.39 (a) Multiple punctate white plaques of Candida that stand out under NBI H180 low magnification. (b) Candida hyphae and occasional yeast forms in surface and desquamated epithelium (PAS stain). (Jonathan Cohen, NYU Langone School of Medicine.)

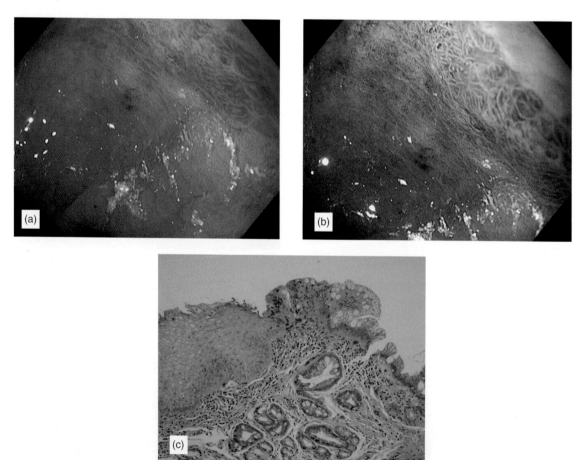

Figure 14.40 (a) Short-segment Barrett's esophagus (SSBE). In this WL H180 view, the villiform Barrett's epithelium is barely discernible proximal to the gastric cardiac epithelium. (b) NBI non-magnified view of SSBE much more clearly delineates the abnormal mucosal pattern than the WL image. (James DiSario, University of Utah Health Sciences Center.) (c) Histopathology from a target biopsy of the suspected Barrett's esophagus seen on the NBI image in (b) confirmed the presence of specialized intestinal-type metaplasia (James DiSario, University of Utah Health Science Center).

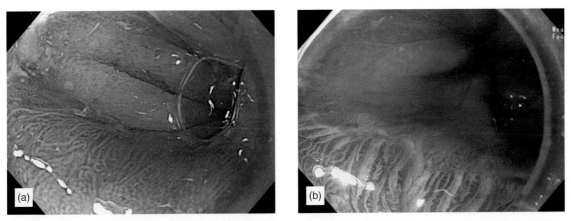

Figure 14.41 (a, b) Thickened linear vessels mark the distal end of the specialized Barrett's epithelium beginning just above the top of the gastric folds: WL and NBI H190 near focus. (Jonathan Cohen, NYU Langone School of Medicine.)

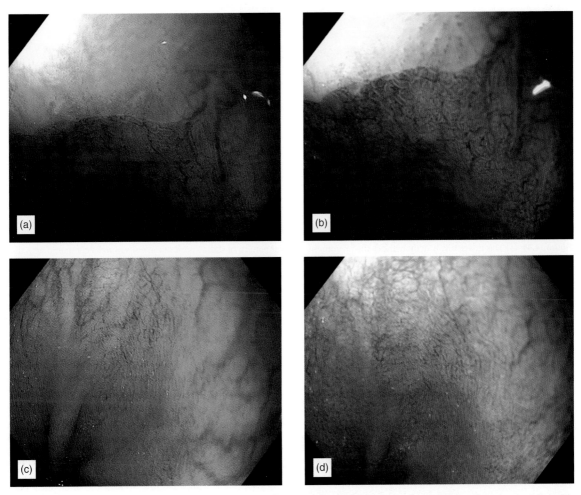

Figure 14.42 (a–d) White light and NBI H190 in low magnification and near focus views of two patients short segment Barrett's esophagus with palisade vessels and long branching vessel pattern. (Jonathan Cohen, NYU Langone School of Medicine.)

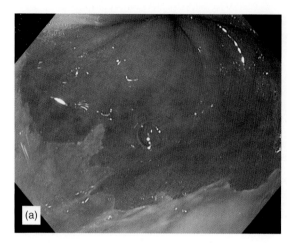
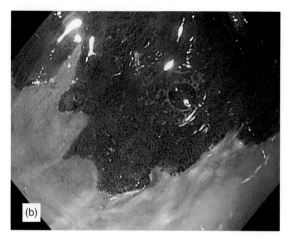

Figure 14.43 (a) High-resolution WL H180 image demonstrating glandular mucosa extending proximally into the tubular esophagus. (b) Close-up high-resolution NBI that nicely demarcates the squamo-columnar junction and short-segment glandular mucosa with normal mucosal vascular and glandular architecture. (Mayo Clinic, Jacksonville.)

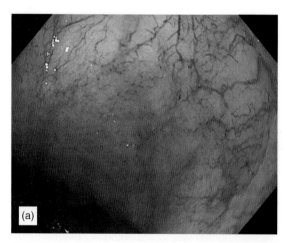
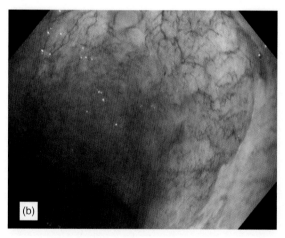

Figure 14.44 (a) This image nicely demonstrates the prominent vascular pattern of short-segment Barrett's mucosa compared with the distal cardiac mucosa and adjacent squamous mucosa H180. (b) NBI highlights the striking vascular pattern of the specialized intestinal metaplasia of Barrett's mucosa compared with the distal cardiac mucosa and adjacent squamous mucosa. (Mayo Clinic, Jacksonville.)

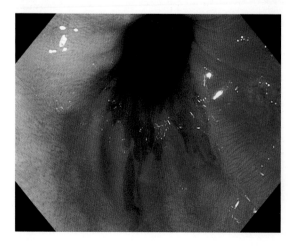

Figure 14.45 NBI H180 image of SSBE. The pink tongues exhibit gyrus/ridge pattern. Type I normal IPCLs and type II elongated IPCLs consistent with reflux are seen in the distal squamous mucosa on the left and right sides of the image, respectively (Johns Hopkins University School of Medicine.)

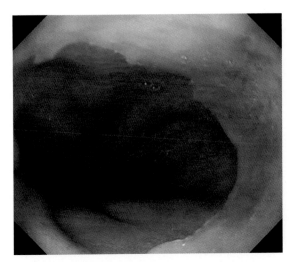

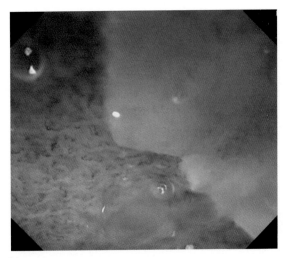

Figure 14.46 SSBE, intestinal metaplasia seen arising just above the top of the gastric folds. On occasion, WL images may be useful in identifying the top of these folds to determine whether the pink mucosa is, in fact, Barrett's esophagus. (Copyright M. Muto, Kyoto University Hospital Cancer Center.)

Figure 14.47 SSBE, intestinal metaplasia. Regular vascular pattern and gyrus mucosal pattern readily discernible on magnification NBI view. (Copyright M. Muto, Kyoto University Hospital Cancer Center.)

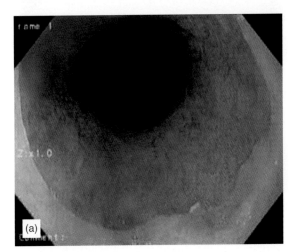

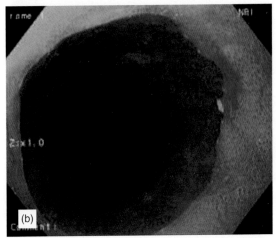

Figure 14.48 (a, b) Long-segment Barrett's esophagus WL H180 view. (Guido Costamagna, Catholic University of the Sacred Heart.)

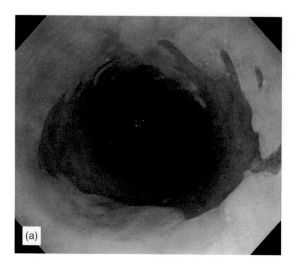
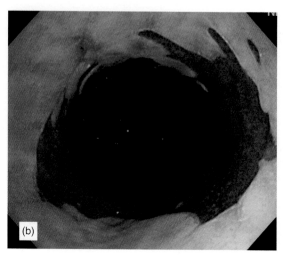

Figure 14.49 (a) Long-segment Barrett's esophagus is clearly evident on this low-magnification WL H180 HRE view. (b) NBI in this case provides sharp contrast between squamous and columnar mucosa but is best utilized here to assess mucosal and vessel patterns with magnification over the Barrett's segment. (University of Amsterdam.)

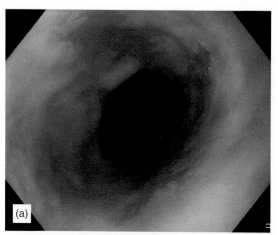
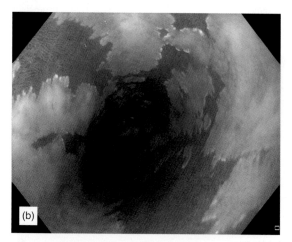

Figure 14.50 (a) Long-segment Barrett's esophagus (190 WLE). WL endoscopy demonstrates tongues of salmon-colored columnar epithelium in the tubular esophagus consistent with Barrett's esophagus. This is in contrast to surrounding normal squamous epithelium, which appears pearly white. (b) NBI image provides better contrast between the areas of Barrett's esophagus mucosa and normal squamous epithelium, allowing better definition of the borders of the Barrett's mucosa. (Neil Gupta, Loyola University Health System.)

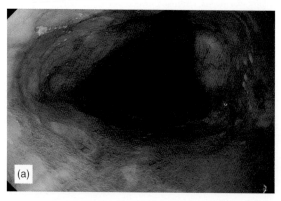
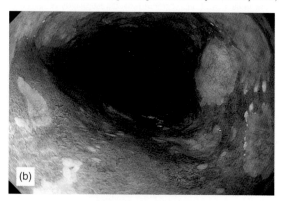

Figure 14.51 (a, b) Long-segment Barrett's esophagus with squamous islands in WL and NBI H190 low magnification. (Krish Ragunath, Queen's Medical Centre, Nottingham.)

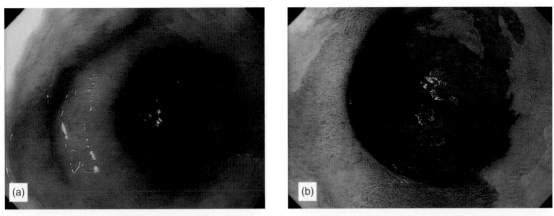

Figure 14.52 (a, b) WL and NBI H190 images of short-segment Barrett's tongue. (Krish Ragunath, Queen's Medical Centre, Nottingham.)

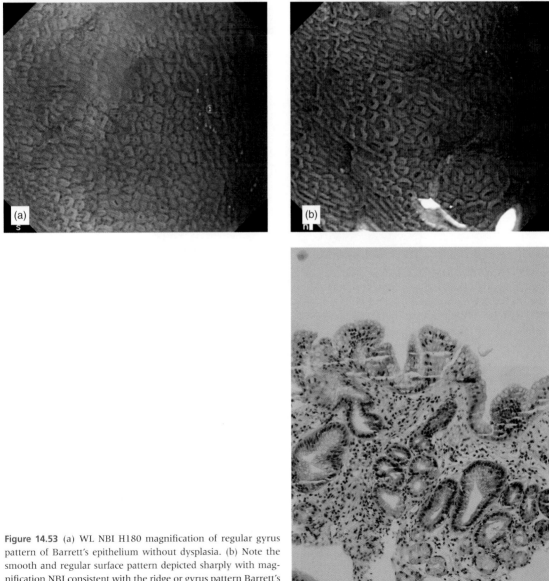

Figure 14.53 (a) WL NBI H180 magnification of regular gyrus pattern of Barrett's epithelium without dysplasia. (b) Note the smooth and regular surface pattern depicted sharply with magnification NBI consistent with the ridge or gyrus pattern Barrett's esophagus. (c) Nondysplastic Barrett's esophagus confirmed by histopathology. (University of Amsterdam.)

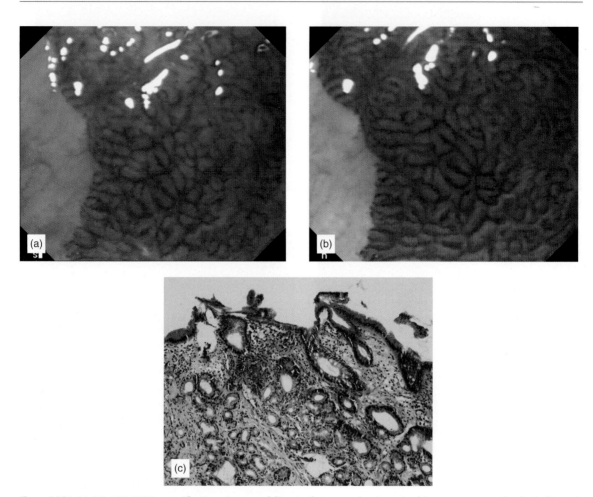

Figure 14.54 (a) WL NBI H180 magnification view can delineate the mucosal pattern in this gyrus-type nondysplastic Barrett's esophagus, though NBI is required to properly analyze the vascular pattern. (b) This is a variation of the ridge or gyrus pattern of nondysplastic Barrett's esophagus that comprises 80% of all cases. NBI H180 magnified view. (c) Intestinal metaplasia of nondysplastic Barrett's esophagus, low-power image. (University of Amsterdam.)

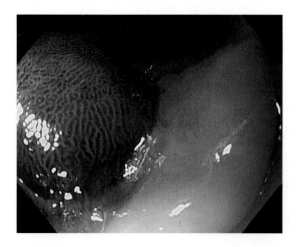

Figure 14.55 NBI H180 view of intestinal metaplasia: regular ridge/villous pattern. (University of Kansas School of Medicine.)

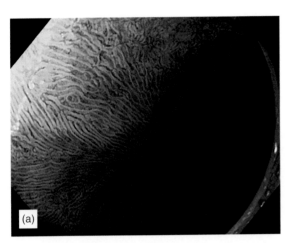

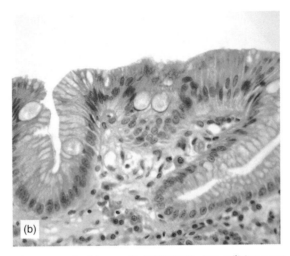

Figure 14.56 (a) Ridge/villous pattern of nondysplastic Barrett's esophagus seen in this magnified NBI H180 view, utilizing a cap fitted to the tip of the endoscope that touches the surface of the mucosa. (b) Histology corresponding to the ridge/villous pattern in the endoscopic photo (a). Intestinal metaplasia is characterized by bluish goblet cells. (University of Kansas School of Medicine.)

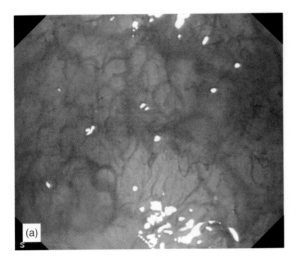

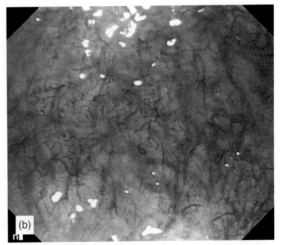

Figure 14.57 (a) This WL magnified image shows flat mucosa with some hint of prominent vessels but no diagnosis of Barrett's esophagus can be made on this basis. (b) NBI H180 magnification provides the necessary contrast and definition of vessels to identify the long branching vessels on flat mucosa that comprises 20% of nondysplastic Barrett's esophagus. (c) Specialized intestinal metaplasia in nondysplastic Barrett's esophagus. (University of Amsterdam.)

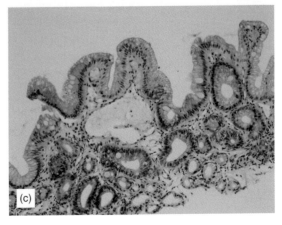

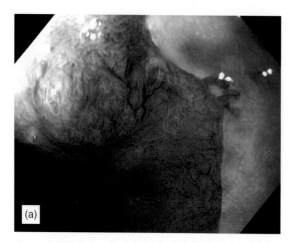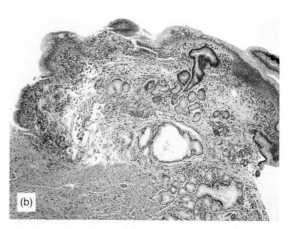

Figure 14.58 (a) Long branching vessel in flat mucosa below the squamo-columnar junction but above the top of the gastric folds indicative of Barrett's esophagus NBI H180. (b) Inflamed columnar mucosa near squamo-columnar junction with ectatic blood vessel corresponding to endoscopic NBI image. Adjacent sections show intestinalized epithelium with goblet cells consistent with Barrett's mucosa. (Jonathan Cohen, NYU Langone School of Medicine.)

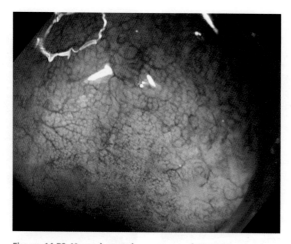

Figure 14.59 Normal vascular pattern of Barrett's esophagus without dysplasia NBI H180. (Prateek Sharma, University of Kansas School of Medicine.)

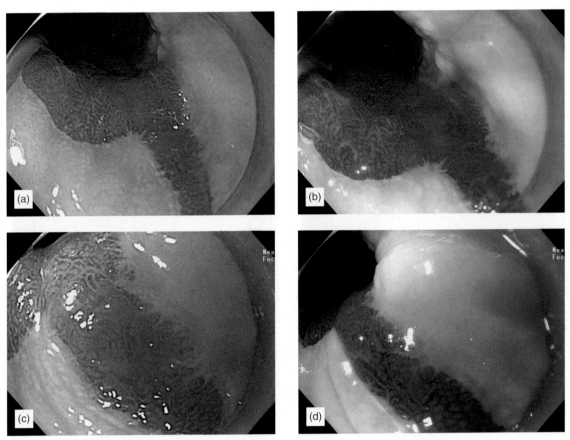

Figure 14.60 (a–d) WL and NBI H190 views in low magnification and near focus in this patient with Barrett's with Prague classification C5 M7. Non dysplastic areas are seen. (Jonathan Cohen, NYU Langone School of Medicine.)

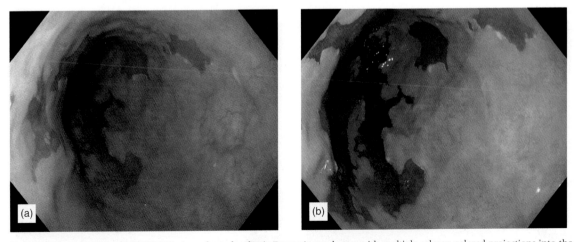

Figure 14.61 (a, b) WL and NBI H190 view of nondysplastic Barrett's esophagus with multiple salmon colored projections into the distal esophagus. (Jonathan Cohen, NYU Langone School of Medicine.)

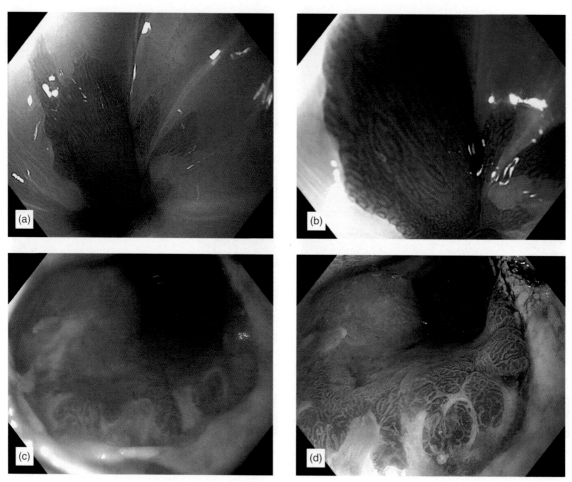

Figure 14.62 (a–d) Two cases of short segment Barrett's esophagus WL and NBI H190 views. (Jonathan Cohen, NYU Langone School of Medicine.)

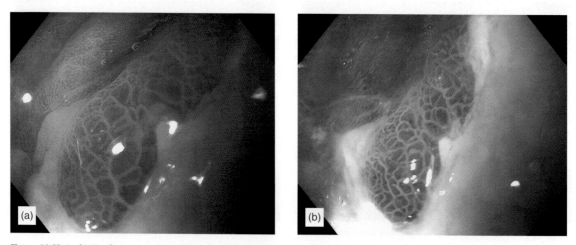

Figure 14.63 (a, b) Single 1 cm projection of salmon colored mucosa with thickened mucosal sulci found to have carditis and intestinal metaplasia within cardia type mucosa WL and NBI H190 low magnification views. (Jonathan Cohen, NYU Langone School of Medicine.)

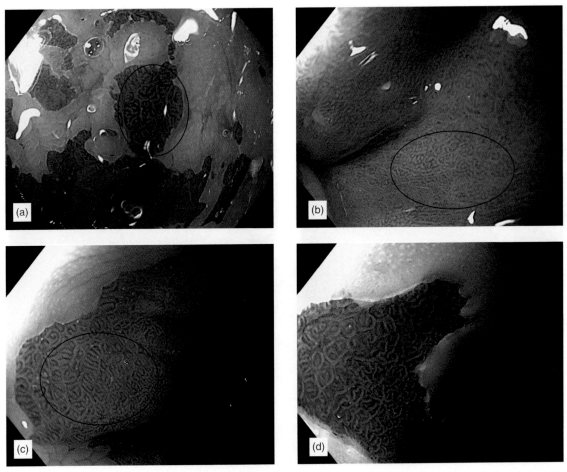

Figure 14.64 (a–d) Nondysplastic Barrett's esophagus: H190 WL and NBI show regular gyrus pattern and normal uniform-caliber vessels. (Prateek Sharma, University of Kansas Medical Center.)

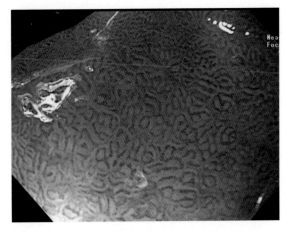

Figure 14.65 Image of NBI H190 near focus highlighting non-dysplastic Barrett's gyrus pattern with uniform vessels in a regular pattern. (Jonathan Cohen, NYU Langone School of Medicine.)

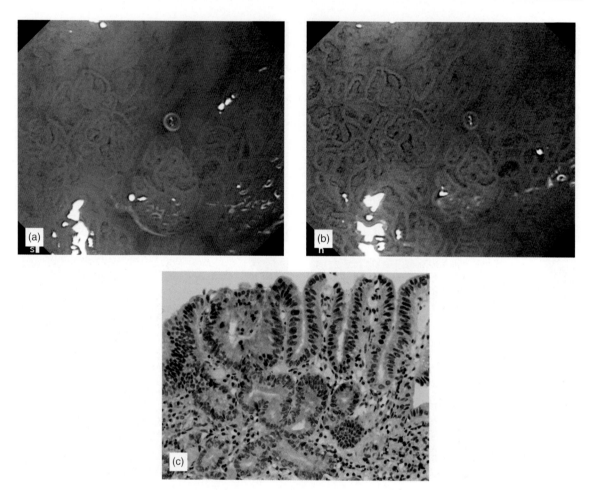

Figure 14.66 (a) Magnification WL H180 HRE view of high-grade dysplasia (HGD) shows abnormal surface morphology, but it is not possible to assess the vascular pattern on this image. (b) NBI magnification view reveals both the irregular mucosal contour and vascular pattern consistent with the optical diagnosis of HGD. (c) HGD is confirmed on histopathology. (University of Amsterdam.)

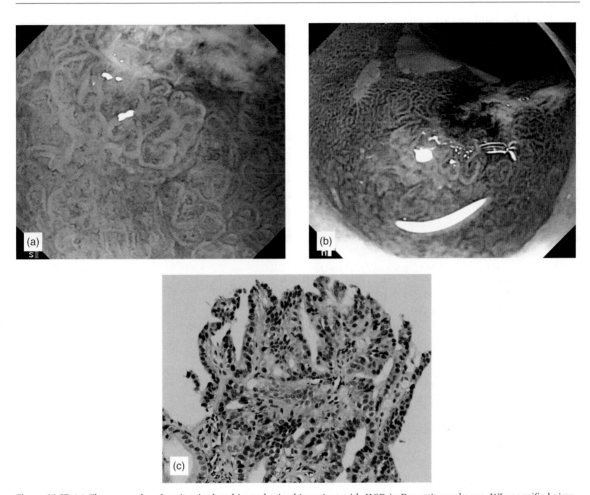

Figure 14.67 (a) The mucosal surface is raised and irregular in this patient with HGD in Barrett's esophagus. WL magnified view. (b) NBI highlights the lesion's topography. Vascular pattern is best seen under magnification. This view is low magnification. (c) HGD suspected on (a) and (b) is confirmed by histopathology. (University of Amsterdam.)

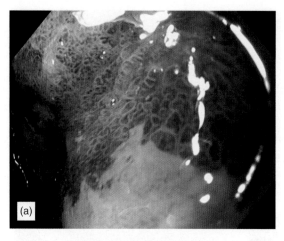

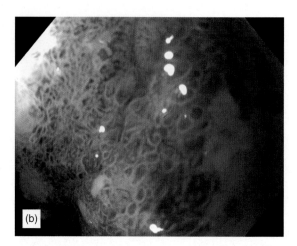

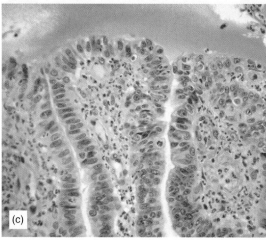

Figure 14.68 (a) Irregular/distorted pattern of mucosa, a key feature of HGD in Barrett's esophagus, is illustrated in this magnified NBI image. (b) The endoscope is pushed closer to the mucosa to gain physical magnification in addition to the digital magnification from this H180 scope. Mucosal irregularities are accentuated. (c) HGD at 100 × showing cytologic atypia, loss of nuclear polarity, full thickness stratification of nuclei, and significantly disordered crypt architecture. (Prateek Sharma, University of Kansas School of Medicine.)

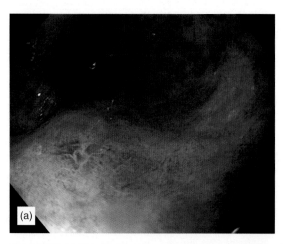

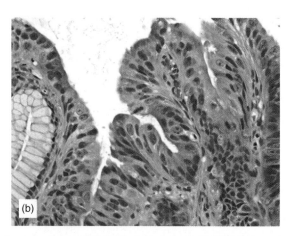

Figure 14.69 (a) Note the irregular surface mucosa evident even in low-magnification NBI H180 of this patient with HGD in Barrett's esophagus. (b) This 40 × high-power image reveals HGD. There is a mitotic figure in the center of the image, high in the epithelium. There is marked nuclear enlargement with vesicular change and prominent nucleoli. (Rob Hawes, Medical University of South Carolina.)

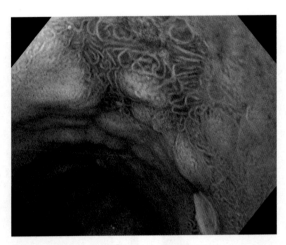

Figure 14.70 Low-magnification NBI HRE H180 view of long-segment Barrett's esophagus with focal HGD. Note the depressed and raised areas, wide sulci arranged in a nonparallel irregular pattern. (Michael Wallace Mayo Clinic, Jacksonville.)

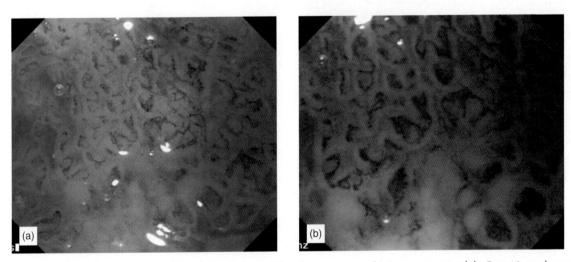

Figure 14.71 (a) WL HRE gives some hint of abnormal vessels but changes seen on this image are very subtle. Barrett's esophagus with HGD. (b) Magnification NBI demonstrates abnormally shaped and thickened blood vessels, a key feature of HGD in Barrett's esophagus. Note the importance of assessing not only the pattern of vessel arrangement, but also the presence of abnormal individual vessels. (University of Amsterdam.)

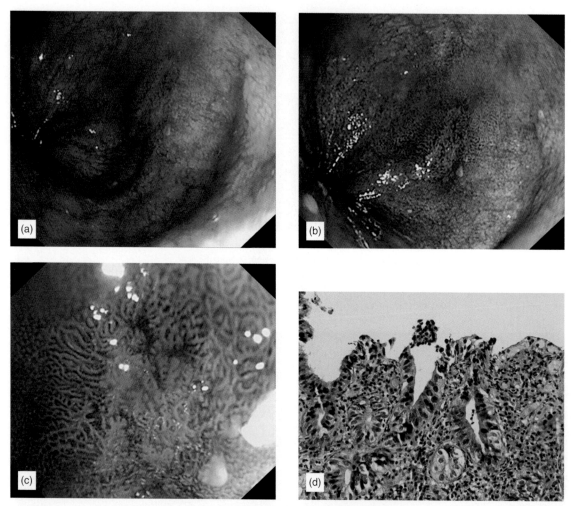

Figure 14.72 (a) This WL H180 image shows what appears may be a simple erosion within Barrett's esophagus; the vascular pattern cannot be determined. (b) HGD in Barrett's esophagus displays both a depressed surface and abnormal vessels where the regular mucosal pattern is disrupted. (c) Magnified NBI view shows abnormal thick vessels in addition to irregular surface pattern. (d) Histopathology confirms the suspected HGD. (University of Amsterdam.)

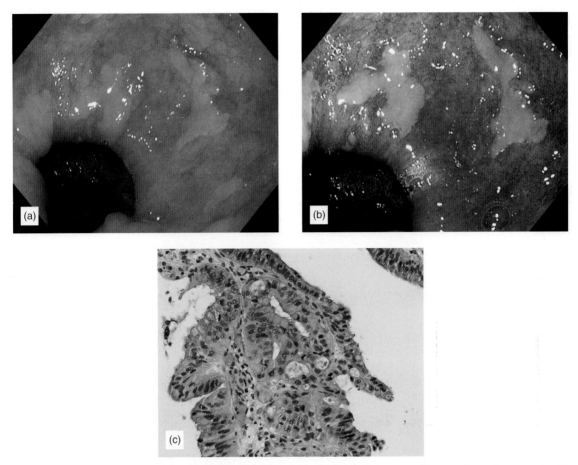

Figure 14.73 (a) Barrett's esophagus with abnormal vessels seen in WL HRE H180 without magnification. (b) NBI improves the ability to detect abnormal vessels in this patient with Barrett's esophagus and HGD over WL even without magnification. (c) Microscopy image demonstrating the special intestinalized metaplasia of Barrett's mucosa with focal areas of HGD. (Mayo Clinic, Jacksonville.)

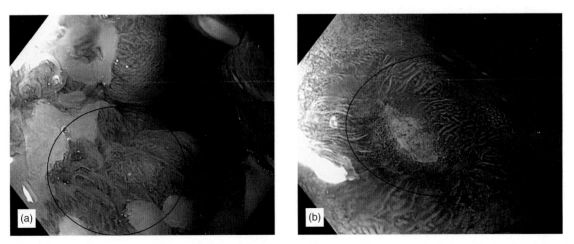

Figure 14.74 (a, b) Barrett's esophagus with thickened irregular vessels: NBI H190 indicates HGD. (Prateek Sharma, University of Kansas Medical Center.)

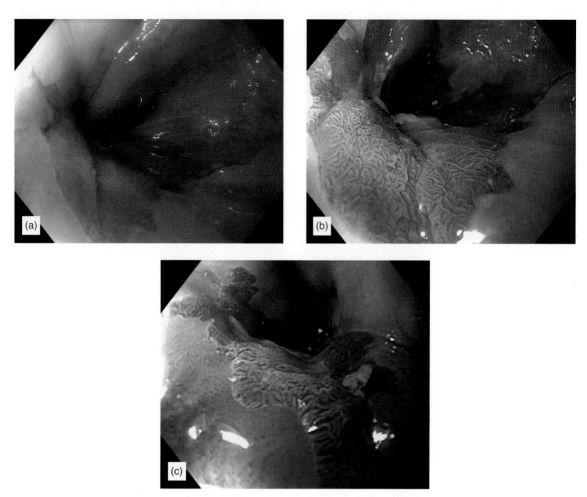

Figure 14.75 (a–c) Villiform but regular appearance on H190 NBI near-focus view of nondysplastic intestinal metaplasia in SSBE. (Jonathan Cohen, NYU Langone School of Medicine.)

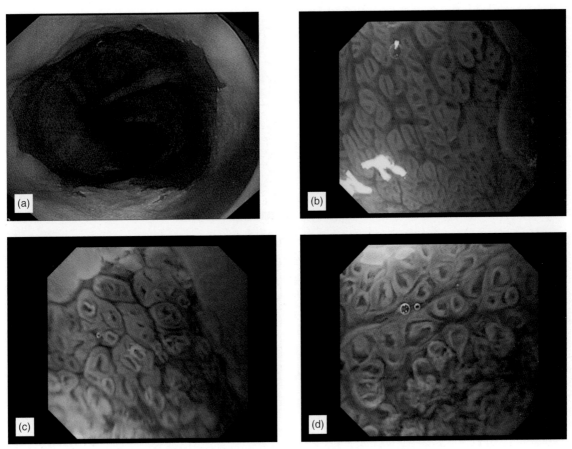

Figure 14.76 (a–g) WL H190 low-magnification overview of a circumferential SSBE. (b) Near-focus magnification WL with acetic acid of one segment with widened sulci from the acetic acid, showing regular nondysplastic pattern. (c) NBI plus acetic acid in this area of nondysplastic Barrett's esophagus. (d) Another area in the same patient in which NBI plus acetic acid shows both irregular mucosal pattern and some thick darker vessels which reflect focal HGD. (Rajvinder Singh, Lyell McEwin Hospital, Adelaide.)

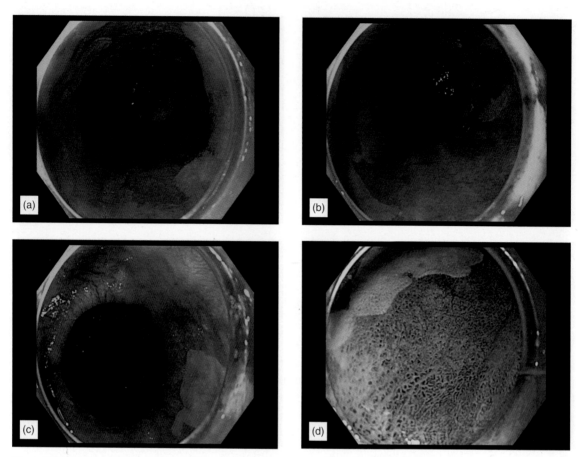

Figure 14.77 (e-g) (a) Long-segment Barrett's esophagus in WL H190 low magnification with 3-mm clear cap on scope to assist in surveillance and stabilize the mucosa during the inspection. (b) Middle portion of the Barrett's WL. (c) Lower portion of the Barrett's. (d) Low-magnification NBI view of upper segment of the Barrett's mucosa.

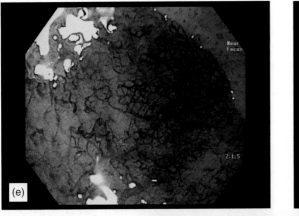

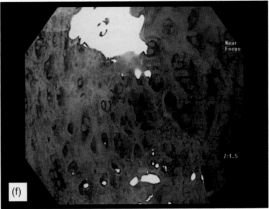

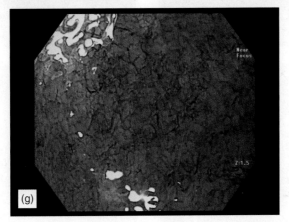

Figure 14.77 (Continued) (e) Near-focus view shows irregular vessels in this segment. (f) High magnification achieved by moving the scope closer to the mucosa in near-focus mode shows highly irregular vessels in area of HGD. (g) Another segment in area of nondysplastic Barrett's esophagus with regular vessels seen on NBI H190 magnification. (Rajvinder Singh, Lyell McEwin Hospital, Adelaide.)

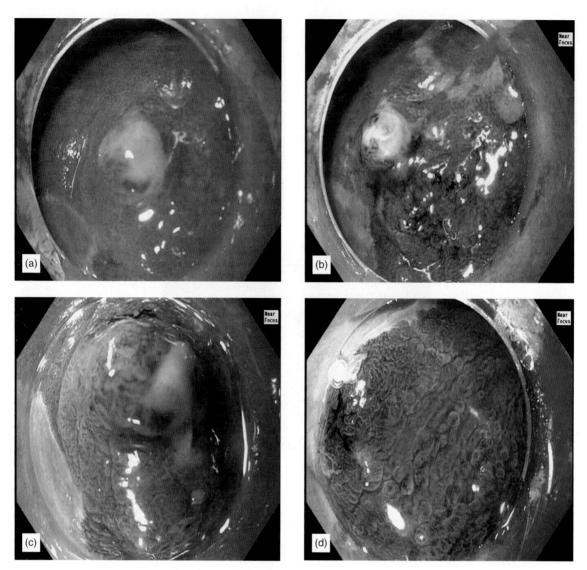

Figure 14.78 (a–d) Barrett's esophagus with T1a intramucosal cancer seen on H190 WL low magnification and near focus NBI views with clear 3 mm cap on the tip of the endoscope. (Michael Wallace, Mayo Clinic, Jacksonville.)

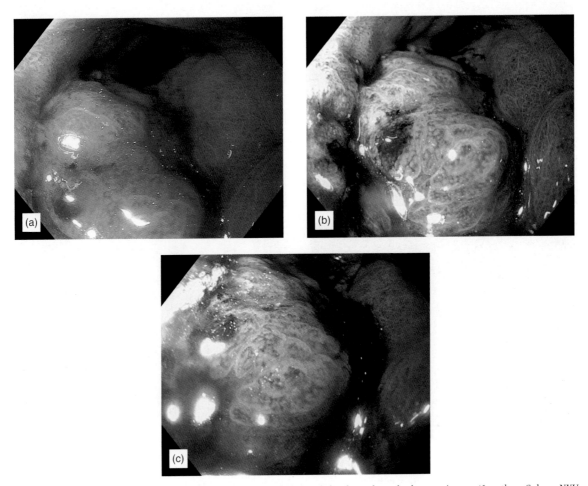

Figure 14.79 (a–c) WL and NBI H190 images of this nodular elevated distal esophageal adenocarcinoma (Jonathan Cohen, NYU Langone School of Medicine.)

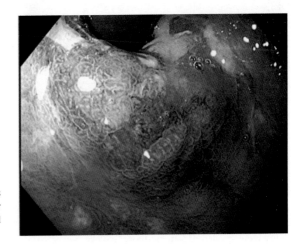

Figure 14.80 NBI H180 view of HGD in Barrett's esophagus demonstrating abnormal thickened vessels in an irregular pattern with a central depression and loss of normal mucosal pattern. (Jonathan Cohen, NYU Langone School of Medicine.)

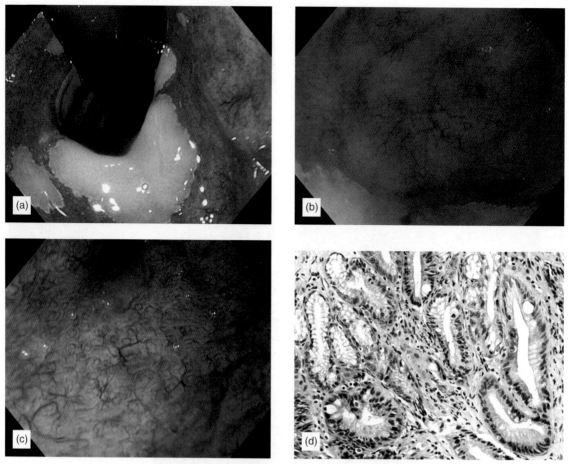

Figure 14.81 (a) This turnaround low-magnification NBI H180 view with prominent vessels to the right of the image within flat mucosa revealed Barrett's esophagus indefinite for dysplasia. (b) WL non-magnified view of this area fails to identify any visible abnormality. The diagnosis would likely have been missed via standard endoscopy. (c) Head-on endoscopic magnification NBI view of this area of Barrett's esophagus, indefinite for dysplasia. (d) Target biopsy within area of Barrett's with abnormal vessel as identified with NBI. Note Barrett's mucosa indefinite for dysplasia. (Jonathan Cohen, NYU Langone School of Medicine.)

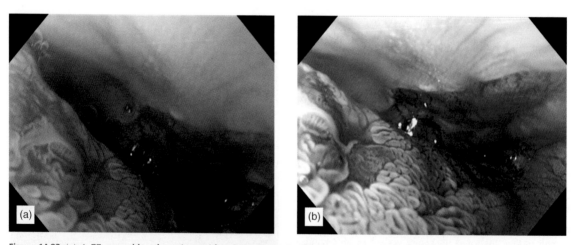

Figure 14.82 (a) A 77-year-old male patient with a 5-cm Barrett's. The Barrett's was stained with 1% acetic acid to clear mucus. 1.5 × magnification with Wl HRE H180. (b) NBI, HRE and 1.5 × digital magnification view. On the left is a "blown-up" pattern, on the right a more "condensed pattern." Histopathology showed low-grade dysplasia in this lesion with abnormal mucosal pattern. (University Medical Center Hamburg Eppendorf.)

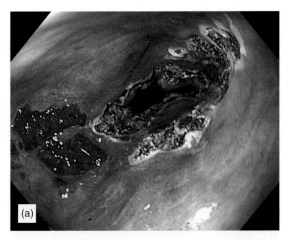 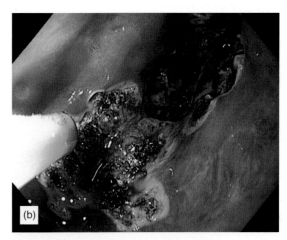

Figure 14.83 (a) NBI H180 view of residual Barrett's after ablation with argon plasma coagulation. Untreated patches remain visible to the left. (b) Argon plasma coagulation to the remaining areas of residual Barrett's, which are easy to detect using NBI under low magnification. (Mayo Clinic, Jacksonville.)

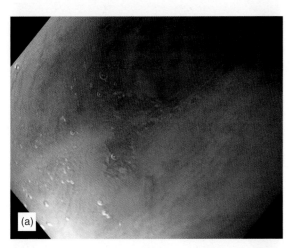 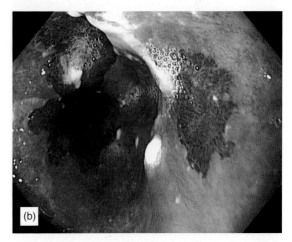

Figure 14.84 (a) WL HRE H180 view of a patient with residual Barrett's esophagus following ablation. (b) NBI much more clearly delineates residual Barrett's following ablation for targeted biopsy or further treatment. (Mayo Clinic, Jacksonville.)

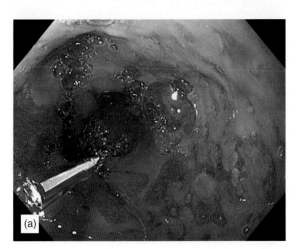 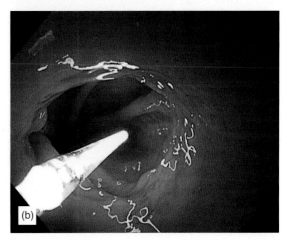

Figure 14.85 (a) WL HRE H180 image of photodynamic therapy for ablation of Barrett's esophagus. (b) While NBI is very useful following photodynamic therapy for assessment of residual Barrett's esophagus, during treatment it has limited added value over WL once the extent and location of the target has been measured. (Mayo Clinic, Jacksonville.)

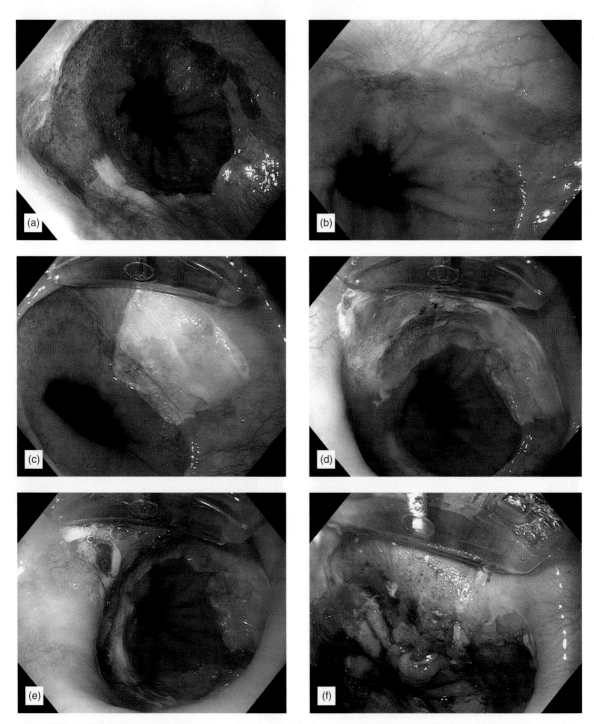

Figure 14.86 (a) NBI H180 low magnification is used to identify this short segment of Barrett's epithelium. (b) This same segment is shown in WL HRE close up prior to Barrx radiofrequency ablation (RFA) of the Barrett's. (c) WL HRE image of HALO 90 RFA after first application with device attached to the tip of the scope positioned at 12 o'clock and seen in the top center of this photo. (Richard Rothstein, Dartmouth Hitchcock Medical Center.) (d) The ablation continues in a counter-clockwise direction. (e) WL HRE image of the entire segment of subsquamous intestinal metaplasia (SSIM) immediately following RFA. (Richard Rothstein, Dartmouth Hitchcock Medical Center.) (f) Chamois-colored area demonstrating change after second RFA application at 12 o'clock position, WL HRE H180 low-magnification view (Richard Rothstein, Dartmouth Hitchcock Medical Center.)

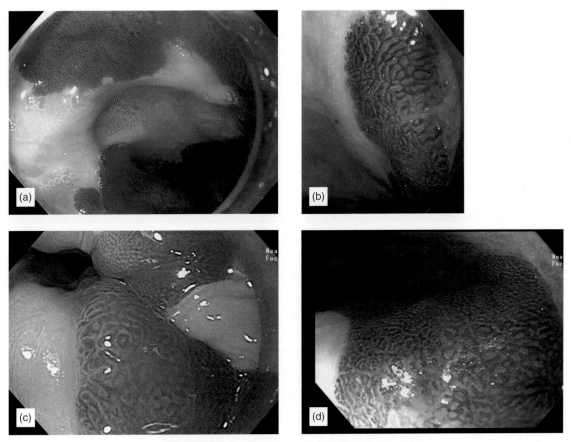

Figure 14.87 (a) NBI H190 view of distal esophagus following multiband EMR of nodular area of HGD shows the treated area to have white neosquamous epithelium with large areas of residual intestinal epithelium clearly demarcated. (b–d) Near-focus NBI and WL close-up views of nondysplastic residual Barrett's esophagus. (Jonathan Cohen, NYU Langone School of Medicine.)

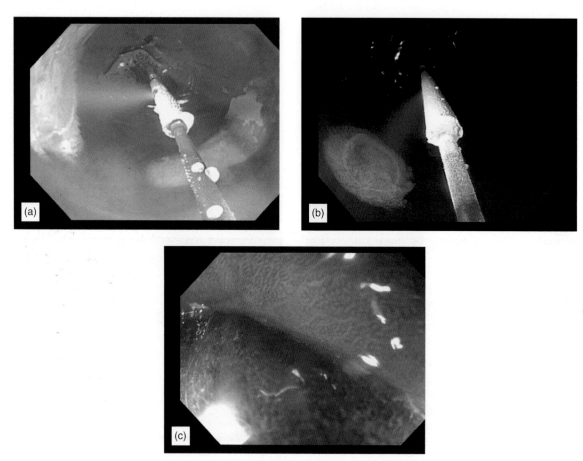

Figure 14.88 (a, b) WL and NBI H190 of focal nitrous oxide cryotherapy delivered via balloon catheter to ablate focal residual tongues of Barrett's epithelium. (c) NBI nicely accentuates the hyperemia resulting in the treated area after the mucosa thaws. (Jonathan Cohen, NYU Langone School of Medicine.)

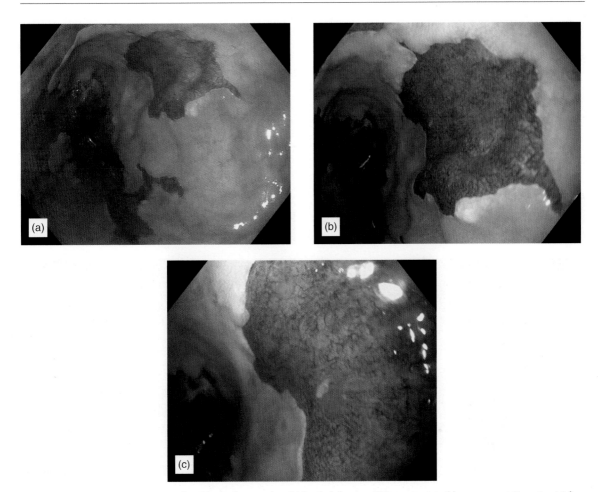

Figure 14.89 NBI H190 assessment of residual salmon colored islands following RFA treatment of long segment Barretts. (a) low magnification WL view. (b, c) Closer examination under NBI with near focus shows no signs of dysplasia. (Jonathan Cohen, NYU Langone School of Medicine.)

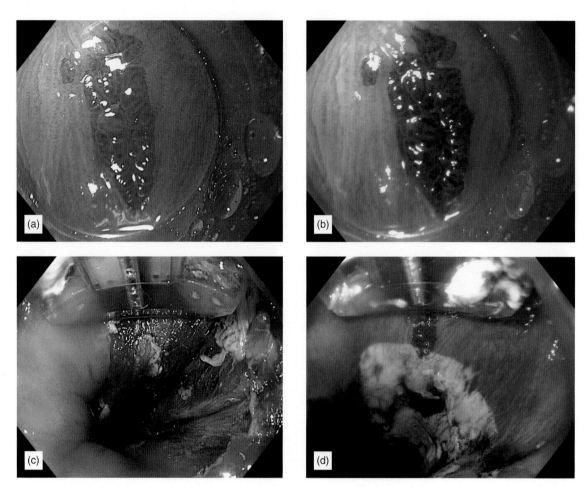

Figure 14.90 (a–d) Use of NBI H190 to direct follow-up RFA sessions to ablate residual Barrett's esophagus. (Jonathan Cohen, NYU Langone School of Medicine.)

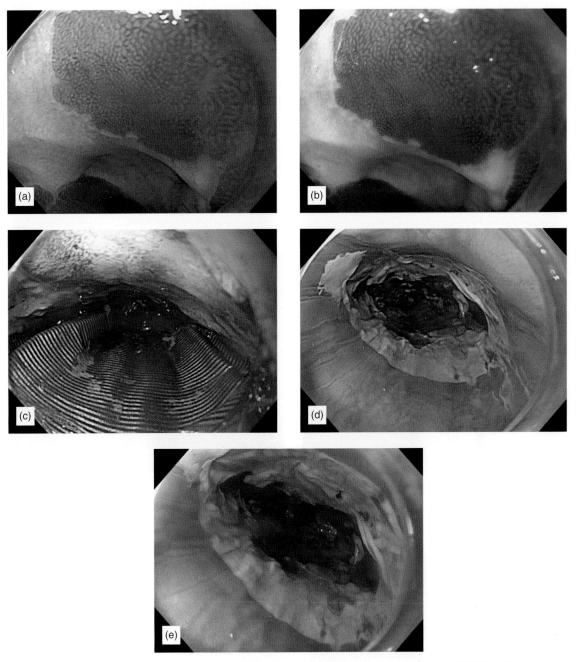

Figure 14.91 (a–e) HALO 360 RFA to wide areas of residual Barrett's following focal EMR for HGD. NBI H190 highlights residual Barrett's and near-focus views show no areas suspicious for flat or raised dysplasia. (Jonathan Cohen, NYU Langone School of Medicine.)

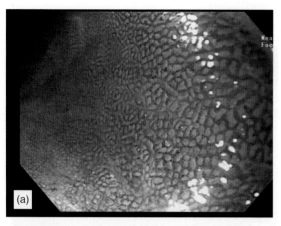

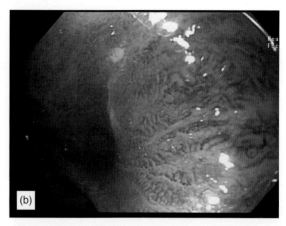

Figure 14.92 Post EMR and ablation residual Barrett's. WL and NBI H190 near-focus assessment for dysplasia in residual Barrett's. (a) Nondysplastic regular vascular network pattern NBI near focus. (b) Area of focus of irregular vessels and scarring corresponding to 1-mm deep glands on volumetric laser endomicroscopy (VLE); biopsy reported as indefinite for dysplasia. (Jonathan Cohen, NYU Langone School of Medicine.)

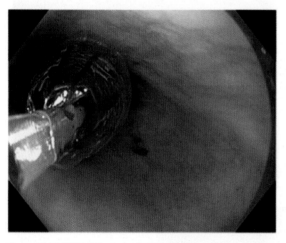

Figure 14.93 H190 WL view of VLE optical coherence tomography balloon catheter in assessment of residual Barrett's esophagus for areas suspicious for dysplasia. (Jonathan Cohen, NYU Langone School of Medicine.)

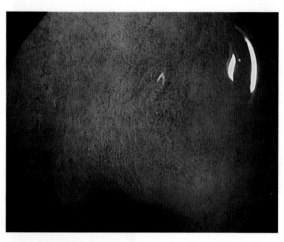

Figure 14.94 Tight circular pattern of normal cardia well delineated on magnification NBI H180 image. (University of Kansas School of Medicine.)

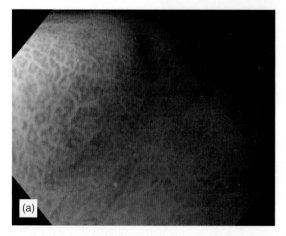

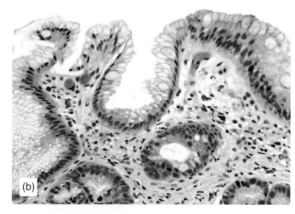

Figure 14.95 (a) NBI H180 close-up 1.5 × magnified view of cardia mucosa just below squamo-columnar junction reveals some thick sulci but round cardia-type mucosal pattern. (b) Histopathology confirms the presence of cardiac mucosa with scant inflammation and intestinal metaplasia negative for dysplasia. (Jonathan Cohen, NYU Langone School of Medicine.)

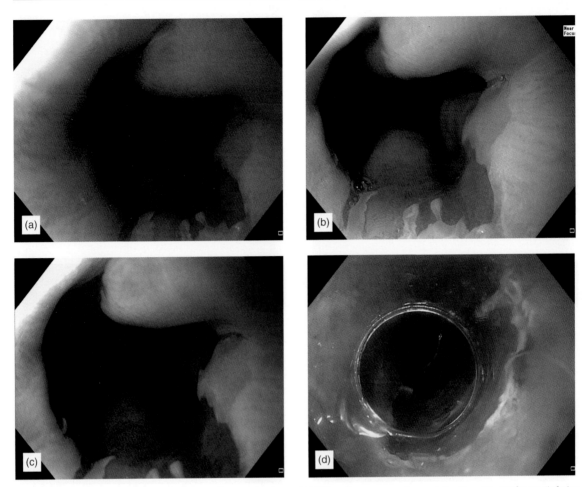

Figure 14.96 (a) Residual Barrett's esophagus following ablation. H190 WL endoscopy reveals remaining Barrett's esophagus (inferior aspect of image between 4 and 6 o'clock positions) following RFA. (b) Near-focus WL endoscopy of the same patient demonstrates residual Barrett's esophagus following RFA. The near-focus resolution allows better visualization of the different mucosal patterns seen between the residual Barrett's esophagus mucosa and cardia of the stomach. (c) NBI of the same patient provides improved contrast between the area of residual Barrett's esophagus and squamous mucosa. (d) Barrett's esophagus following band EMR. A clear outline of the resected esophageal lining is evident in this WL image. Examination of the base of the resection site reveals an intact layer of muscularis propria with no residual mucosa or submucosa throughout the entire resection site. (Neil Gupta, Loyola University Health System.)

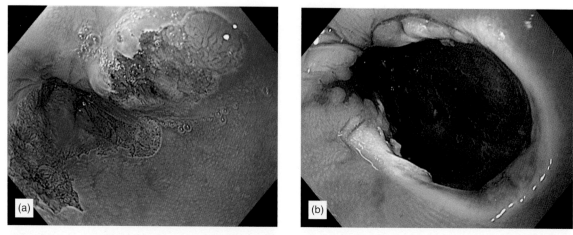

Figure 14.97 (a) This area of focal irregular raised and erythroplastic mucosa in Barrett's esophagus is shown here in NBI low-magnification view H180. (b) WL HRE H180 view of this area following cap EMR of what was found to be a superficial adenocarcinoma. (Thierry Ponchon, Edouard Herriot Hospital).

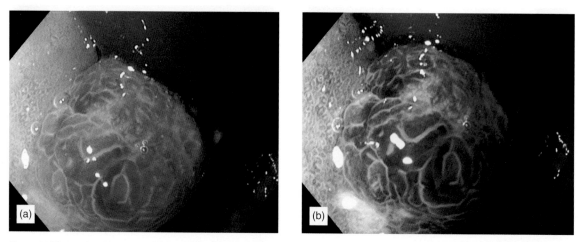

Figure 14.98 (a) View in retroversion of mucosal adenocarcinoma in Barrett's on WL H180. (b) Mucosal cancer of the cardia arising from Barrett's esophagus with grossly irregular gyrus mucosal pattern on NBI view. (University Medical Center Hamburg Eppendorf.)

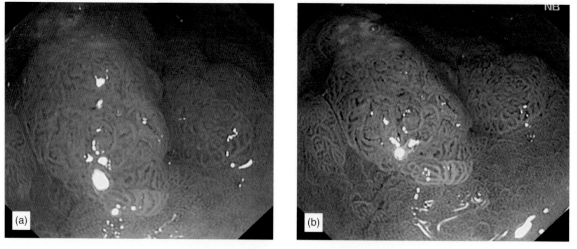

Figure 14.99 (a) WL magnified HRE H180 outlines the abnormal mucosal topography of this adenocarcinoma of the cardia. (b) NBI magnification view both accentuates the abnormal topography apparent under WL a and reveals the irregular thickened vessels arranged in an abnormal pattern. (University of Amsterdam.)

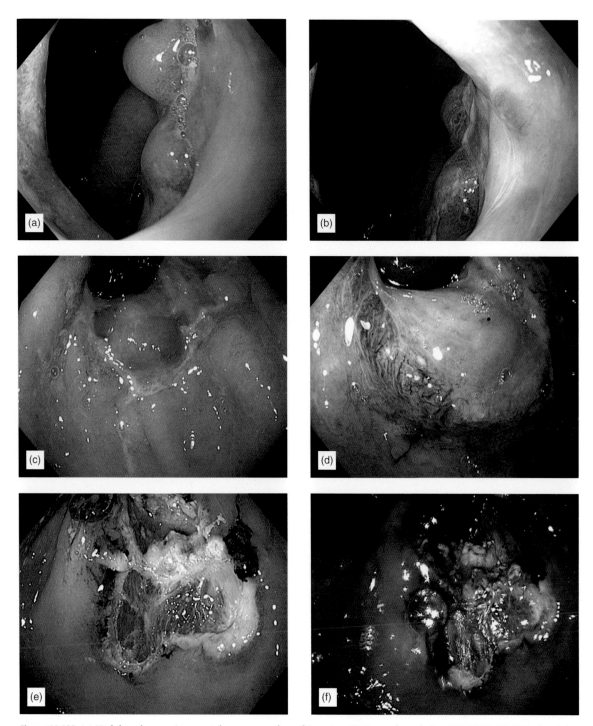

Figure 14.100 (a) Nodular adenocarcinoma at the gastroesophageal junction (GEJ): esophageal view WL H180. (b) NBI of nodular GEJ carcinoma from distal esophagus. (c) Nodular GEJ carcinoma, retroflexed view from the cardia. (d) NBI of GEJ nodular carcinoma, retroflexed view from the cardia shows much greater definition of the lesion, its vessels, and its margins. (e) HRE image after band EMR, view from the cardia. (f) NBI of nodular carcinoma after EMR. NBI is particularly useful in examining for any residual tumor or polyp following resection. (Mayo Clinic, Jacksonville.)

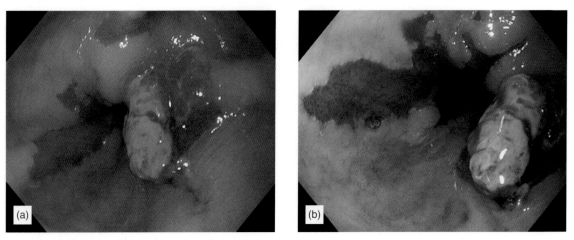

Figure 14.101 (a) White raised esophageal adenocarcinoma arising in Barrett's esophagus here seen in WL H180 on low magnification. (b) NBI low-magnification view of this lesion is well demarcated, but does not add much over this clearly discernible lesion. (Rob Hawes, Medical University of South Carolina.)

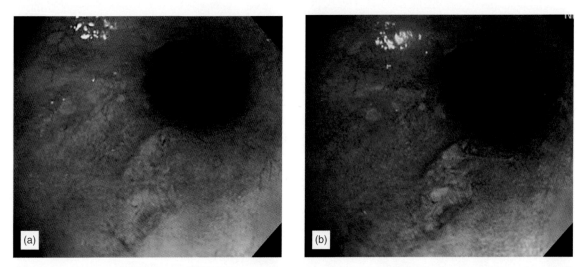

Figure 14.102 (a) WL HRE H180 image of this esophageal adenocarcinoma detects an abnormality but the appearance is not well distinguished from a benign erosion in this view. (b) NBI of this adenocarcinoma. The lesion demonstrates depressed irregular mucosa and irregular vessel pattern. (University of Amsterdam.)

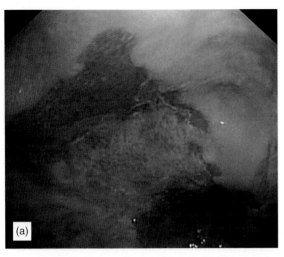
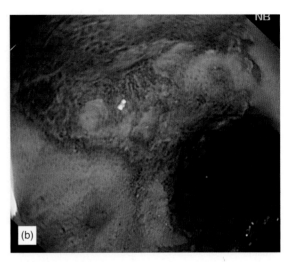

Figure 14.103 (a) This WL HRE H180 image of an adenocarcinoma clearly shows Barrett's esophagus with some apparent squamous re-epithelialization. The abnormal morphology is much better appreciated with NBI. (b) This adenocarcinoma arising out of Barrett's esophagus displays marked abnormal morphology with focal depression and irregular vessel pattern even on low-magnification view. (University of Amsterdam.)

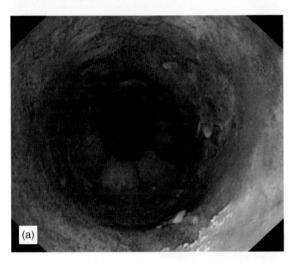
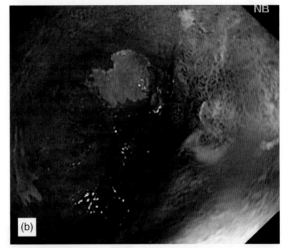

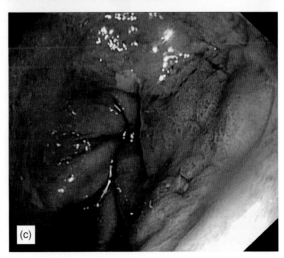

Figure 14.104 (a) An early esophageal adenocarcinoma discernible in this WL H180 low-magnification image as a flat discoloration and slightly irregular surface at 3 o'clock. (b) NBI more clearly defines the lesion by highlighting the mucosal surface change and increased vessel density. (c) Chromoendoscopy reveals pit pattern and more clearly defines the neoplastic lesion. (University of Amsterdam.)

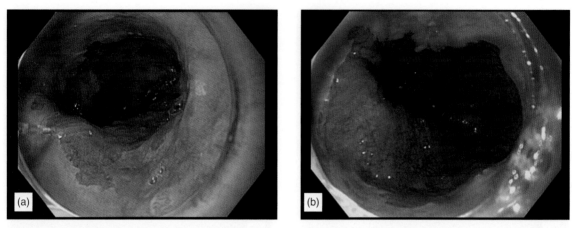

Figure 14.105 H190 WL and NBI views of nondysplastic SSBE. (a) WL endoscopy in this patient shows salmon-colored mucosa in the distal esophagus consistent with SSBE. Determining the precise borders of abnormal mucosa with WL endoscopy alone in patients such as this one can be difficult. (b) NBI of the same patient highlights the contrast between a short segment of Barrett's esophagus in the distal esophagus and the surrounding normal mucosa. NBI is particularly useful for delineating Barrett's in such patients where WL endoscopy alone may be insufficient. (Neil Gupta, Loyola University Health System.)

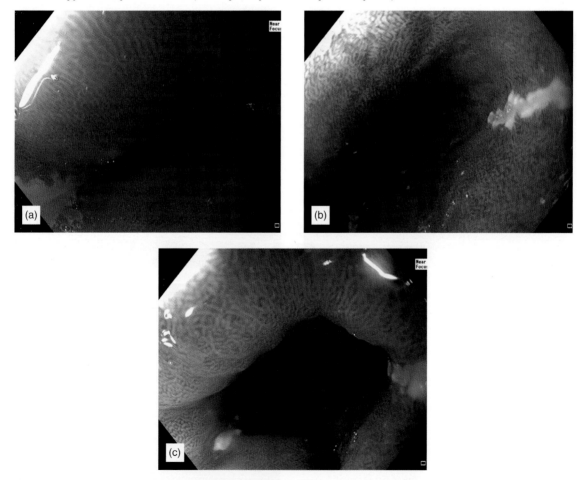

Figure 14.106 (a) H190 WL near-focus endoscopy reveals Barrett's esophagus with a ridged villous mucosal pattern. Pathology would reveal nondysplastic changes. (b) NBI highlights the ridged villous mucosal pattern of the same patient's nondysplastic Barrett's esophagus. (c) NBI near-focus view of the same patient again shows a ridged villous mucosal pattern consistent with nondysplastic Barrett's esophagus. (Neil Gupta, Loyola University Health System.)

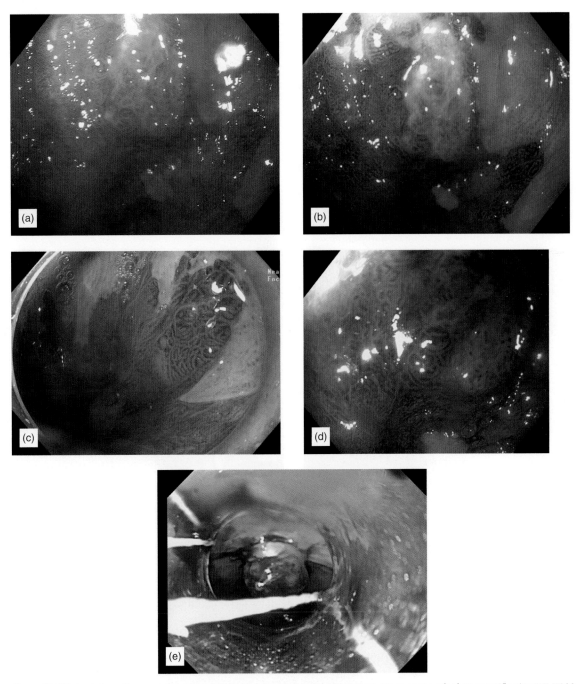

Figure 14.107 (a–e) Surveillance examination showed focal area of nodularily in Barrett's mucosa under low magnification WL H190 and NBI (a, b); (c) After washing off mucous and near focus examination, area suspicious for high grade dysplasia is identified and confirmed with biopsy. Band EMR to this focal area performed. (Jonathan Cohen, NYU Langone School of Medicine.)

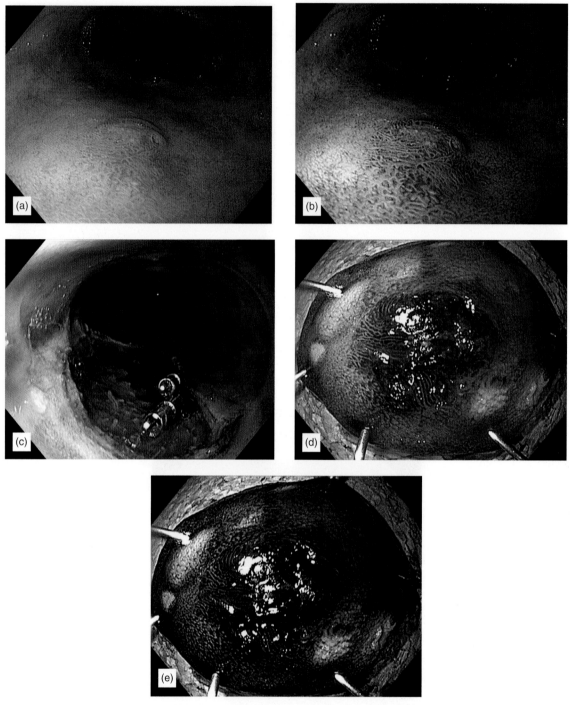

Figure 14.108 (a) A raised irregular superficial lesion is seen in this esophagus under WL low magnification H180. (b) NBI low-magnification image of this nodular superficial carcinoma (Paris Type 0 IIa lesion) arising in Barrett's esophagus. Improved delineation of margins and characterization of surface morphology over WL is demonstrated. (c) WL image of lesion immediately following EMR. Clips have been applied to control bleeding. (d) Magnified WL examination of the resection specimen. (e) NBI of completely resected lesion with margins. (Thierry Ponchon, Edouard Herriot Hospital.)

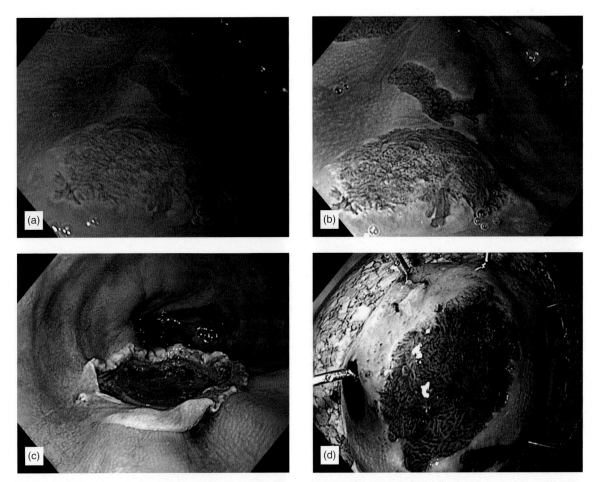

Figure 14.109 (a) WL low-magnification H180 view of nodular isolated superficial carcinoma arising in Barrett's esophagus. (b) NBI low-magnification image provides more precise characterization. The surface appears irregular and contrasts with the normal Barrett's tongue at the top of the photo (loss of the regular villous or gyrus pattern of nondysplastic Barrett's esophagus). (c) NBI is used to assess for any residual tissue following successful EMR of this lesion. (d) NBI examination of the fully resected superficial carcinoma. (Thierry Ponchon, Edouard Herriot Hospital.)

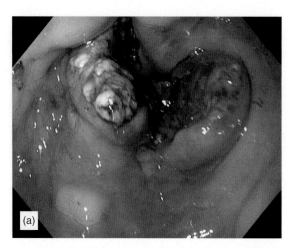

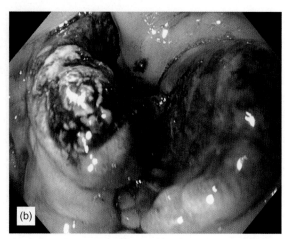

Figure 14.110 (a) Special contrast is not needed to diagnose this near-obstructing esophageal carcinoma seen here in low-magnification WL H180. (b) Obstructing esophageal adenoarcinoma, NBI view with markedly abnormal vessels and macroscopic appearance consistent with invasive malignant disease. (Mayo Clinic, Jacksonville.)

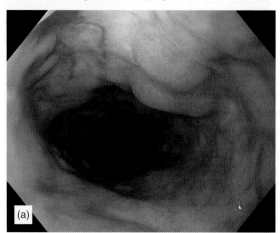

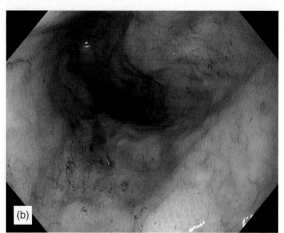

Figure 14.111 (a) WL HRE H180 low-magnification image of a patient with esophageal varices. Note the one prominent column in the 1 o'clock position. (b) Esophageal varices, seen on NBI light without obvious advantage over WL view. (Mayo Clinic, Jacksonville.)

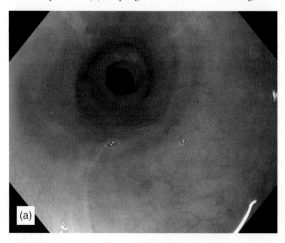

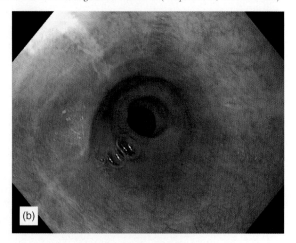

Figure 14.112 (a) Normal magnification WL H180 provides a good assessment of this smooth benign esophageal stricture. (b) Benign esophageal stricture, NBI low-magnification view. The surface structure and vascular pattern appears normal. (Mayo Clinic, Jacksonville.)

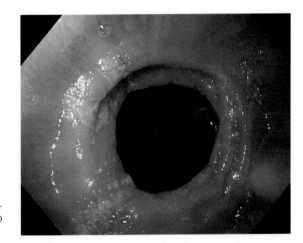

Figure 14.113 Rings in distal esophagus in patient with confirmed eosinophilic esophagitis, WL non-magnified view H180 (Jonathan Cohen, NYU Langone School of Medicine.)

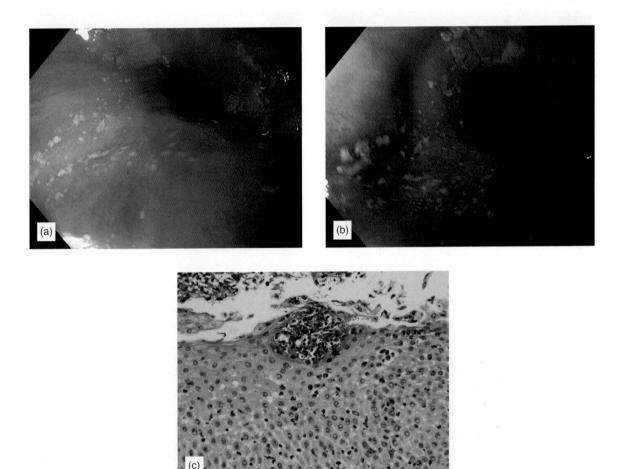

Figure 14.114 (a) Multiple tiny white plaques suggesting candidiasis actually represent eosinophilic esophageal microabscesses. WL non-magnified view H180. (b) Eosinophilic esophagitis, NBI non-magnified view. (c) Eosinophilic esophagitis. Numerous eosinophils are distributed throughout the epithelium, with aggregates forming microabscesses at the surface. (Jonathan Cohen, NYU Langone School of Medicine.)

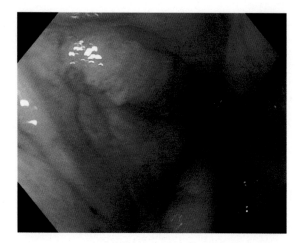

Figure 14.115 Pediatric patient with a clinical presentation of dysphagia found to have eosinophilic esophagitis. NBI low-magnification view H180 (Johns Hopkins University School of Medicine.)

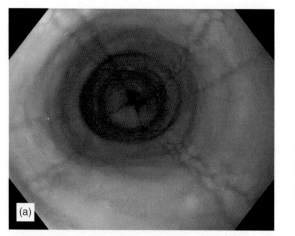
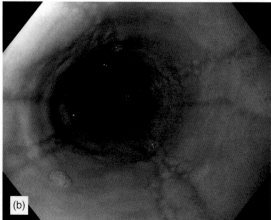

Figure 14.116 Linear grooves and subtle rings seen in (a) WL and (b) NBI in patient with eosinophilic esophagitis H190. (Jonathan Cohen, NYU Langone School of Medicine.)

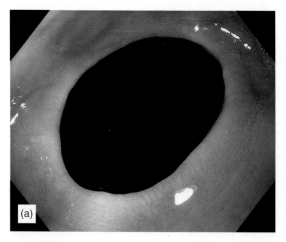
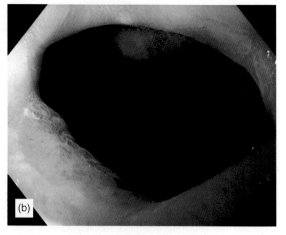

Figure 14.117 (a, b) WL and NBI H190 image of Schatski ring. (Jonathan Cohen, NYU Langone School of Medicine.)

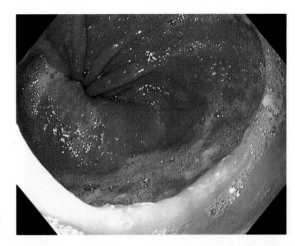

Figure 14.118 NBI H190 non-magnified view of Schatski ring. (Jonathan Cohen, NYU Langone School of Medicine.)

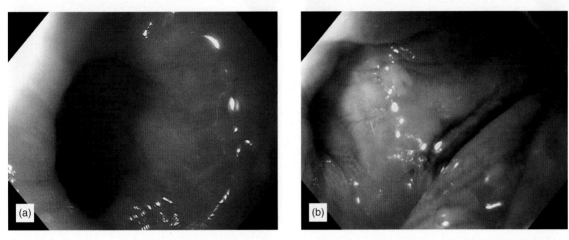

Figure 14.119 (a, b) WL and NBI H190 view of epiphrenic diverticulum. (Jonathan Cohen, NYU Langone School of Medicine.)

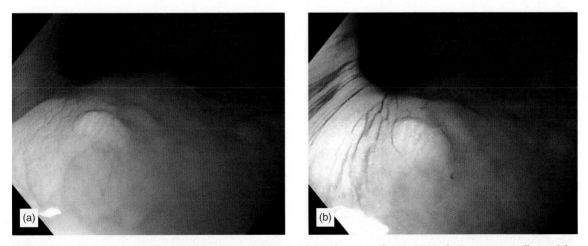

Figure 14.120 (a) Squamous papilloma of the esophagus viewed with WL, low magnification H180. (b) Squamous papilloma of the esophagus viewed with NBI light. Note the confluent color of the mucosa and the papilloma. (James DiSario, University of Utah Health Sciences Center.)

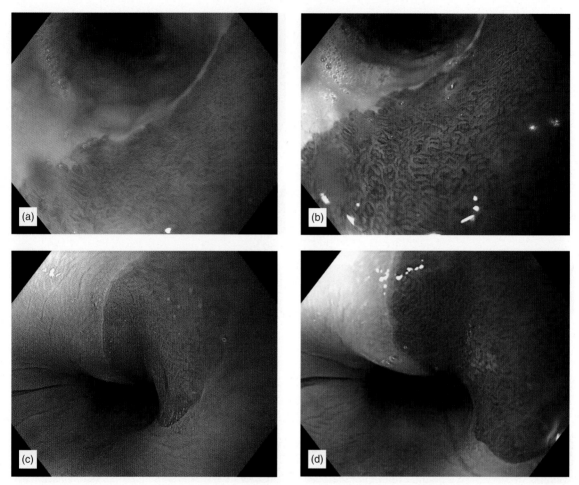

Figure 14.121 (a–d) Inlet patch, WL and NBI H190. (Jonathan Cohen, NYU Langone School of Medicine.)

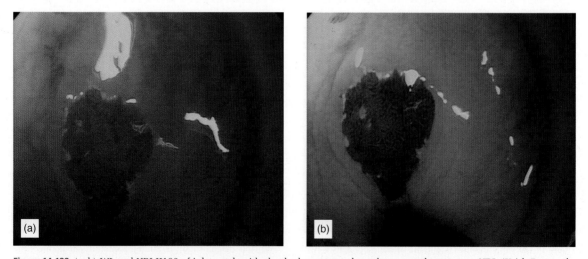

Figure 14.122 (a, b) WL and NBI H190 of inlet patch with clearly demonstrated regular mucosal pattern on NBI. (Krish Ragunath, Queen's Medical Centre, Nottingham.)

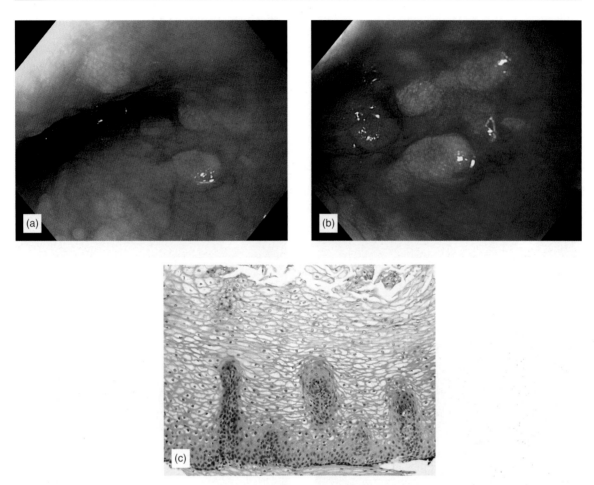

Figure 14.123 (a) WL non-magnifying image H180 of esophageal glycogen deposits. (b) NBI view of esophageal glycogen deposits. (c) The supra-basal squamous cells are distended with barely visible eosinophilic cytoplasm due to glycogen accumulation. (Jonathan Cohen, NYU Langone School of Medicine.)

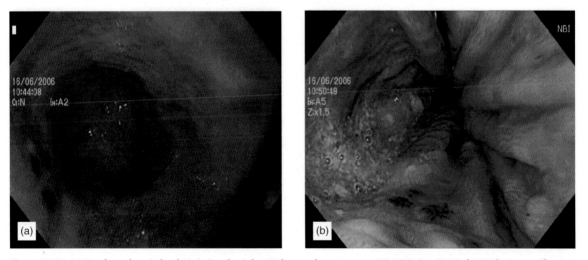

Figure 14.124 (a) Esophageal angiodysplasia in Rendu–Osler–Weber syndrome seen on WL HRE view H180. (b) NBI low-magnification view of esophageal angiodysplasia in Rendu–Osler–Weber syndrome. (Guilherme Macedo, Hospital Sao Marcos.)

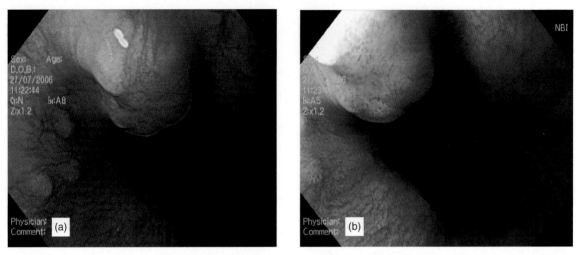

Figure 14.125 (a) Esophageal leiomyoma seen here with WL HRE H180 without magnification. (b) Low-magnification NBI view of this esophageal leiomyoma. (Guilherme Macedo, Hospital Sao Marcos.)

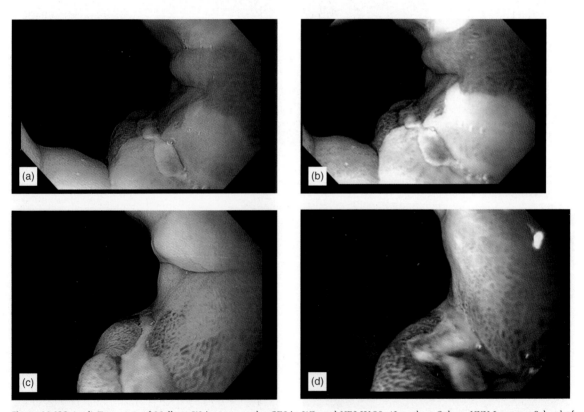

Figure 14.126 (a–d) Two cases of Mallory–Weiss tears at the GEJ in WL and NBI H190. (Jonathan Cohen, NYU Langone School of Medicine.)

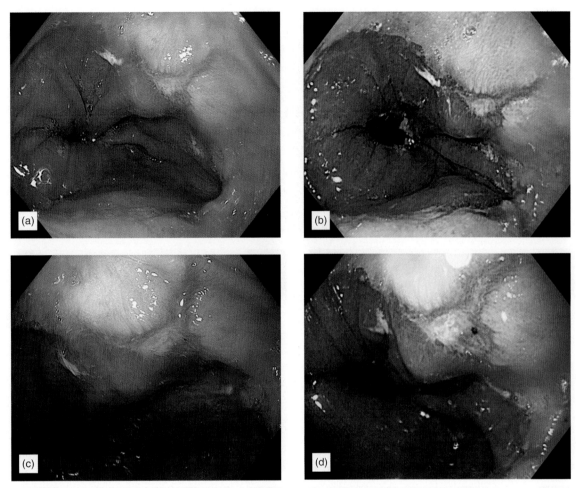

Figure 14.127 (a–d) WL and NBI H190 views of erosive esophagitis, LA grade A. (Jonathan Cohen, NYU Langone School of Medicine.)

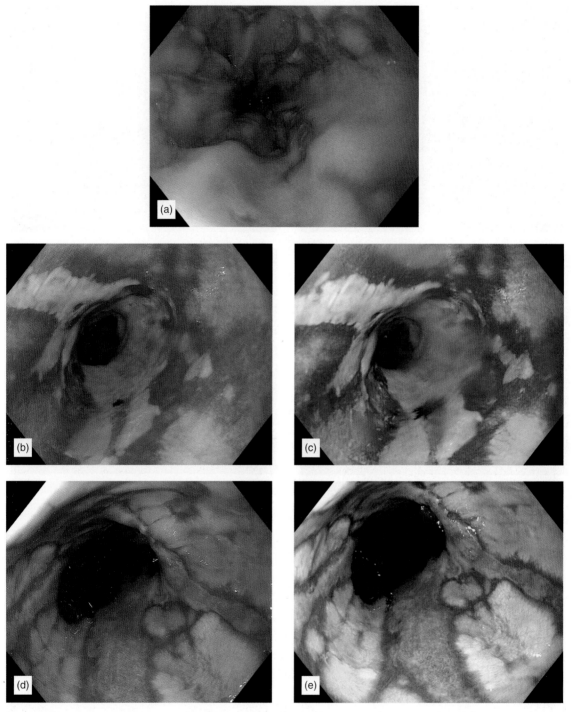

Figure 14.128 (a–e) (a) H190 WL view of grade 4 erosive esophagitis. (b, c) WL and NBI view of circumferential severe peptic esophagitis. (d, e) Similar views in another patient with the same degree of mucosal damage. (Jonathan Cohen, NYU Langone School of Medicine.)

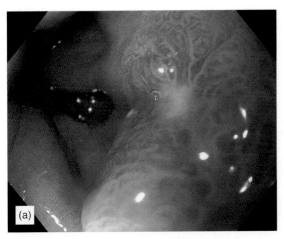

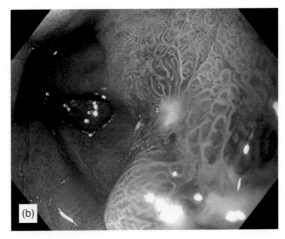

Figure 14.129 Focal ulcer in distal esophagus. Regular but inflamed and thickened surrounding folds seen in NBI H190 near focus suggest benign process, but limited examination for possible Barrett's or dysplasia in the setting of active ulcerative esophagitis. (Jonathan Cohen, NYU Langone School of Medicine.)

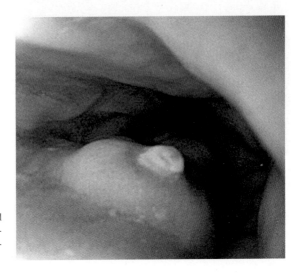

Figure 14.130 WL H180 view of platelet plug on esophageal varix the so-called "nipple sign" indicating high risk for imminent rebleeding. (Dennis Jensen, David Geffen School of Medicine at UCLA.)

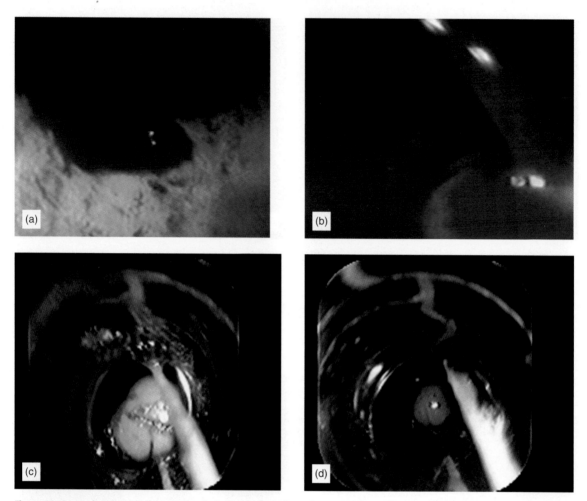

Figure 14.131 (a–d) WL H180 images of actively bleeding esophageal varix before and after band ligation. (Dennis Jensen, David Geffen School of Medicine at UCLA).

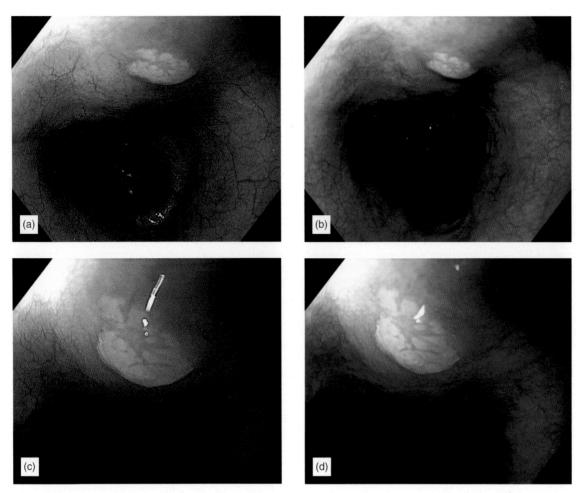

Figure 14.132 (a–d) Esophageal lymphangiectasia WL and NBI H190 low magnification and near focus (Jonathan Cohen, NYU Langone School of Medicine.)

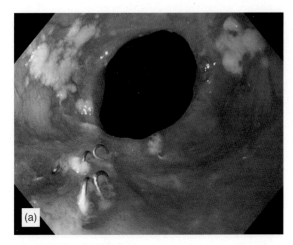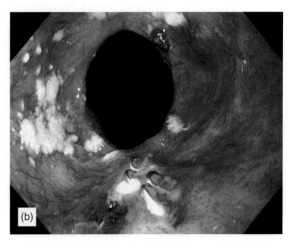

Figure 14.133 (a) Esophageal–gastric anastomosis with staples and yeast, WL HRE H180 low-magnification view. (b) NBI image here easily detects abnormalities on the surface in low magnification in this narrow lumen where there is sufficient light for its contrast to be effective in scanning the mucosa for lesions. (Mayo Clinic, Jacksonville.)

ABBREVIATIONS

EMR	endoscopic mucosal resection
GEJ	gastroesophageal junction
GERD	gastroesophageal reflux disease
HGD	high-grade dysplasia
HRE	high-resolution endoscopy
IPCL	intraepithelial papillary capillary loop
NBI	narrowband imaging
PAS	periodic acid–Schiff
RFA	radiofrequency ablation
SCC	squamous cell carcinoma

SSBE	short-segment Barrett's esophagus
VLE	volumetric laser endomicroscopy
WL	white light

Video clips to accompany this book can be found in the online material at www.wiley.com/go/cohen/NBI

The following video relates specifically to this chapter:
Video 88 POEM and submucosal tunnel vessels on white light and NBI

Stomach atlas

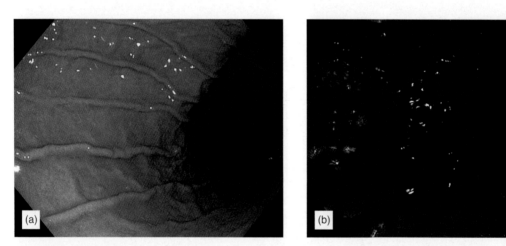

Figure 15.1 (a) WL H180 HRE image of the folds of the gastric body, greater curvature. (b) NBI image of the same view is far too dark to reveal mucosal detail; the gastric lumen is too wide to utilize NBI as a screen for lesion detection in contrast to narrower lumen organs such as the esophagus or colon. (Jonathan Cohen, NYU Langone School of Medicine.)

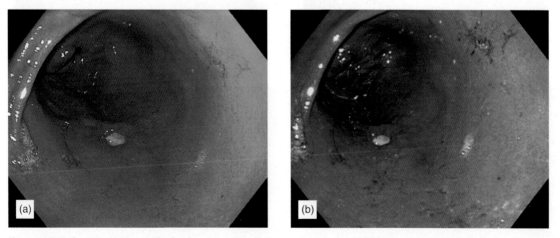

Figure 15.2 (a, b) NBI H190 provides brighter image to allow examination in NBI light even within the wide lumen of the gastric antrum and body. In this pair of WL and NBI H190 images a small benign appearing ulcer is seen in the antrum at a distance. (Jonathan Cohen, NYU Langone School of Medicine.)

Comprehensive Atlas of High-Resolution Endoscopy and Narrowband Imaging, Second Edition. Edited by Jonathan Cohen.
© 2017 John Wiley & Sons, Ltd. Published 2017 by John Wiley & Sons, Ltd.
Companion website: www.wiley.com/go/cohen/NBI

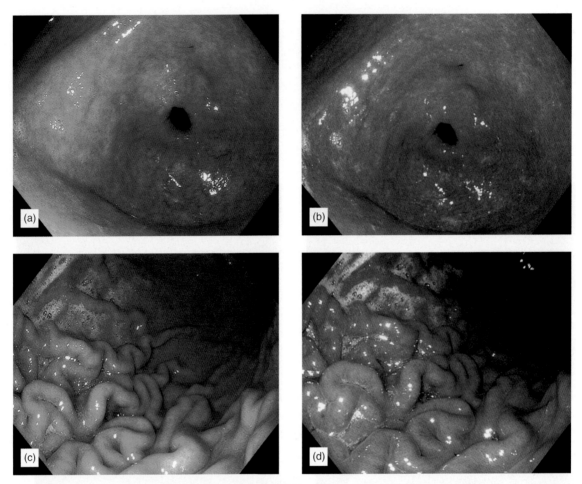

Figure 15.3 (a, b) Normal gastric antrum, WL and NBI views. H190 images have sufficient brightness to enable wide-view inspection in the stomach, as compared with earlier 180 models which could only allow close-up NBI inspection of areas identified as abnormal on WL view. (c, d) Normal rugal folds of gastric body, WL and NBI views. (Jonathan Cohen, NYU Langone School of Medicine.)

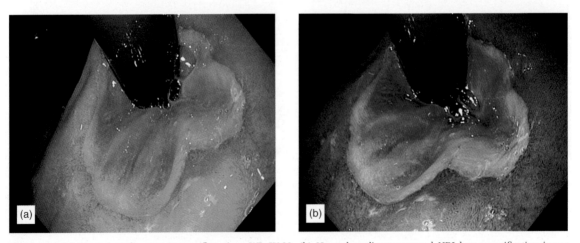

Figure 15.4 (a) Normal cardia seen in retroflex view, WL H180. (b) Normal cardia turnaround NBI low-magnification image. (Jonathan Cohen, NYU Langone School of Medicine.)

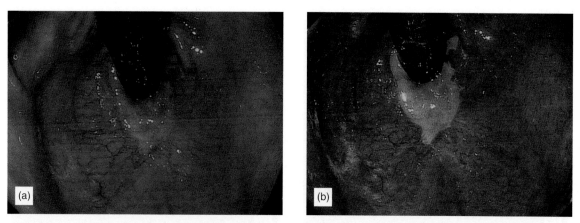

Figure 15.5 (a, b) Retroflexion view of normal cardia and gastroesophageal junction (GEJ), WL and NBI H190. (Krish Ragunath, Queen's Medical Centre, Nottingham.)

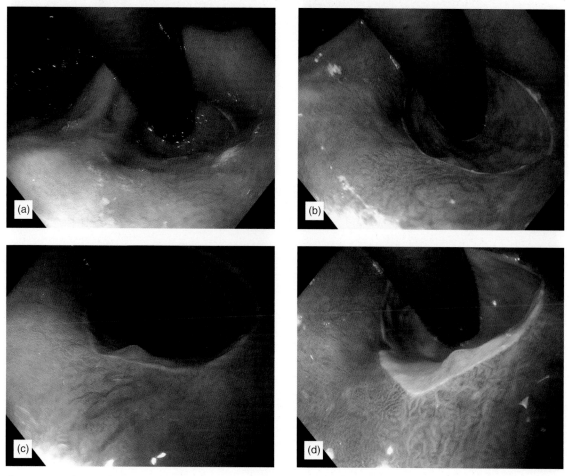

Figure 15.6 (a–d) Retroflexion view in the stomach of small sliding hiatal hernia. WL and NBI inspection of Z line and cardia vessels and mucosal pattern in two patients. (Jonathan Cohen, NYU Langone School of Medicine.)

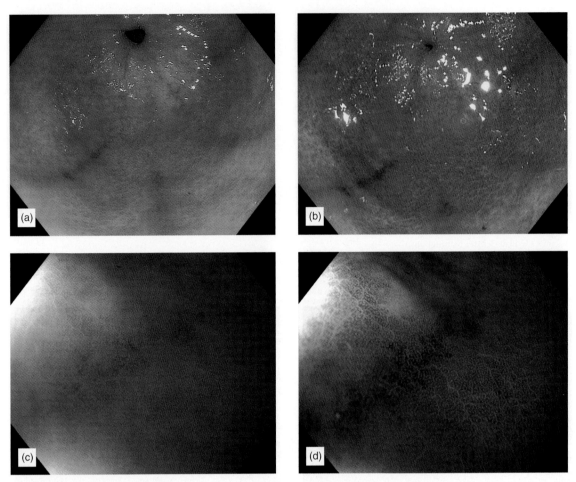

Figure 15.7 (a–d) Linear antral erythema and superficial erosions H190 WL and NBI, low magnification and near focus. (Jonathan Cohen, NYU Langone School of Medicine.)

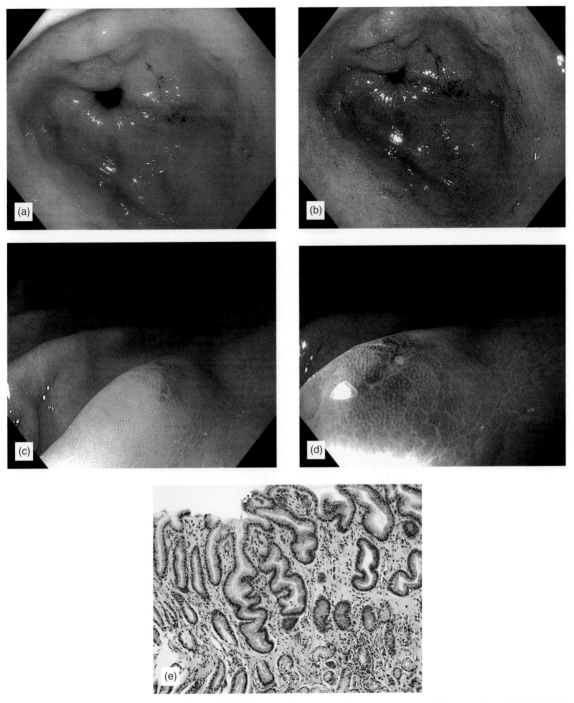

Figure 15.8 (a–d) Antral erosive gastritis. WL and NBI H190 views in a patient taking nonsteroidal anti-inflammatory drugs (NSAIDs). (e) Reactive gastropathy: the gastric mucosa is hyperplastic with tortuous glands, diminished mucin in the foveolar epithelium, and muscularization of the lamina propria. (Jonathan Cohen, NYU Langone School of Medicine.)

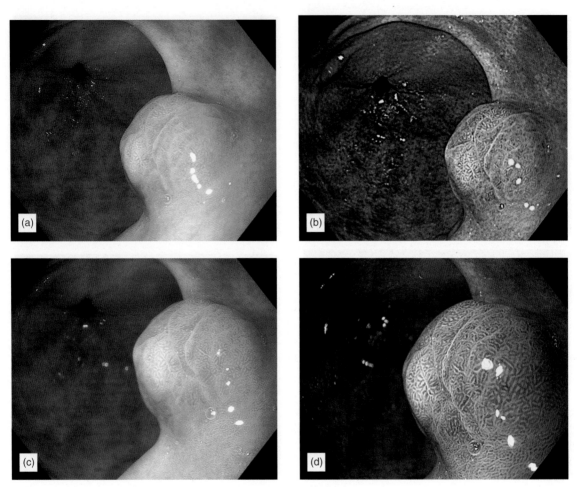

Figure 15.9 (a–d) Erosive gastritis with hyperplastic polyp, WL and NBI H190 low magnification and near focus views. (Jonathan Cohen, NYU Langone School of Medicine.)

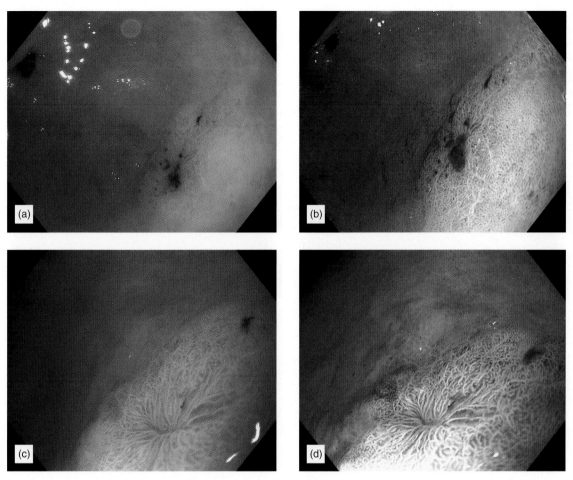

Figure 15.10 (a–d) Gastric erosion. WL and NBI views without magnification with evidence of recent minor bleeding and near-focus views after washing. (Jonathan Cohen, NYU Langone School of Medicine.)

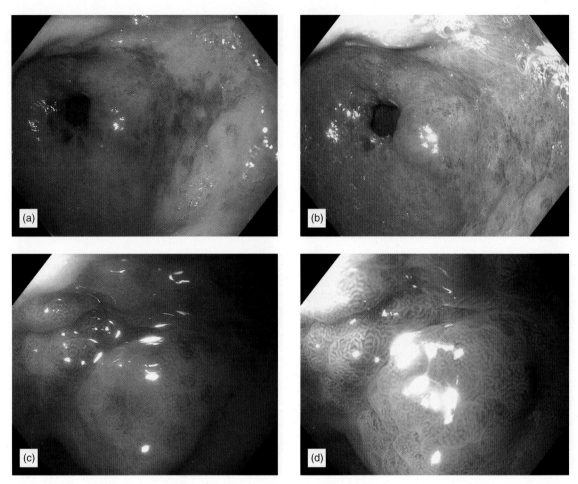

Figure 15.11 (a, b) Moderate antral erosive gastritis, WL and NBI normal magnification. H190 view much brighter than H180 view and allows good visualization at distance in NBI mode. (c, d) Near-focus WL and NBI reveal normal vessel pattern and no loss of mucosal pattern, reducing suspicion for neoplasia. (Jonathan Cohen, NYU Langone School of Medicine.)

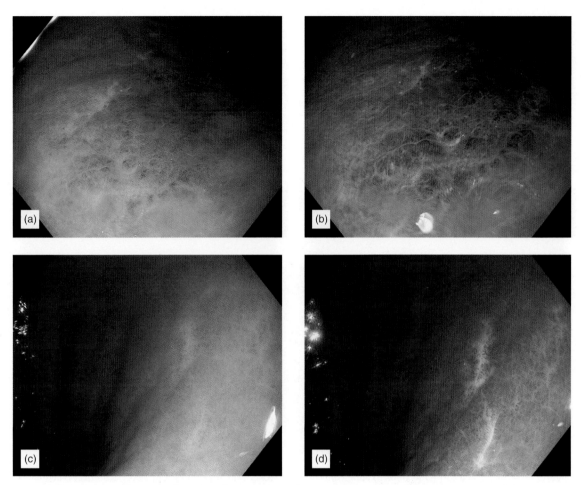

Figure 15.12 (a–d) WL and NBI H190 low magnification and near focus views of moderate diffuse gastritis with nodularity and scarring. (Jonathan Cohen, NYU Langone School of Medicine.)

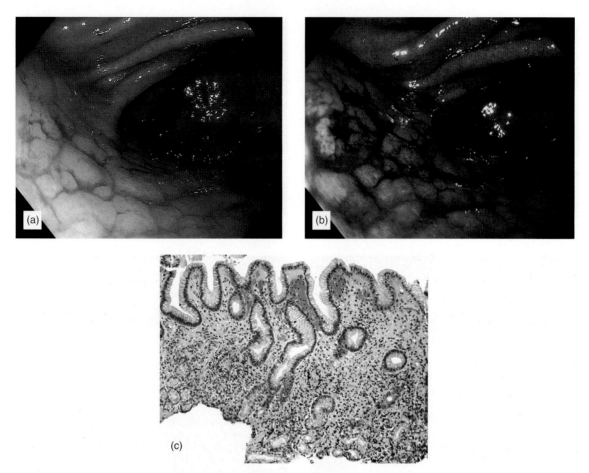

Figure 15.13 (a, b) WL and NBI H180 views of bumpy mucosa of stomach. Note that blood from biopsy accentuates the nodular mucosal pattern in this patient with *Helicobacter pylori* gastritis. (c) *Helicobacter*-associated active chronic antral gastritis. (Jonathan Cohen, NYU Langone School of Medicine.)

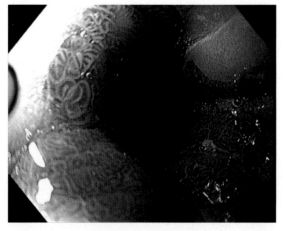

Figure 15.14 NBI H180 image of carditis. Note the thickened round mucosal pattern of inflamed cardia mucosa. (Jean-François Rey, Institut Arnault Tzanck.)

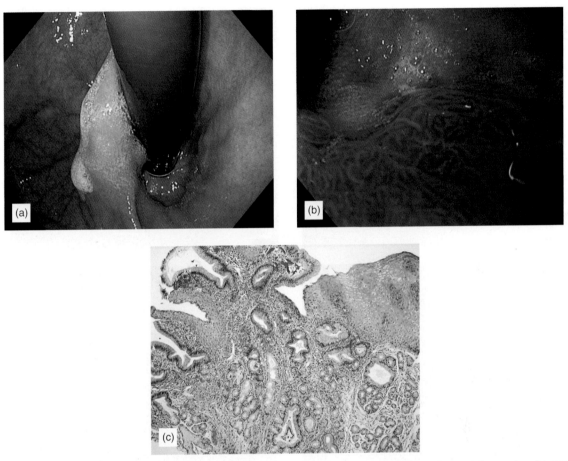

Figure 15.15 (a) Retroflex WL H180 low-magnification view of cardia with pathology-confirmed chronic inflammation. (b) NBI 1.5× magnified view in turnaround of chronic inflammation of cardia mucosa. (c) Reflux carditis. There is intense acute and chronic inflammation of the cardia mucosa at the squamo-columnar junction. (Jonathan Cohen, NYU Langone School of Medicine.)

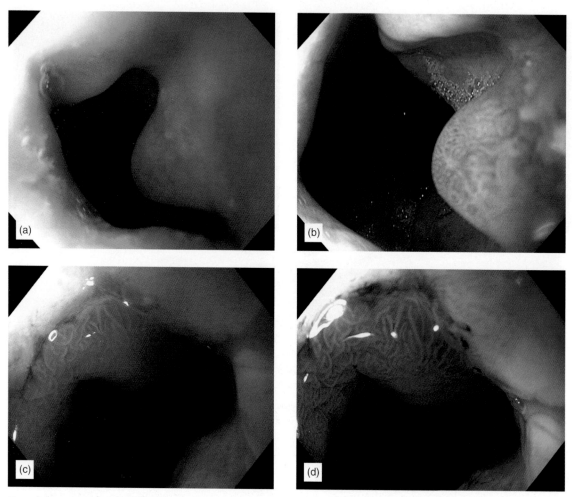

Figre 15.16 (a–d) WL and NBI H190 images of carditis. Thickened and darker but regular and round pattern of vessels seen on NBI view just below the GEJ. (Jonathan Cohen, NYU Langone School of Medicine.)

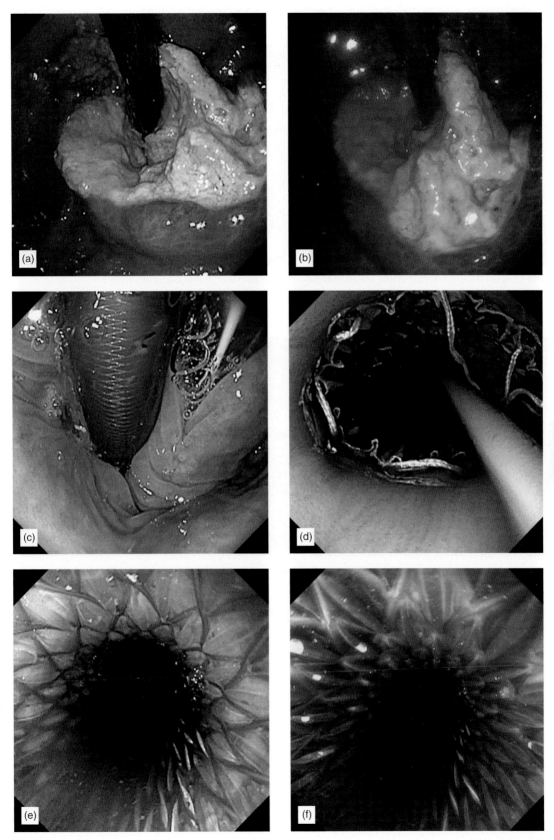

Figure 15.17 (a–f) Retroflexion in WL and NBI H190 views after traversing an ulcerated esophageal cancer extending to the cardia and view from lumen of subsequently placed partly uncovered esophageal stent. (Jonathan Cohen, NYU Langone School of Medicine.)

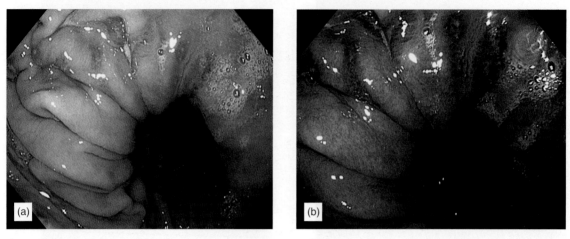

Figure 15.18 Cameron lesions. (a) WL H180 HRE low-magnification view. (b) NBI view. (Mayo Clinic, Jacksonville.)

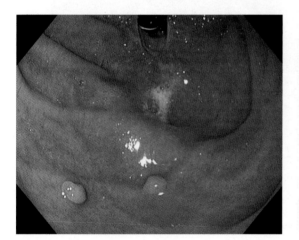

Figure 15.19 WL H180 HRE low-magnification image of normal fundus with two small fundic gland polyps and hiatal hernia seen in turnaround view. (Mayo Clinic, Jacksonville.)

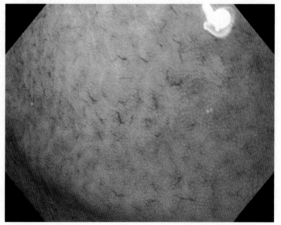

Figure 15.20 This magnification H180 NBI image of the fundic mucosa reveals normal vascular pattern and surface pattern. Corresponding histopathology confirmed normal mucosa. (Jonathan Cohen, NYU Langone School of Medicine.)

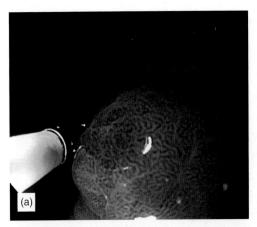
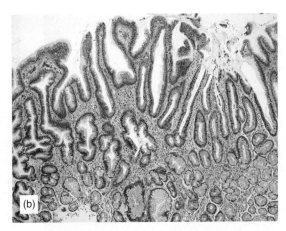

Figure 15.21 (a) Raised area of antral mucosa without erosion in this patient taking NSAIDs NBI H180 view. (b) Histopathology of this lesion shows reactive gastropathy. Elongated tortuous antral glands are lined by epithelium with mild reactive atypia. Consistent with chemical gastritis. (Jonathan Cohen, NYU Langone School of Medicine.)

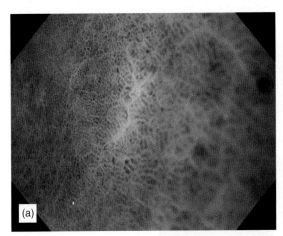
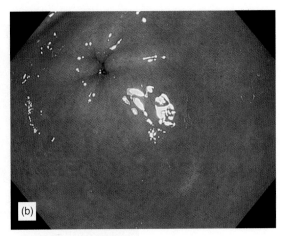

Figure 15.22 (a) Antral scar representing healed erosion, *Helicobacter pylori* negative, H180 NBI 1.5× magnification view. (b) Antrum in patient with healed erosion not apparent in WL low-magnification view. (Jonathan Cohen, NYU Langone School of Medicine.)

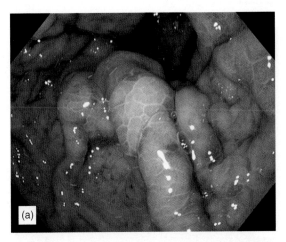
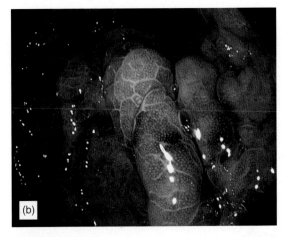

Figure 15.23 Fundic varices (a) H180 WL HRE view, (b) NBI view. (Mayo Clinic, Jacksonville.)

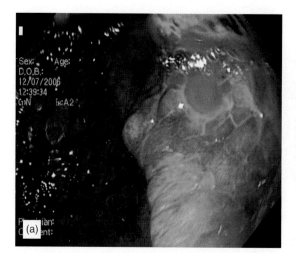
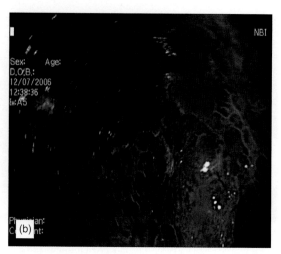

Figure 15.24 Severe portal hypertensive gastropathy (a), WL H180 low-magnification view, (b) NBI low-magnification view demonstrating leopard-skin appearance. In this case, due to the darker images in the stomach related to the larger lumen, WL better illustrates the finding. (Guilherme Macedo, Hospital Sao Marcos.)

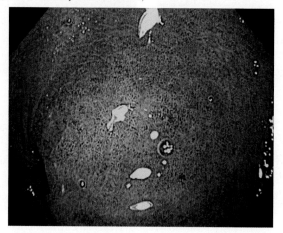

Figure 15.25 Subepithelial hemorrhages in portal hypertensive gastropathy, H180 NBI view low magnification. (Jean-François Rey, Institut Arnault Tzanck.)

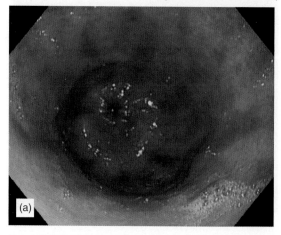
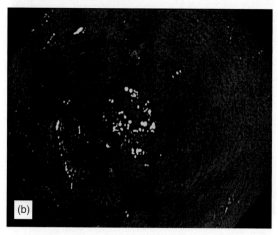

Figure 15.26 (a) WL H180 HRE low-magnification view of portal hypertensive gastropathy, gastric antral vascular ectasia (GAVE) pattern. (b) Portal hypertensive gastropathy with GAVE pattern, NBI low-magnification view. (Jean-François Rey, Institut Arnault Tzanck.)

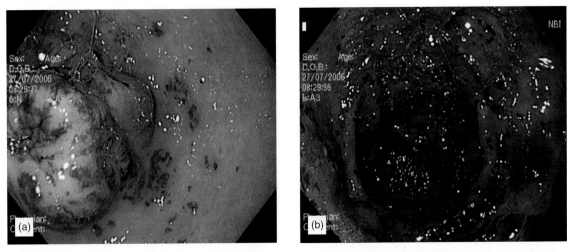

Figure 15.27 (a) GAVE pattern, H180 HRE low-magnification view, (b) NBI HRE low-magnification view. (Guilherme Macedo, Hospital Sao Marcos.)

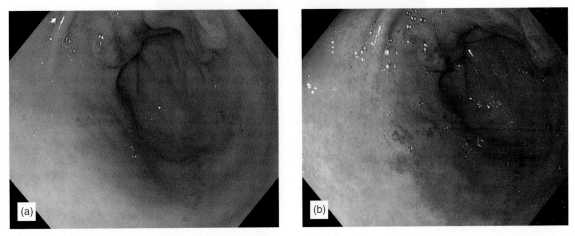

Figure 15.28 (a) Subtle changes of GAVE pattern on WL H180 HRE, (b) More evident on NBI. (Gregory Haber, Lenox Hill Hospital.)

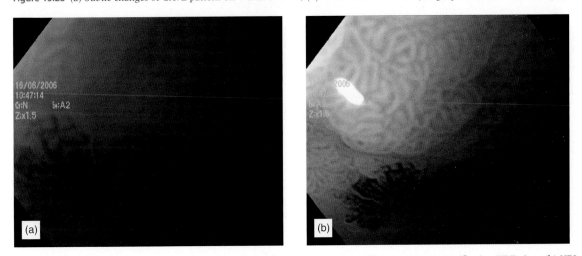

Figure 15.29 (a) Gastric angiodysplasia in Rendu–Osler–Weber syndrome seen well in WL H180 magnification HRE view. (b) NBI magnified view of the same lesion, now black in appearance instead of red. (Guilherme Macedo, Hospital Sao Marcos.)

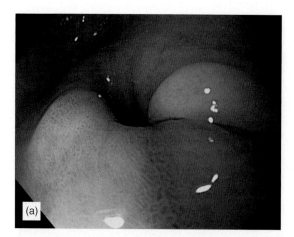

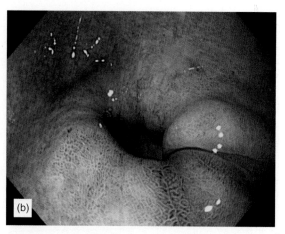

Figure 15.30 Pyloric erosion (a) faintly visible on WL H180 HRE, (b) More easily seen on NBI low-magnification view than on WL. (Jacques Deviere, Erasmus University Hospital.)

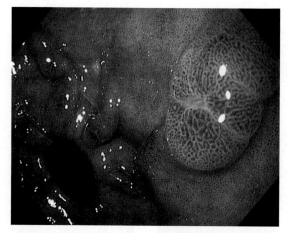

Figure 15.31 Focal antral erosion in patient with portal hypertension taking NSAIDs, NBI H180 1.5× magnification. (Jonathan Cohen, NYU Langone School of Medicine.)

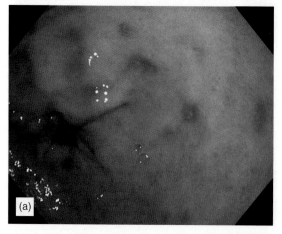

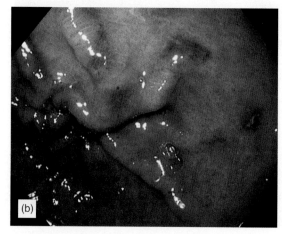

Figure 15.32 Multiple antral gastric erosions related to NSAIDs, (a) WL H180 HRE non-magnified view, (b) NBI low-magnification view. (Mayo Clinic, Jacksonville.)

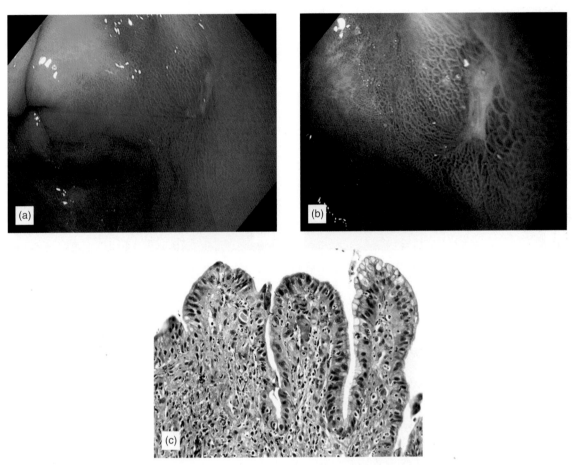

Figure 15.33 Benign-appearing chronic gastric ulcer, (a) WL H180, (b) NBI non-magnified view. Pathology demonstrated foveolar hyperplasia, active chronic gastritis, and focal intestinal metaplasia. (c) Acutely inflamed mucosa of benign gastric ulcer with marked reactive epithelial atypia present at the ulcer edge. (Jonathan Cohen, NYU Langone School of Medicine.)

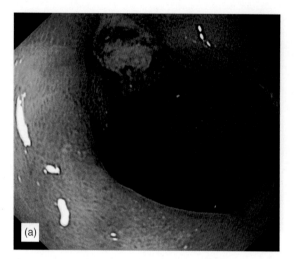
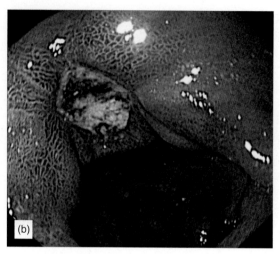

Figure 15.34 (a) Non-magnified WL H180 view of benign-appearing gastric ulcer with smooth regular borders. (b) Well-demarcated NBI image of benign solitary gastric ulcer, non-magnified view. The flat nature of the pigmented spot is clearly seen. (Jean-François Rey, Institut Arnault Tzanck.)

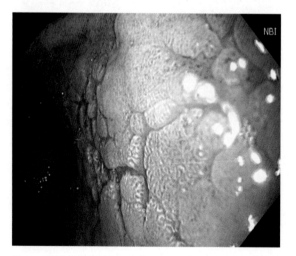

Figure 15.35 NBI H180 HRE low-magnification view of gastric intestinal metaplasia. (Guilherme Macedo, Hospital Sao Marcos.)

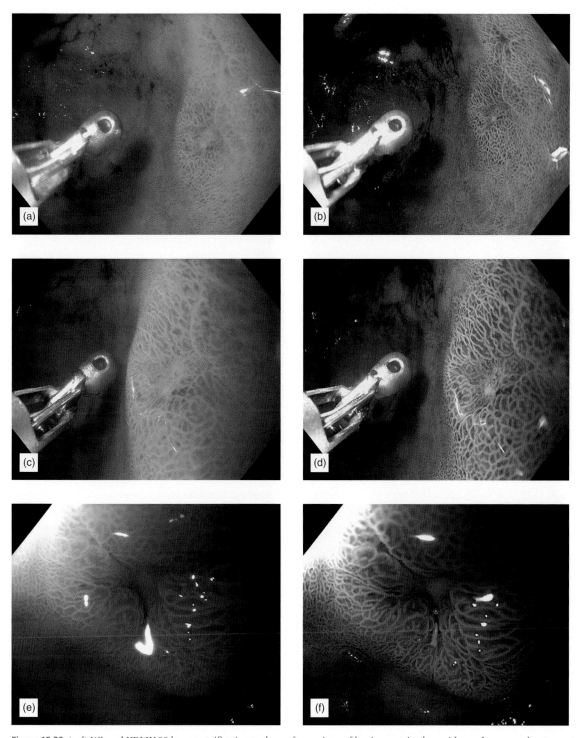

Figure 15.36 (a–f) WL and NBI H190 low magnification and near focus views of benign gastric ulcer with regular mucosal pattern at borders; no abnormal vessels seen. (Jonathan Cohen, NYU Langone School of Medicine.)

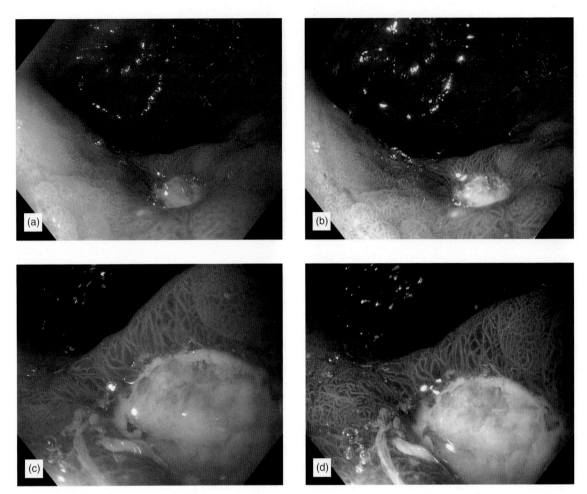

Figure 15.37 (a–d) Benign gastric ulcer with clean base in WL and NBI H190 and near-focus views. (Jonathan Cohen, NYU Langone School of Medicine.)

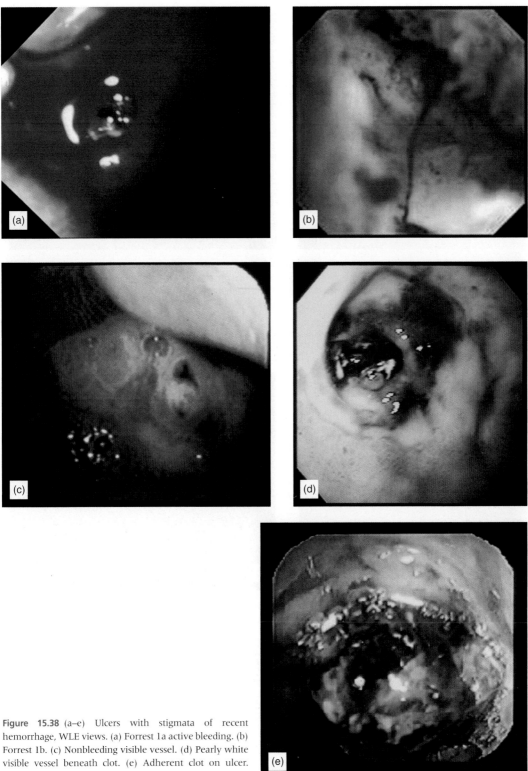

Figure 15.38 (a–e) Ulcers with stigmata of recent hemorrhage, WLE views. (a) Forrest 1a active bleeding. (b) Forrest 1b. (c) Nonbleeding visible vessel. (d) Pearly white visible vessel beneath clot. (e) Adherent clot on ulcer. (Dennis Jensen, David Geffen School of Medicine at UCLA.)

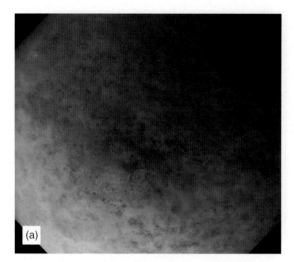
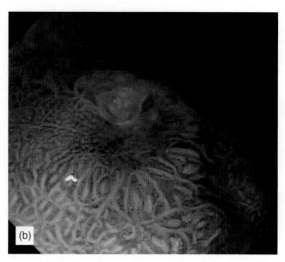

Figure 15.39 (a) Chronic inflammation. This raised red lesion might raise suspicions for early cancer on first glance. (b) Magnification NBI image shows it to be an erosion due to chronic inflammation; notice the regular surrounding mucosal pattern and while the central area loses this pattern, there are no abnormal microvessels. (Copyright M. Muto, Kyoto University Hospital Cancer Center.)

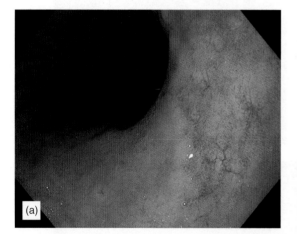
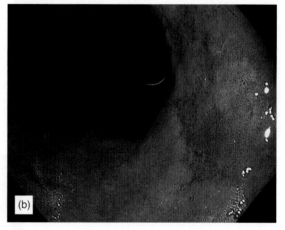

Figure 15.40 (a) Low-grade dysplasia under WL H180 low-magnification view. The lesion is slightly depressed with a reddened color. (b) NBI close-up image is more valuable than WL view in assessing for low-grade dysplasia. (Gregory Haber, Lenox Hill Hospital.)

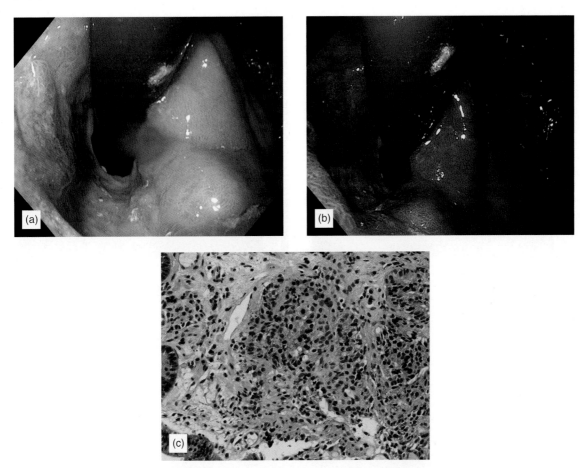

Figure 15.41 (a) Hiatal hernia with intramucosal carcinoma in the cardia, WL H180 HRE low-magnification image. (b) NBI low-magnification view more clearly delineates the abnormal area. Magnification is required to assess the microvascular pattern. (c) Histologic section from cardia demonstrating high-grade dysplasia suspicious for intramucosal carcinoma. (Mayo Clinic, Jacksonville.)

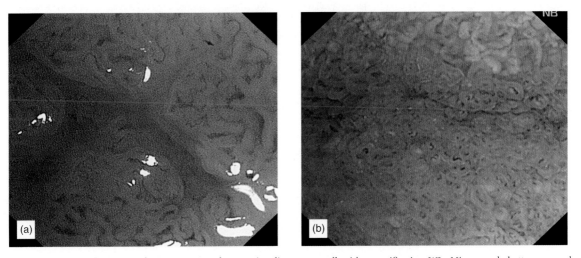

Figure 15.42 (a) Delineation of gastric cancer, demarcation line seen well with magnification WL. Microvessels better assessed with NBI. (b) Delineation of early gastric cancer with sharp demarcation line at loss of mucosal pattern, NBI magnification view. (University of Amsterdam.)

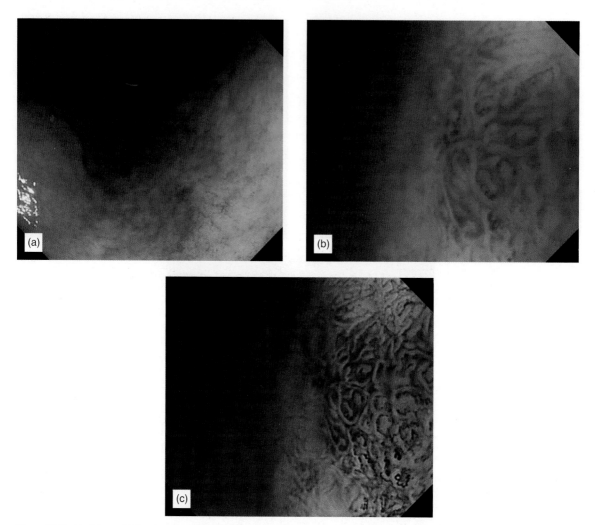

Figure 15.43 (a) This small discoloration in the upper stomach could reflect a benign erosion, a telangiectasia, or an early neoplasm. (b) Magnification demonstrates no erosion to mucosal surface, which has a regular pattern. (c) This is a gastric telangiectasia. While there are a few abnormal microvessels, there is no demarcation line, an indication that this is a non-neoplastic lesion. (Copyright M. Muto, Kyoto University Hospital Cancer Center.)

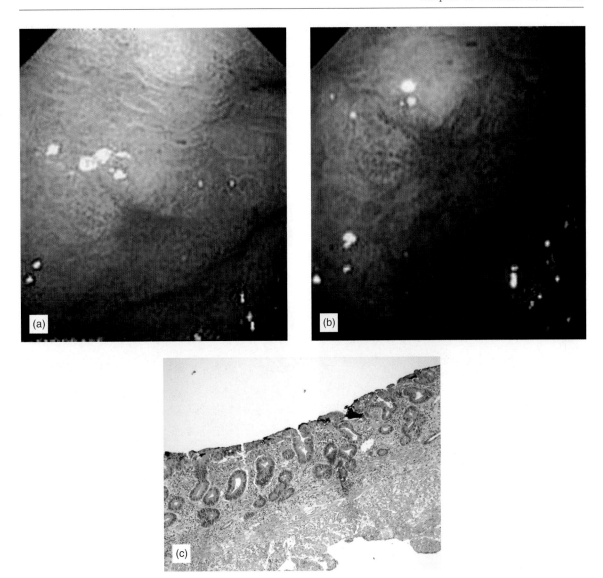

Figure 15.44 (a) Endoscopic view of a superficial IIa-IIc lesion in the gastric antrum. (b) NBI H180 view; vascular pattern more discernible in depressed portion. (c) Endoscopic mucosal resection (EMR) specimen showing moderately differentiated adenocarcinoma limited to the epithelial layer. (Guido Costamagna, Catholic University of the Sacred Heart.)

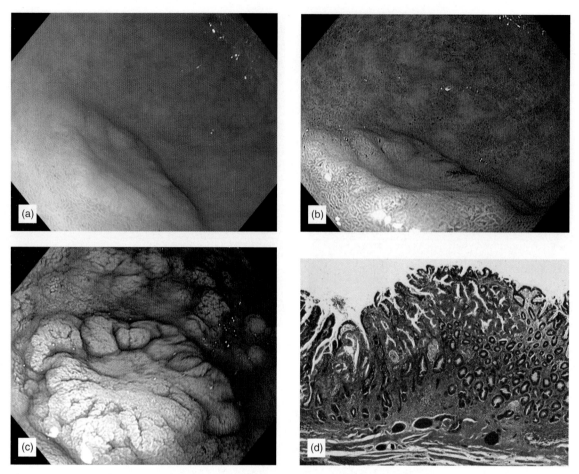

Figure 15.45 (a) Superficial gastric carcinoma on the greater curvature IIa–IIc mixed raised and depressed lesion, seen in WL H180 low-magnification view. (b) The lesion appears whitish and is better delineated than with WL. (c) With indigocarmine: the lesion is better delineated than with NBI, especially in terms of the surface assessment of the raised portion. Indigo > NBI > WL. (Edouard Herriot Hospital). (d) Early gastric cancer, in this case confined to the mucosa. (Thierry Ponchon, Edouard Herriot Hospital.)

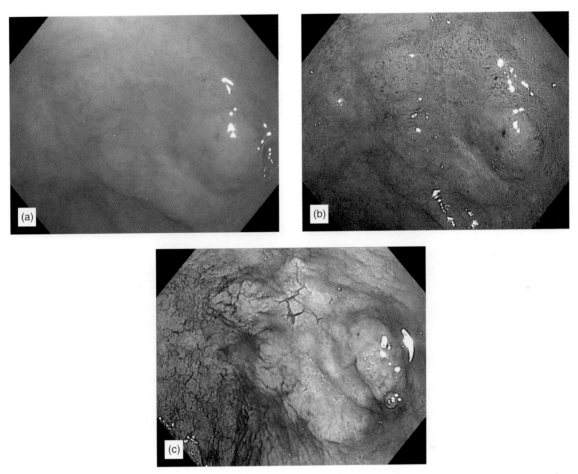

Figure 15.46 (a) This gastric superficial carcinoma IIa-IIc appears on WL H180 view as discoloration and slightly irregular surface. (b) The lesion appears whitish and is better delineated than with WL. Better assessment of microvessels requires magnification. (c) With indigocarmine. Margins seen more easily for this raised lesion than with NBI. (Thierry Ponchon, Edouard Herriot Hospital.)

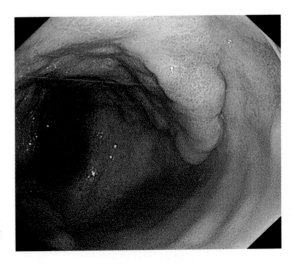

Figure 15.47 WL HRE view of an early gastric carcinoma on a background of intestinal metaplasia and atrophy. (University of Amsterdam.)

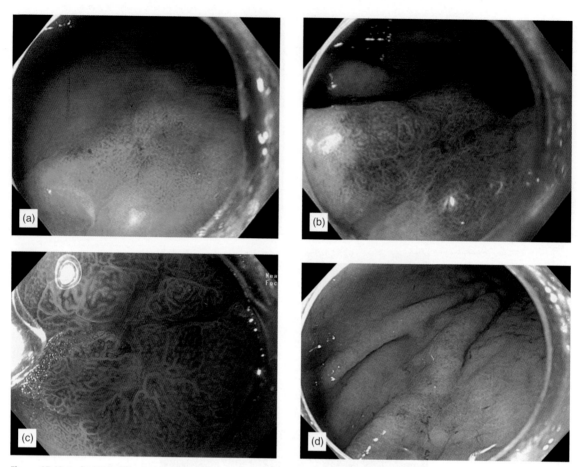

Figure 15.48 (a–h) Well-differentiated superficial gastric adenocarcinoma detected on WL H190 (a) only as an atypical red area. (b) NBI and (c) NBI near-focus views show loss of mucosal pattern. (d, e) Chromoendoscopy and

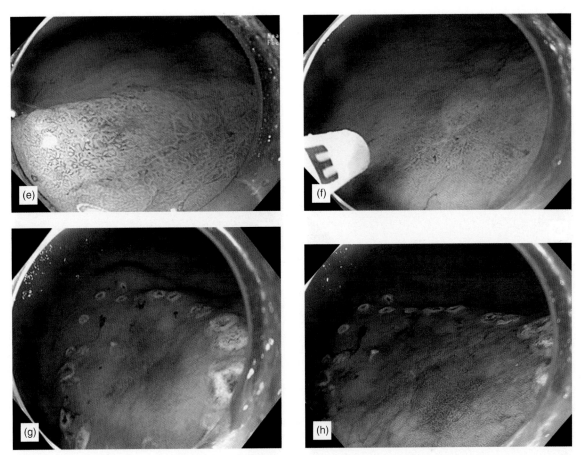

Figure 15.48 (Continued) (f) magnification chromoendoscopy best delineates the lesion margin. (g, h) Margin marked with argon plasma coagulation (APC) seen on WL and NBI views prior to endoscopic submucosal dissection (ESD). (Jonathan Cohen, NYU Langone School of Medicine.)

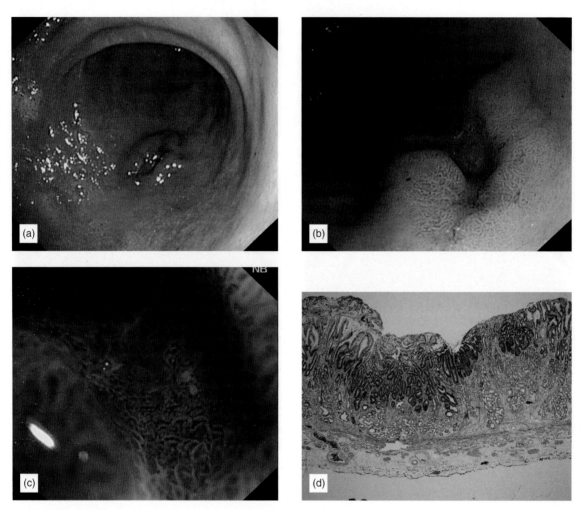

Figure 15.49 (a) Intramucosal carcinoma, intestinal type, of the antrum. At a distance this WL H180 view raises suspicions of a malignant-appearing ulcer. (b) Intramucosal carcinoma, intestinal type, of the antrum. Close-up WL view of the malignant-appearing lesion depicted in (b). (c) Detailed view of the center of type IIa-IIc intramucosal carcinoma of the antrum. Mesh pattern of microvessels with loss of mucosal structure predicts well-differentiated tumor and possible candidacy for ESD. (d) High-grade dysplasia/well-differentiated intramucosal adenocarcinoma (intestinal type). No penetration of the muscularis mucosae, confirming the optical diagnosis made in (c) using magnification NBI. (University of Amsterdam.)

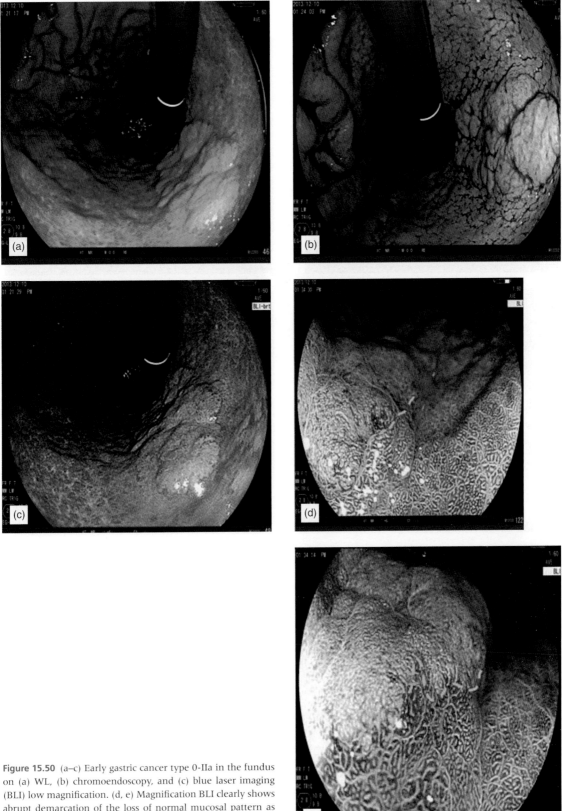

Figure 15.50 (a–c) Early gastric cancer type 0-IIa in the fundus on (a) WL, (b) chromoendoscopy, and (c) blue laser imaging (BLI) low magnification. (d, e) Magnification BLI clearly shows abrupt demarcation of the loss of normal mucosal pattern as indicated by the yellow dashed lines. (Copyright Dr. Nobuaki Yagi, Kyoto Prefectural University of Medicine.)

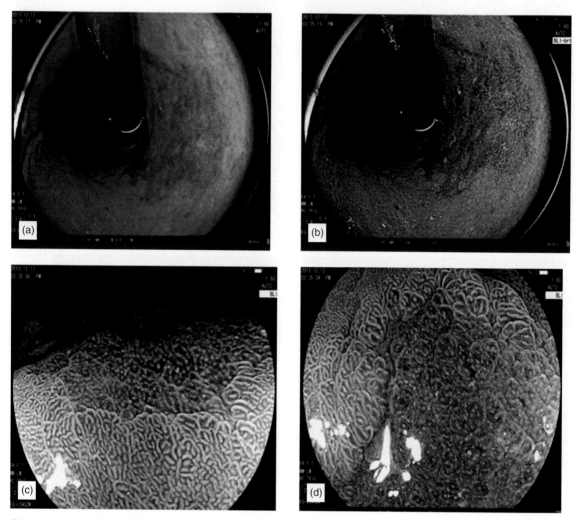

Figure 15.51 Type 0-IIc gastric adenocarcinoma: (a) WL; (b) Fuji Intelligent Chromoendoscopy (FICE); (c, d) BLI magnification views. (Copyright Dr. Nobuaki Yagi, Kyoto Prefectural University of Medicine.)

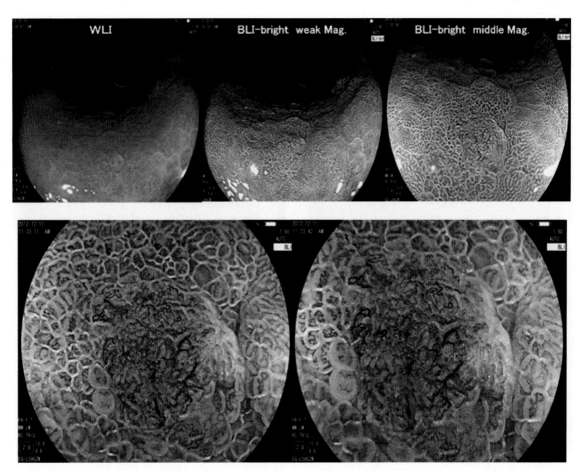

Figure 15.52 BLI with optical magnification views of early gastric cancer type 0-IIa. High magnification shows loss of normal mucosal pattern with sharp demarcation and a fine network pattern of vessels consistent with well-differentiated adenocarcinoma. (Reproduced from Yagi N *et al.* Nippon Rinsho 2014;72(Suppl 1):266–271.)

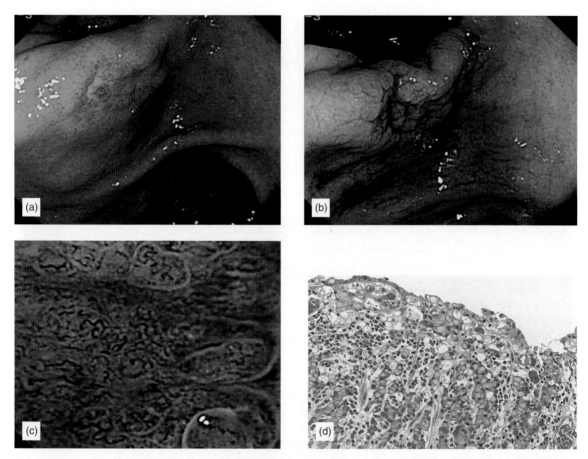

Figure 15.53 (a) WL HRE image of small depressed lesion in the gastric angularis suspicious for a type 0-IIc carcinoma. (b) Chromoendoscopy highlights the mucosal pattern of this depressed lesion that consists of poorly differentiated carcinoma. (c) NBI magnification of this lesion reveals loss of mucosal pattern in the depressed area with abnormal microvessels in the corkscrew pattern consistent with poorly differentiated adenocarcinoma. (d) Histopathology: high-power view confirms the diagnosis of poorly differentiated carcinoma predicted by NBI analysis of the microvessel pattern. (Copyright M. Kaise, T. Nakayoshi, and H. Tajiri, Jikei University School of Medicine.)

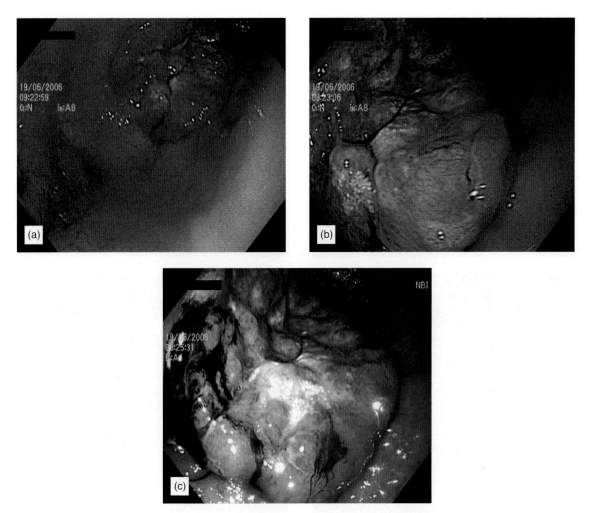

Figure 15.54 (a) Malignant gastric ulcer in distal body, low-magnification NBI H180 view. (b) Magnified WL view of malignant gastric ulcer with irregular borders and necrotic center. (c) NBI magnified view of this large raised lesion that grossly suggests sm2 invasion or greater. (Guilherme Macedo, Hospital Sao Marcos.)

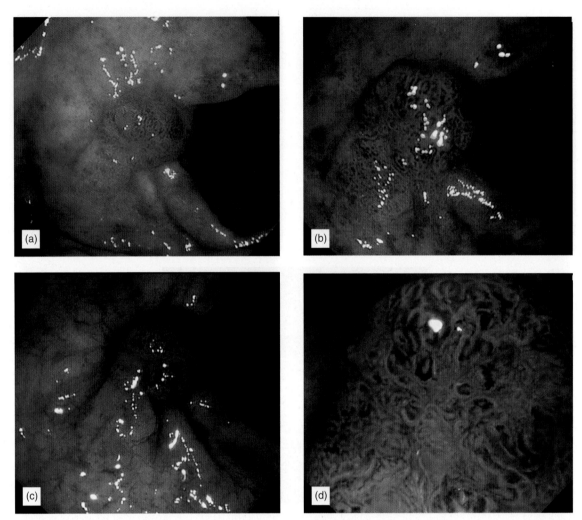

Figure 15.55 (a) WL HRE low-magnification view of local recurrence after EMR for superficial gastric cancer. (b) NBI clearly shows worrisome features not apparent on WL even without magnification. This case underscores the rationale for consideration of ESD for larger superficial lesions to reduce the risk of local recurrence. (c) Chromoendoscopy view of local recurrence after EMR for gastric cancer. (d) Magnification NBI shows both abnormal disrupted pit pattern and abnormal vessels in this recurrent cancer. (Copyright M. Muto, Kyoto University Hospital Cancer Center.)

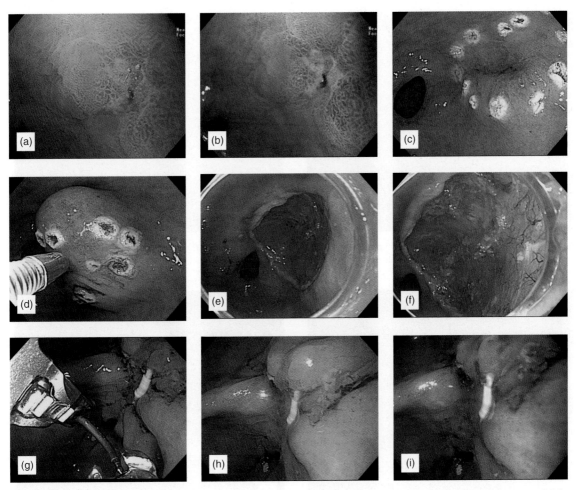

Figure 15.56 (a–i) Well-differentiated 0-IIa+c antral adenocarcinoma: WL H190, near focus, NBI, marking, ESD specimen, and defect before and aftere suture closure. (Jonathan Cohen, NYU Langone School of Medicine.)

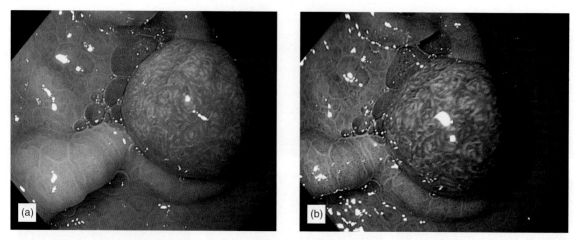

Figure 15.57 (a) Inflamed fundic gastric polyp seen here in WL H180 HRE view. (b) NBI view of the lesion with clearly delineated regular pit pattern. (Mayo Clinic, Jacksonville.)

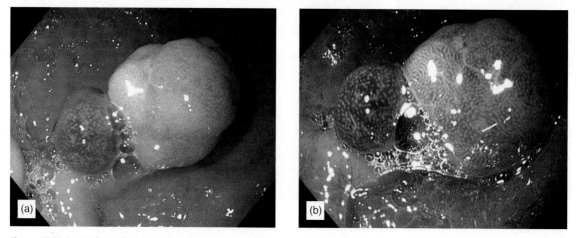

Figure 15.58 (a) High-resolution WL H180 image of unusual-appearing fundic gland polyps in the body of the stomach of varying size and degree of inflammation. (b) NBI of unusual-appearing fundic gland polyps in the body of the stomach of varying size and degree of inflammation. Pathology confirmed this as a fundic gland polyp with hyperplastic and inflammatory fibroid polypoid features. (Mayo Clinic, Jacksonville.)

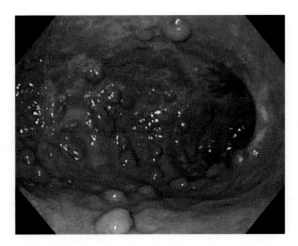

Figure 15.59 Multiple fundic gland polyps, WL H180 non-magnified view. (Jean-François Rey, Institut Arnault Tzanck.)

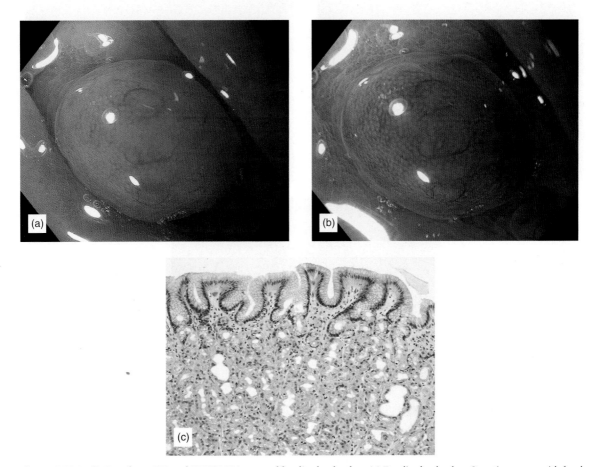

Figure 15.60 (a, b) Near-focus WL and NBI H180 images of fundic gland polyp. (c) Fundic gland polyp. Oxyntic mucosa with focal cystic dilation of the glands. (Jonathan Cohen, NYU Langone School of Medicine.)

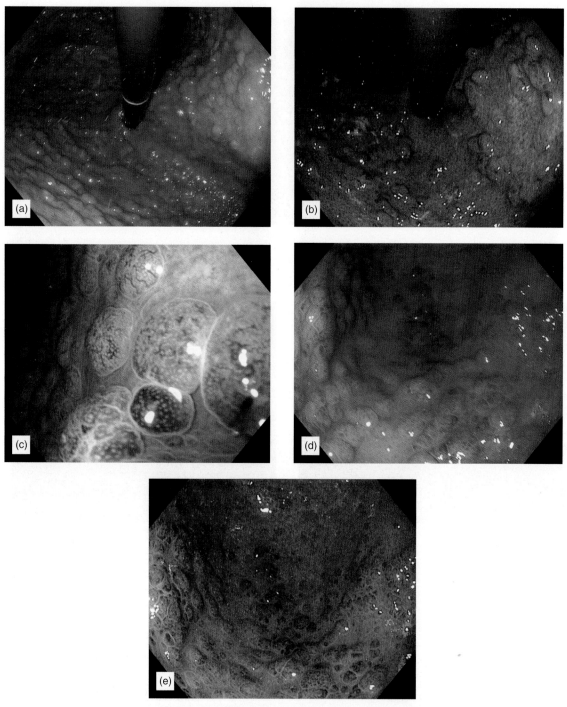

Figure 15.61 (a) WL H180 view of multiple small sessile fundic gland polyps in familial adenomatous polyposis. Note the lack of detail of the polyp mucosa and the similar color of the polyps and gastric mucosa. (b) NBI view of multiple small sessile fundic gland polyps in familial adenomatous polyposis. Note that the polyps are darker than the mucosa and the polyp mucosa has a larger and more pronounced reticulated pattern. (c) NBI magnified view of fundic gland polyps. Note that the small blood vessels and pitted surface of the polyps are clearly seen. (d) WL view of fundic gland polyps with a similar color to the gastric mucosa, a nodular appearance, and scant mucosal detail. (e) NBI view of fundic gland polyps accentuated with a darker color than the gastric mucosa, a clearly defined nodular appearance, and precise mucosal detail. (James DiSario, University of Utah Health Sciences Center.)

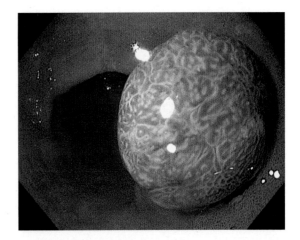

Figure 15.62 Hyperplastic antral polyp seen here in NBI H180 low-magnification view. Note the regular round surface mucosal pattern. (Thierry Ponchon, Edouard Herriot Hospital).

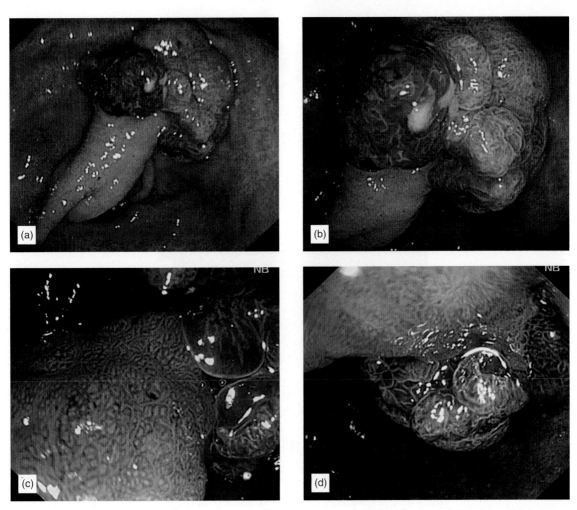

Figure 15.63 (a) Hamartomatous polyp, indefinite for dysplasia H180 WL view. (b) Magnified WL image. (b) Magnified WL H180 image. (c) NBI magnification view highlights the transition of the mucosal patterns from the stalk to the darker, more villous appearing area to the right of the image. (d) Inflamed-appearing tip of the large gastric polyp with pathologic findings indefinite for dysplasia. (University of Amsterdam.)

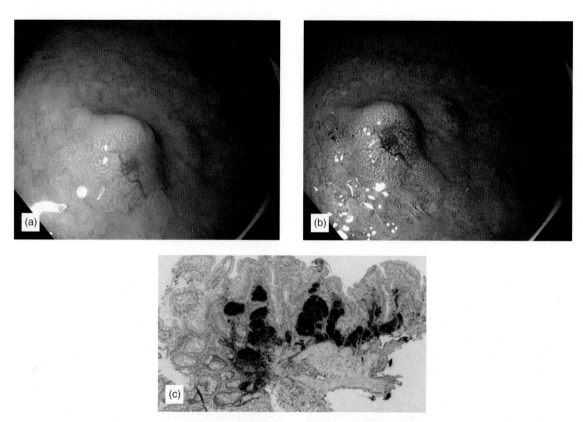

Figure 15.64 (a) Corpus greater curvature, larger proximal and smaller distal lesion positive for carcinoid, WL H180 HRE. (b) NBI HRE low-magnification view of gastric carcinoid tumors in the body, greater curvature. (c) Gastric carcinoid arising in a setting of atrophic gastritis and intestinal metaplasia. (University Medical Center Hamburg Eppendorf.)

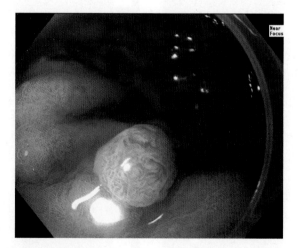

Figure 15.65 NBI H190 near focus image of gastric carcinoid tumor. (Jonathan Cohen, NYU Langone School of Medicine.)

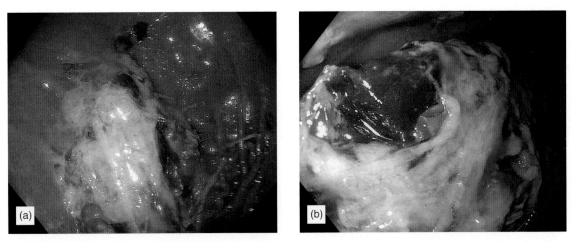

Figure 15.66 (a, b) WL H190 image of phytobezoar in stomach. (Jonathan Cohen, NYU Langone School of Medicine.)

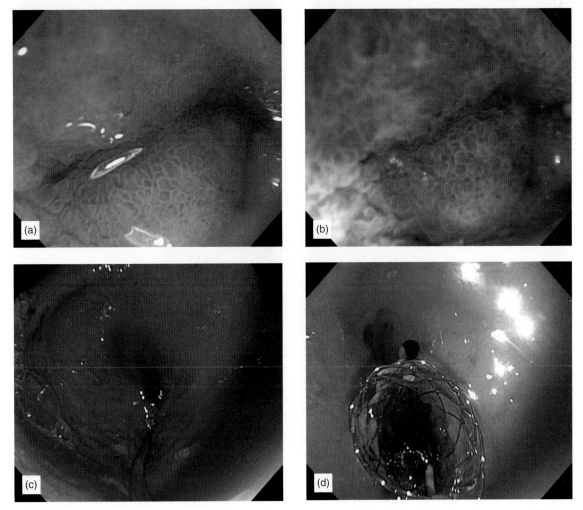

Figure 15.67 (a–d) WL and NBI H190 images of duodenal obstruction due to malignant tumor arising from the pancreas with placement of uncovered enteral self-expanding metal stent. (Jonathan Cohen, NYU Langone School of Medicine.)

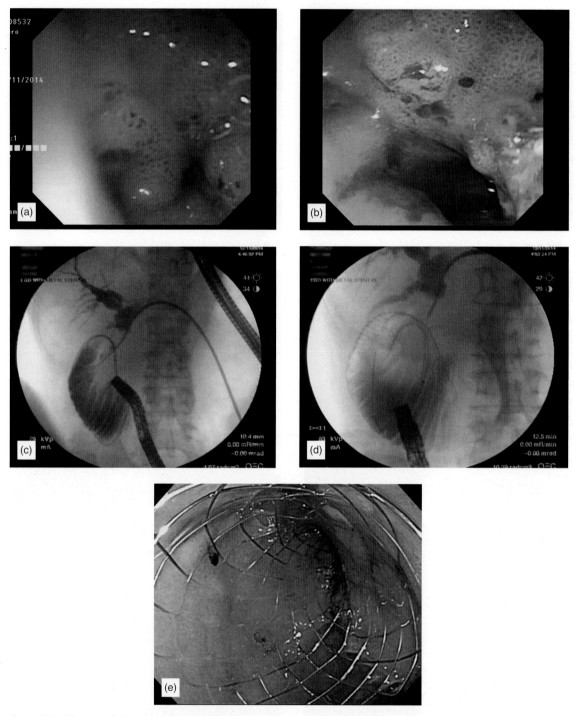

Figure 15.68 The view of the pylorus shows a tight narrowing due to duodenal compression in a patient presenting with symptoms of gastric outlet obstruction and biliary obstruction preventing ERCP. A combined percutaneous transhepatic cholangiogram and endoscopy with concurrent placement of a duodenal self-expanding metal stent and a biliary metal stent anterograde thought the mesh of the duodenal stent is performed. (a,b) appearance of narrowing at the pyloric outlet. (c, d) Fluoroscopic images of cholangiogram and dilated duodenum distal to the obstruction prior to and following deployment of the duodenal stent. (e) WL HRE view of the proximal end of the duodenal stent in the antrum. (Jonathan Cohen, NYU Langone School of Medicine.)

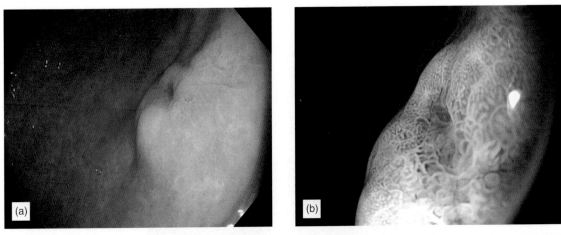

Figure 15.69 Gastric carcinoid. (a) WL H180 low-magnification view in the antrum, posterior wall. Biopsies from the center as well as from the margin of the lesion were positive for carcinoid. (b) Close-up HRE NBI image. (University Medical Center Hamburg Eppendorf.)

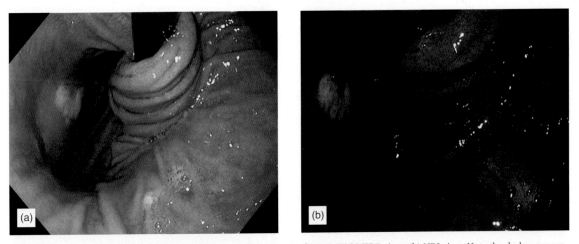

Figure 15.70 Nissen-type fundoplication, (a) with wrap well intact in this WL H180 HRE view; (b) NBI view. Note the darker appearance due to the large lumen that makes NBI H180 less useful for general use in the stomach and most appropriate for close-up magnification of suspicious lesions. (Mayo Clinic, Jacksonville.)

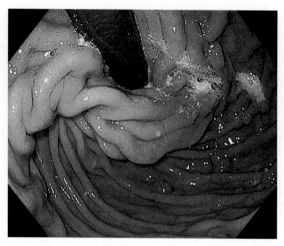

Figure 15.71 HRE H190 WL retroflex view of a patient with a prior fundoplication. (Jonathan Cohen, NYU Langone School of Medicine.)

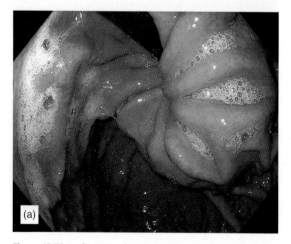

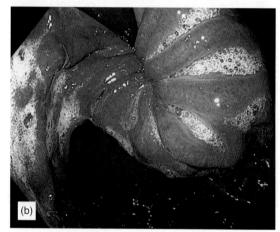

Figure 15.72 (a, b) WL and H190 NBI images of retroflexion view in the stomach following lap band surgery without complication. Here the H190 NBI is sufficiently bright to examine the area using NBI, in contrast to earlier H180 endoscopes. (Jonathan Cohen, NYU Langone School of Medicine.)

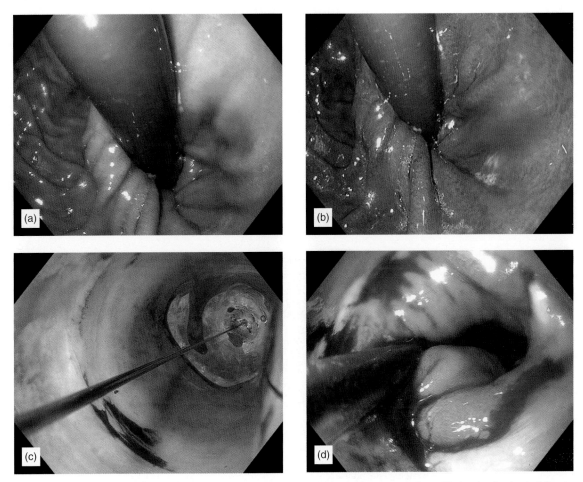

Figure 15.73 (a, b) Fundoplication retroflexion view in WL and NBI H190. (c, d) 20-mm balloon dilation for dysphagia following operation and view post dilation. (Jonathan Cohen, NYU Langone School of Medicine.)

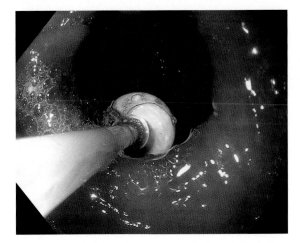

Figure 15.74 Deployment of video capsule through the pylorus via gastroscope in a patient unable to swallow the capsule WL H190 view. (Jonathan Cohen, NYU Langone School of Medicine.)

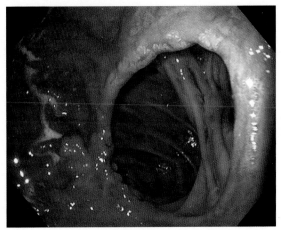

Figure 15.75 WL H180 HRE image provides a sharp view of this gastrojejunal anastomosis. A Billroth II gastrectomy had been performed in this patient 53 years previously for recurrent ulcers. (University Medical Center Hamburg Eppendorf.)

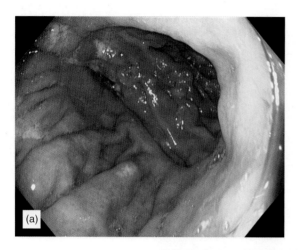

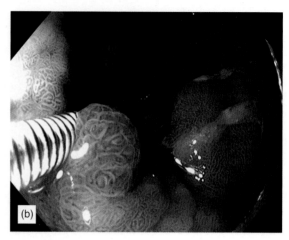

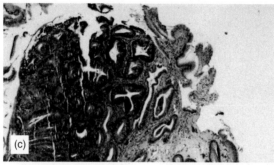

Figure 15.76 (a) Low-magnification WL H180 HRE of asymptomatic 71-year-old female 50 years following Billroth II gastrectomy. From a distance in WL, no suspicious lesion is seen. (b) Close-up with HRE and NBI of low-grade intraepithelial neoplasia (LGIN) at the Billroth II anastomosis with 0.8-mm diameter biopsy forceps as scale. The wide sulci and irregular mucosal pattern on NBI raises the suspicion for dysplasia and allows for target biopsy of the lesion. (c) 10× H&E image shows LGIN in the area of a Billroth II anastomosis. (University Medical Center Hamburg Eppendorf.)

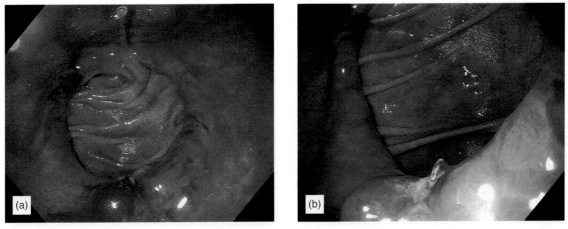

Figure 15.77 (a, b) Gastrojejunal anastomosis following a Whipple resection revealed a benign small area of ulceration WL H190 view. (Jonathan Cohen, NYU Langone School of Medicine.)

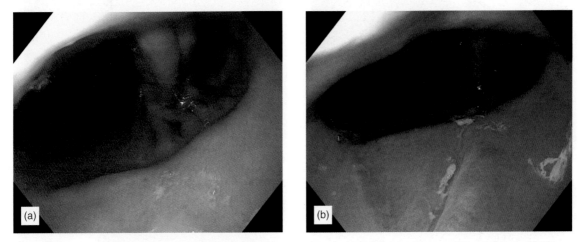

Figure 15.78 (a, b) WL and NBI H190 views of a dilated gastrojejunal anastomosis following Roux-en-Y gastric bypass (RYGB) surgery in a patient evaluated for weight regain. (Jonathan Cohen, NYU Langone School of Medicine.)

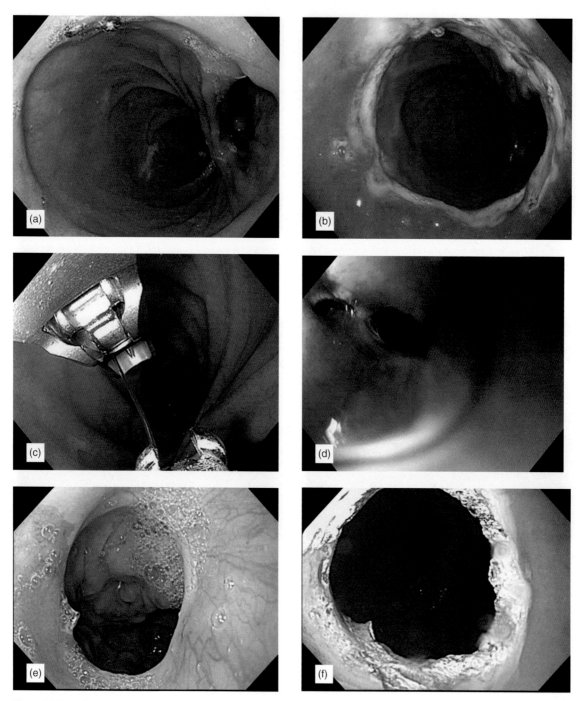

Figure 15.79 (a–d) Gastrojejunostomy with dilated anastomosis associated with weight regain. NBI view following circumferential APC ablation at anastomosis. Overstitch suture stoma reduction. (e–k) Similar revision of dilated gastrojejunal anastamosis for weight regain is shown. In (j) a small balloon is used to dilate the narrow anastomosis after the suture is fastened to ensure the opening is not too narrow. (Jonathan Cohen, NYU Langone School of Medicine.)

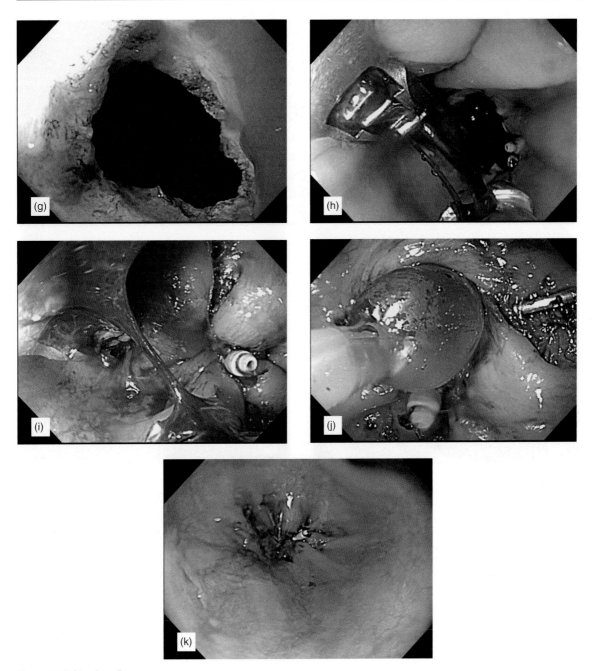

Figure 15.79 (Continued)

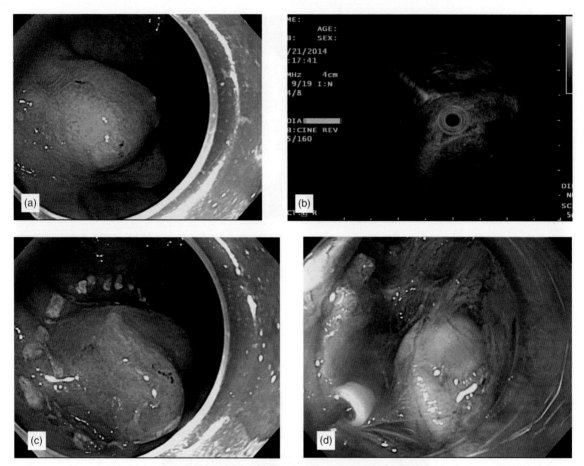

Figure 15.80 (a–h) Gastrointestinal stromal tumor in fundus: ESD full-thickness endoscopic resection in WL H190 views, retrieval of specimen and 2-month follow-up inspection of the site, which had been sutured closed. (Jonathan Cohen, NYU Langone School of Medicine.)

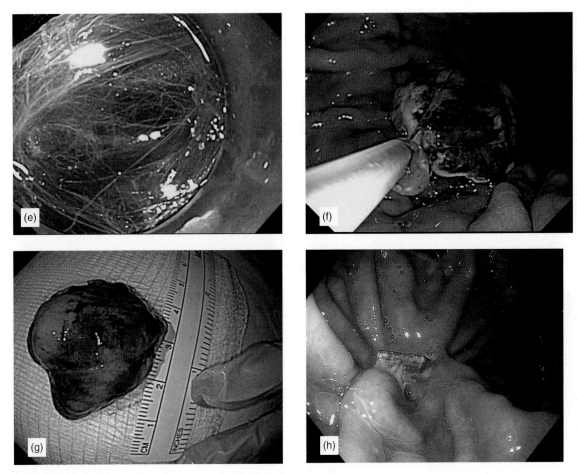

Figure 15.80 (Continued)

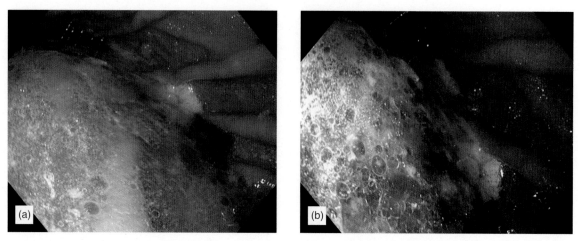

Figure 15.81 (a) WL H180 HRE of retained contents in gastric remnant after esophagectomy. (b) Low-magnification NBI view shows the oily remnants which now appear pink instead of yellow. (Mayo Clinic, Jacksonville.)

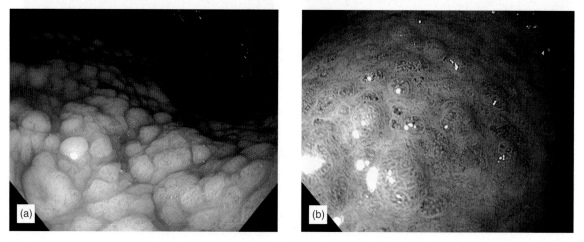

Figure 15.82 (a) WL H180 HRE low-magnification view of micronodular appearance of rare entity of collagenous gastritis (fundus). (b) NBI of micronodular fundic folds in collagenous gastritis (Mayo Clinic, Jacksonville.)

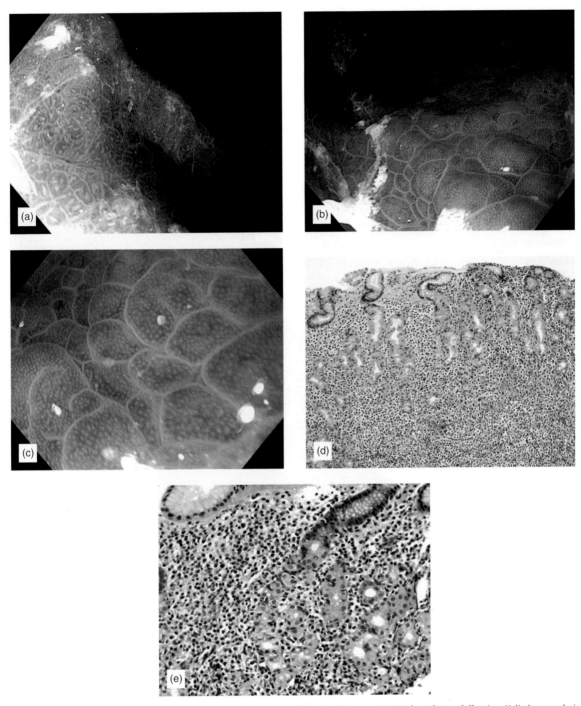

Figure 15.83 (a) Gastric fundus in patient with mucosa-associated lymphoid tissue (MALT) lymphoma following *Helicobacter pylori* eradication and 1 month of Rituxan therapy, NBI H180 low-magnification view. (b) Prominent bumps and grooves in gastric body in patient with MALT lymphoma following *Helicobacter pylori* eradication and 1 month of Rituxan therapy, (b) NBI low-magnification view, (c) NBI magnification view. (d) A dense infiltrate of atypical lymphoid cells expands the mucosa and destroys gastric glands. (e) High-power view; there is invasion and destruction of gastric gland epithelium by neoplastic lymphocytes ("lymphoepithelial lesion"). (Jonathan Cohen, NYU Langone School of Medicine.)

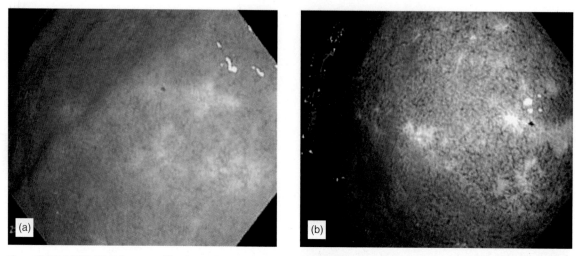

Figure 15.84 (a) WL H180 low-magnification endoscopic view of gastric MALT hyperplasia. (b) NBI low-magnification view. (Guido Costamagna, Catholic University of the Sacred Heart.)

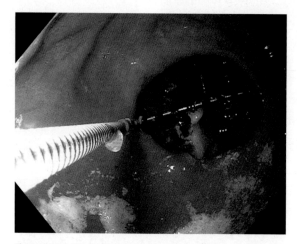

Figure 15.85 WL H180 HRE image shows use of the Olympus measuring catheter to demonstrate an enlarged gastrojejunal stoma following gastric bypass surgery. (Richard Rothstein, Dartmouth Medical School.)

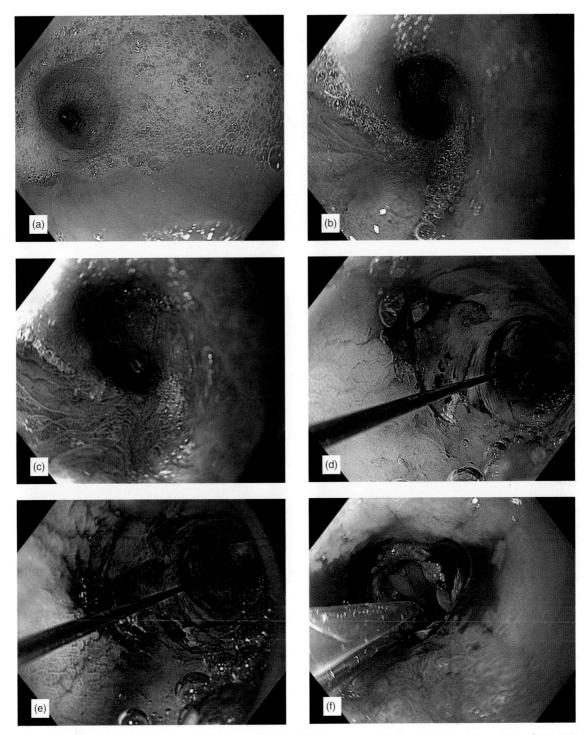

Figure 15.86 (a–f) Stenosis of gastrojejunal anastomosis following RYGB surgery with balloon dilation to 10 mm, WL and NBI H190 views. (Jonathan Cohen, NYU Langone School of Medicine.)

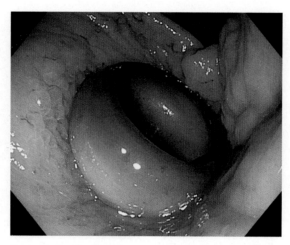

Figure 15.87 WL H190 view of percutaneous endoscopic gastrostomy (PEG) bumper in stomach. (Jonathan Cohen, NYU Langone School of Medicine.)

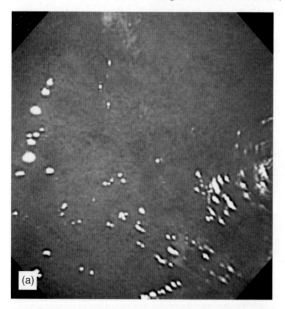

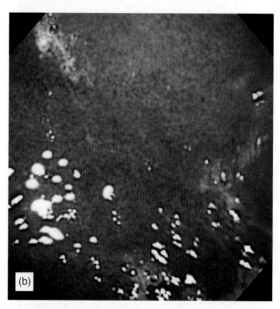

Figure 15.88 (a) WL H180 low-magnification image in this patient initially notable only for somewhat uneven surface contour without significant erythema or erosions. (b) Magnified NBI image of the gastric antrum in this child showed nonspecific congestion of vessels seen here as patches of darker areas. Biopsies revealed eosinophilic gastritis. (Johns Hopkins University School of Medicine.)

ABBREVIATIONS

APC	argon plasma coagulation
BLI	blue laser imaging
EMR	endoscopic mucosal resection
ESD	endoscopic submucosal dissection
FICE	Fuji Intelligent Chromoendoscopy
GAVE	gastric antral vascular ectasia
GEJ	gastroesophageal junction
HRE	high-resolution endoscopy
LGIN	low-grade intraepithelial neoplasia

MALT	mucosa-associated lymphoid tissue
NBI	narrowband imaging
NSAID	nonsteroidal anti-inflammatory drug
PEG	percutaneous endoscopic gastrostomy
RYGB	Roux-en-Y gastric bypass
WL	white light

 Video clips to accompany this book can be found in the online material at www.wiley.com/go/cohen/NBI

16 Small intestine atlas

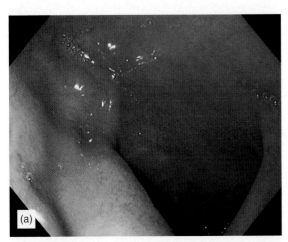 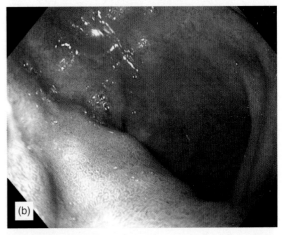

Figure 16.1 WL H180 image of a normal duodenal bulb. The villiform architecture is indistinct. (b) NBI low-magnification image of a normal duodenal bulb. The villiform architecture is accentuated by the NBI imaging. (James DiSario, University of Utah Health Sciences Center.)

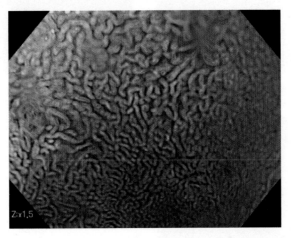

Figure 16.2 Normal mucosal appearance in the bulb, H180 NBI view 1.5× magnification. (Jacques Deviere, Erasmus University Hospital.)

Comprehensive Atlas of High-Resolution Endoscopy and Narrowband Imaging, Second Edition. Edited by Jonathan Cohen.
© 2017 John Wiley & Sons, Ltd. Published 2017 by John Wiley & Sons, Ltd.
Companion website: www.wiley.com/go/cohen/NBI

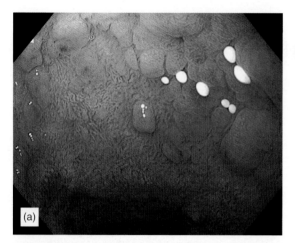
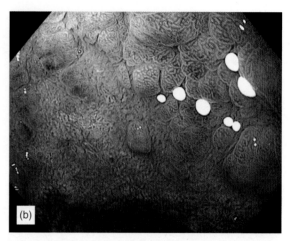

Figure 16.3 (a) Nodular mucosa in the duodenal bulb of Brunner's glands viewed with high-resolution WL. (b) Nodular mucosa in the duodenal bulb of Brunner's glands viewed with high-resolution NBI H180 (note the white medication granules). (Mayo Clinic, Jacksonville.)

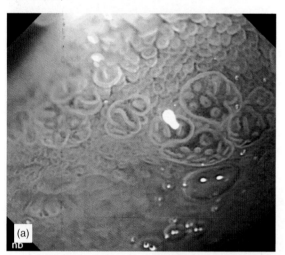
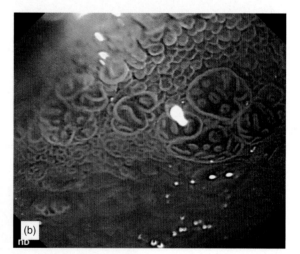

Figure 16.4 (a) Brunner's gland hyperplasia of the duodenal bulb seen in WL HRE H180 magnification view. (b) High-magnification NBI image provides excellent definition of these Brunner's glands. (Jean-François Rey, Institut Arnault Tzanck.)

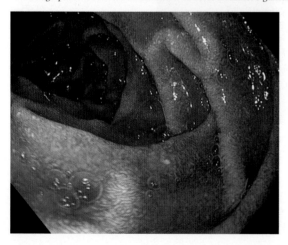

Figure 16.5 NBI H180 light view of a normal duodenal fold. The villiform architecture is readily discernible. (Rob Hawes, Medical University of South Carolina.)

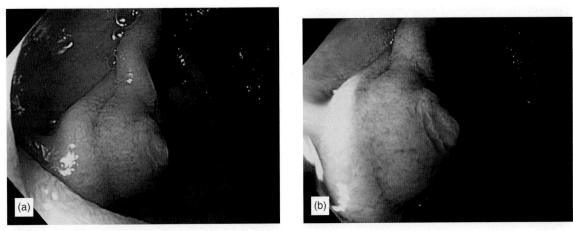

Figure 16.6 (a) Normal major papilla H180 WL view. (b) Under NBI low magnification. (Jacques Deviere, Erasmus University Hospital.)

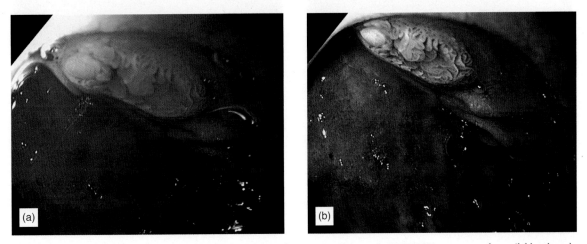

Figure 16.7 (a) WL Q180V view of major papilla 1.2× magnification. Duodenoscope NBI HDTV not currently available, though such high definition of ampulla could one day facilitate endoscopic retrograde cholangiopancreatography (ERCP). (b) NBI non-magnification view of normal major papilla. (Jonathan Cohen, NYU Langone School of Medicine.)

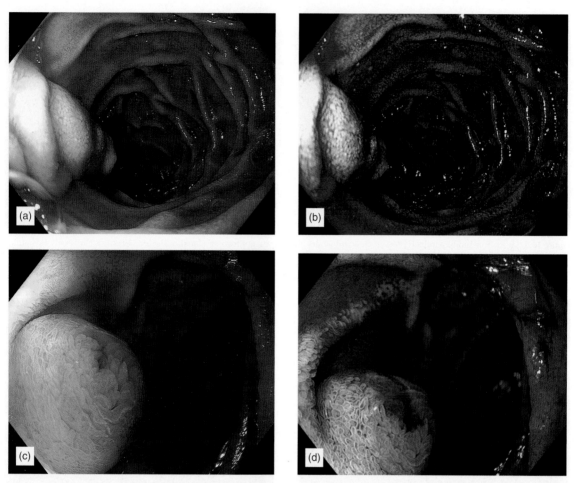

Figure 16.8 (a, b) Major papilla, WL and NBI with H190 gastroscope. (c, d) Bile, which appears pink on NBI view (d), is seen emerging from the biliary orifice. (Jonathan Cohen, NYU Langone School of Medicine.)

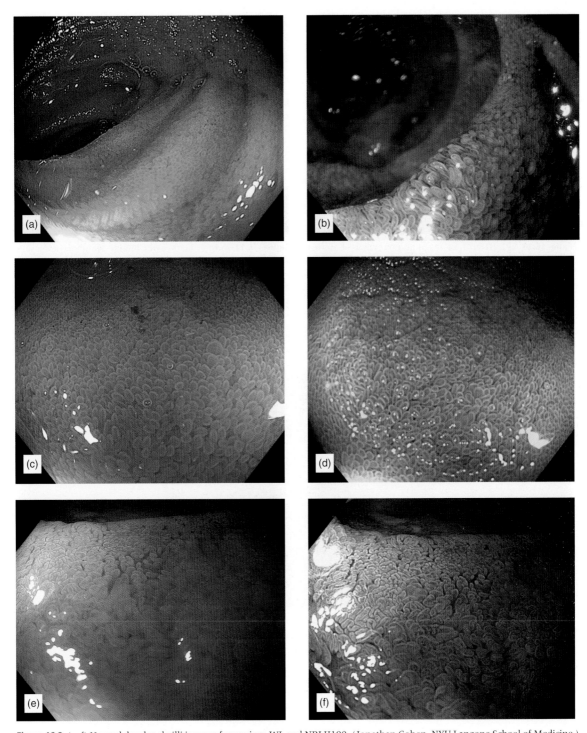

Figure 16.9 (a–f) Normal duodenal villi in near-focus view, WL and NBI H190. (Jonathan Cohen, NYU Langone School of Medicine.)

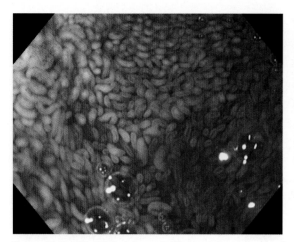

Figure 16.10 NBI H180 1.5× magnification view of normal duodenal villi. (Jonathan Cohen, NYU Langone School of Medicine.)

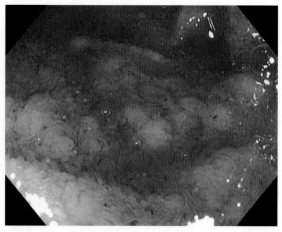

Figure 16.11 Normal ileum with bumpy lymphoid tissue and clearly discernible villi well visualized on low-magnification NBI view. In addition to the thin brownish superficial capillaries, one can appreciate some deeper vessels that appear green, such as one at the top middle of the photograph. (Jonathan Cohen, NYU Langone School of Medicine.

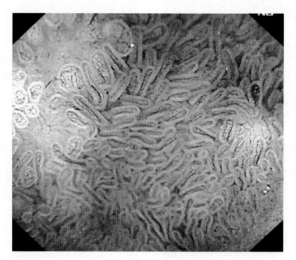

Figure 16.12 NBI with magnification of terminal ileal villi showing capillary loops and plexuses within individual villi. (James East, St Mark's Hospital.)

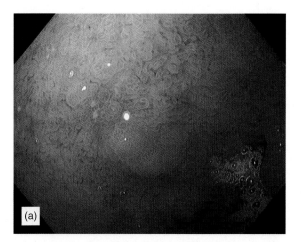 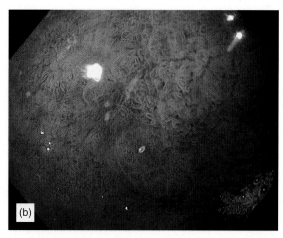

Figure 16.13 (a) Subtle inflammation of duodenal bulb on WL non-magnified view. (b) Subtle erosions and inflammation in duodenal bulb indicated on NBI non-magnified view. The contrast under NBI between the dark inflamed mucosa and the white erosion may make subtle findings such at these easier to detect. (Jonathan Cohen, NYU Langone School of Medicine.)

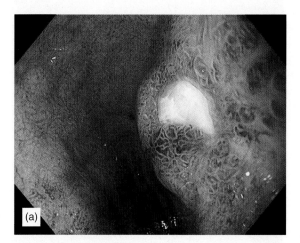 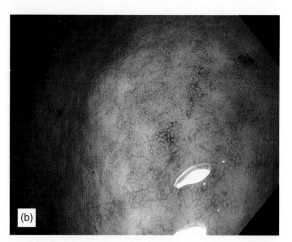

Figure 16.14 (a) This duodenal bulb ulcer was found in a patient taking baby aspirin following one episode of melena without abdominal pain. It is not known whether NBI will enhance detection of subtle stigmata. This HRE H180 image clearly defines the ulcer as clean based. (b) The antrum of the patient in (a) shows prominent lymphoid follicles and the histopathology confirmed active *Helicobacter pylori* gastritis. (Jonathan Cohen, NYU Langone School of Medicine.)

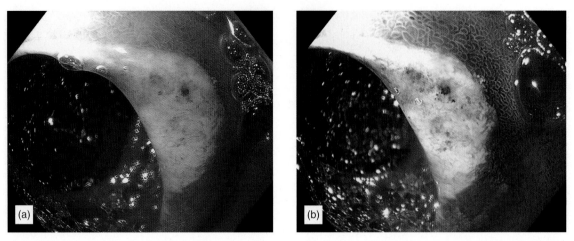

Figure 16.15 Large but superficial duodenal ulcer in (a) WL H190 and (b) NBI with flat dark spot. Copyright Jonathan Cohen, NYU Langone School of Medicine.

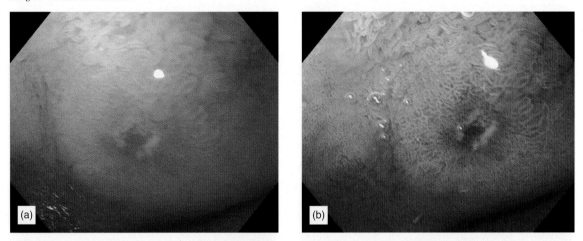

Figure 16.16 (a) Duodenal erosion faintly visible on WL H180 view seen here in 1.5× magnification. (b) Small duodenal erosion seen clearly with low-magnification NBI. (Jonathan Cohen, NYU Langone School of Medicine.)

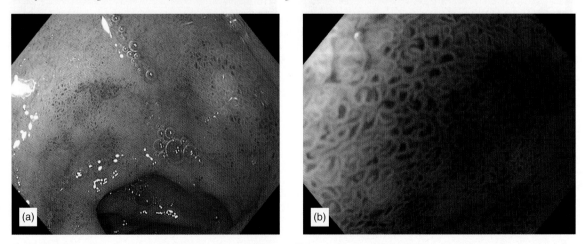

Figure 16.17 (a) Moderate peptic duodenitis under WL low magnification. (b) Magnified NBI view of moderate duodenitis of the bulb. Note the prominent though uniform vessels and preservation of normal mucosal pattern. H190 images. (Jonathan Cohen, NYU Langone School of Medicine.)

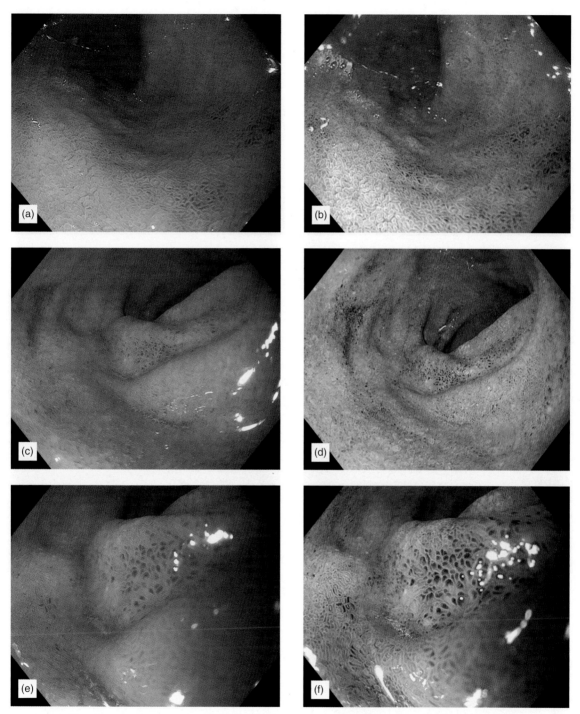

Figure 16.18 (a, b) Mild duodenitis of the bulb, WL and NBI H190 in low magnification. Mucosal pattern is preserved with no erosions though inflammation is clearly present. (c–f) Moderate duodenitis WL and NBI normal magnification and near focus views (e, f) identifying the patchy hyperemia without mucosal breaks. (Jonathan Cohen, NYU Langone School of Medicine.)

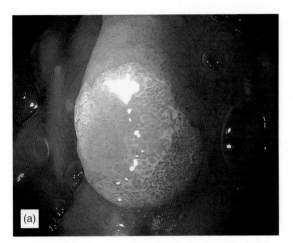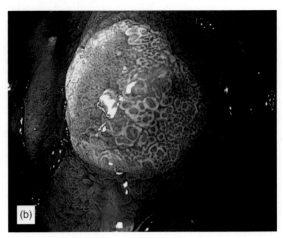

Figure 16.19 (a, b) WL and NBI H190 images of flat raised lesion in the duodenal bulb. The white tufted appearance on NBI raises suspicion for a duodenal adenoma. (Jonathan Cohen, NYU Langone School of Medicine.)

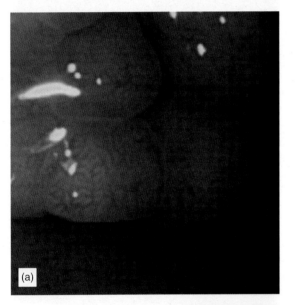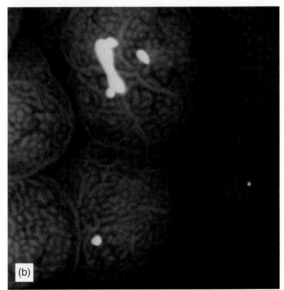

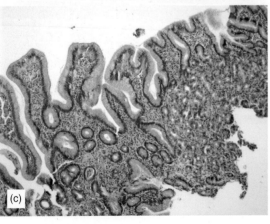

Figure 16.20 (a) Duodenal bulb hyperplastic polyp, WL H180 low magnification. (b) NBI view of gastric polyp located in the duodenal bulb. Regular gastric-type pit pattern seen well. (c) Oxyntic-type gastric crypts in the lamina propria (bottom right) and the lack of goblet and Paneth cells in the superficial epithelium are consistent with fundic-type gastric heterotopic epithelium. (Guido Costamagna, Catholic University of the Sacred Heart.)

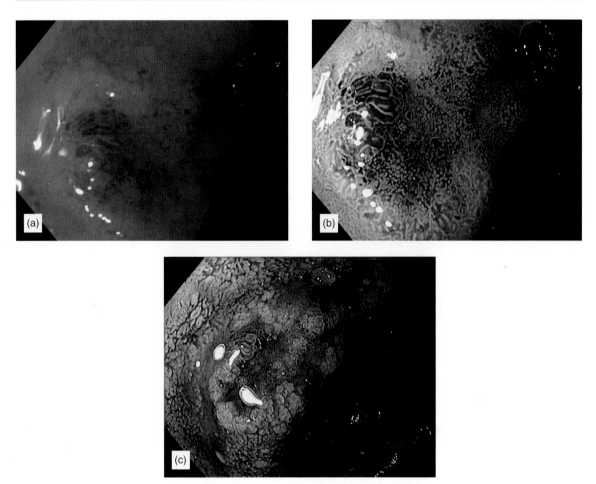

Figure 16.21 (a) This duodenal red slightly raised area here seen in low-magnification WL H180 might be mistaken for an area of duodenitis; however, note the irregularity of the vessels in comparison to the images of duodenitis in Figures 16.17 and 16.18. (b) On NBI, the gyrus mucosal surface pattern and vascular pattern more readily identify this lesion as an adenoma. (c) Indigocarmine view of the same lesion; NBI appears to provide better delineation of this adenoma. (Thierry Ponchon, Edouard Herriot Hospital.)

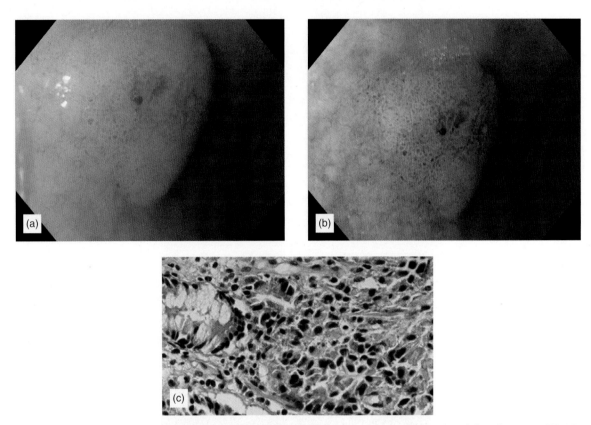

Figure 16.22 (a) Flat duodenal polyp; pathology revealed undifferentiated adenocarcinoma with invasion of the submucosa, HRE WL H180. (b) NBI low-magnification view of this flat duodenal bulb adenocarcinoma highlights abnormal surface contour and irregular vessels. (c) Poorly differentiated duodenal adenocarcinoma. (University Medical Center Hamburg Eppendorf.)

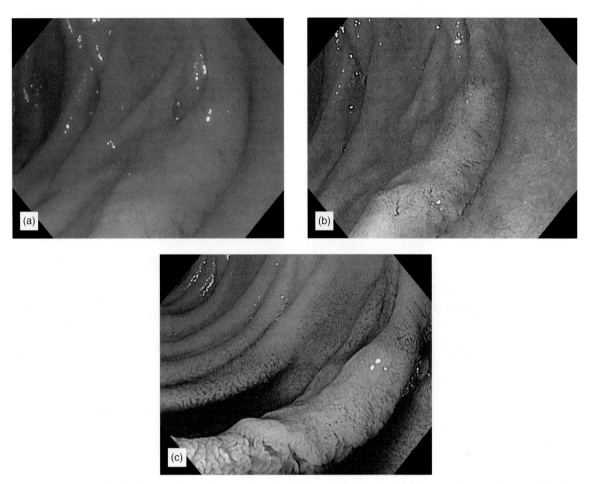

Figure 16.23 (a) Duodenal adenoma detected as an irregular fold on WL low magnification H180. (b) NBI low-magnification view of duodenal adenoma: the lesion appears whitish whereas the normal background is pink. Easier to be detected than WL. (c) Indigocarmine image provides similar image to NBI; NBI appears as easier replacement to chromoendoscopy. (Thierry Ponchon, Edouard Herriot Hospital).

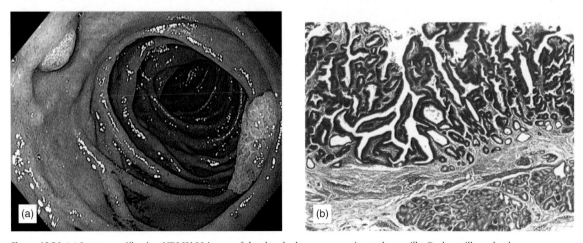

Figure 16.24 (a) Low-magnification NBI H180 image of duodenal adenoma opposite to the papilla. Both papilla and polyp appear gray and normal duodenal mucosa appears pink. (b) Duodenal adenoma. The normal mucosa is replaced by a tubulovillous proliferation lined by hyperchromatic dysplastic epithelium. (Thierry Ponchon, Edouard Herriot Hospital.)

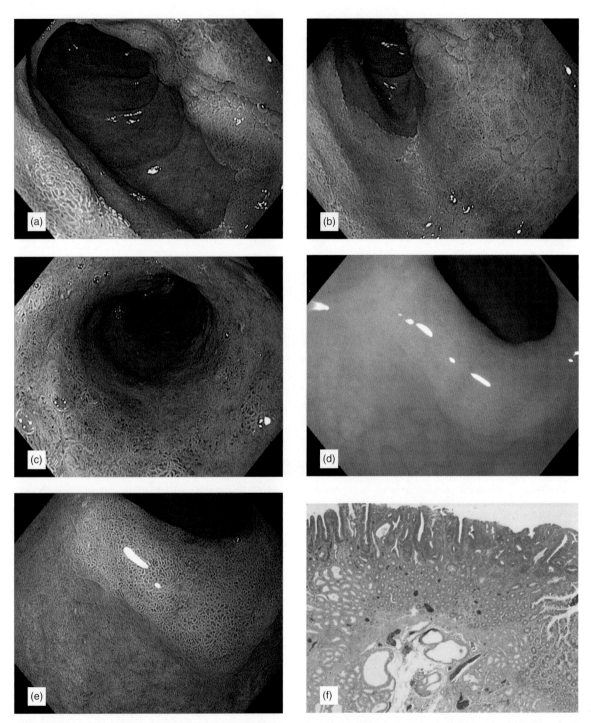

Figure 16.25 (a) Extensive circumferential duodenal adenoma from the pylorus to D3. Lower margin in D3 is very clearly discerned using NBI with low magnification H180. (b) NBI view of lower end of adenoma; notice the irregular surface pattern and vasculature highlighted by NBI. (c) NBI low-magnification view of middle of this lateral spreading adenoma. (d) Extensive duodenal adenoma from the pylorus to D3. View from the antrum: irregular pattern on the pylorus. WL non-magnified image. (e) Low-magnification NBI view from the antrum greatly accentuates the margin of the lesion compared to WL view shown in (c). (f) Duodenal adenoma. Dysplastic epithelium has replaced the duodenal epithelium in the upper half of the mucosa and spread widely, forming an extensive flat carpet of dysplasia. (Thierry Ponchon, Edouard Herriot Hospital).

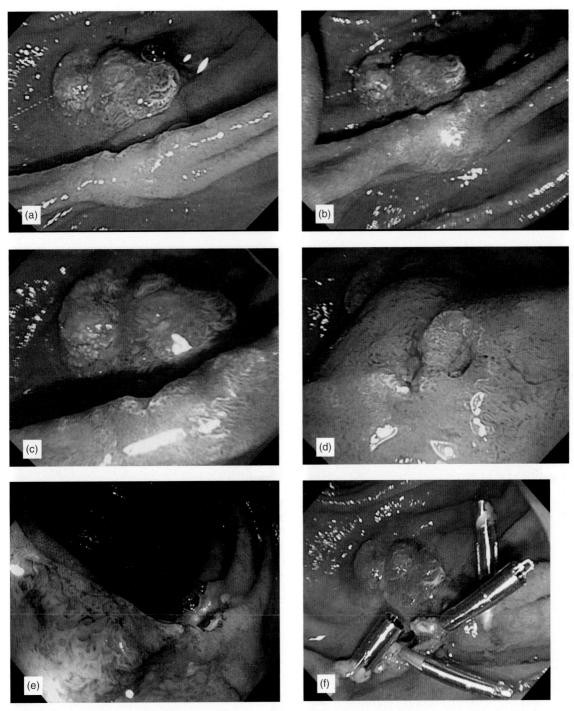

Figure 16.26 Periampullary adenoma image with duodenoscope. (a, b) Flat lesion with white tufted edges on fold WL view. (d) Post-injection lift with saline, dilute epinephrine and methylene blue. (e) NBI shows residual polyp to the left of the image. (f) Post resection with clip closure. (Jonathan Cohen, NYU Langone School of Medicine.)

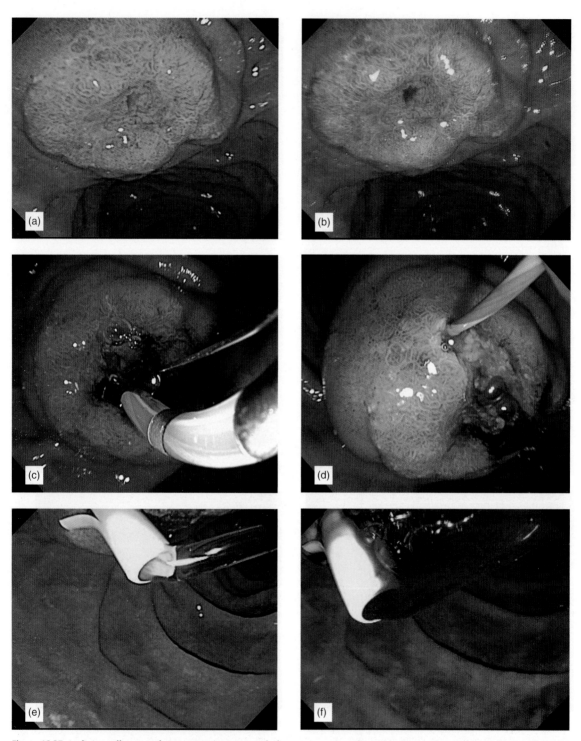

Figure 16.27 (a–f) Ampullary neoplasm presenting as post-cholecystectomy jaundice. Firm appearance and irregular vessels on NBI raise suspicion for advanced histology prompting sampling, sphincterotomy and plastic stenting pending results and consideration of surgical management, as shown.

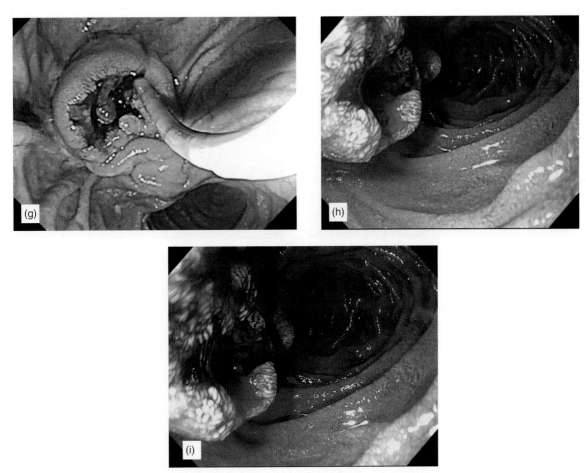

Figure 16.27 (Continued) (g–i) Repeat look in 2 months for stent change in this patient not resected due to significant co-morbidity more clearly demonstrates growing ampullary cancer. (Jonathan Cohen, NYU Langone School of Medicine.)

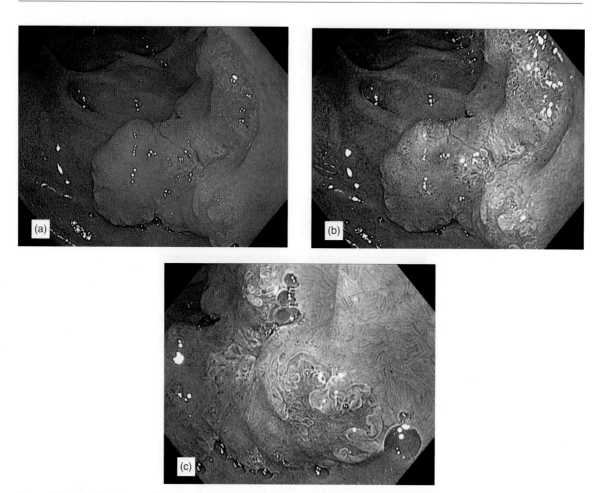

Figure 16.28 (a) WL low-magnification HRE H180 view of large sessile duodenal adenoma. (b) NBI low-magnification view of large sessile duodenal adenoma: better delineation and characterization with NBI. (c) This closer view with the same magnification illustrates the physical zoom property of HDTV endoscopy; image sharpness is not reduced when the scope tip is pushed closer to the lesion. (Thierry Ponchon, Edouard Herriot Hospital.)

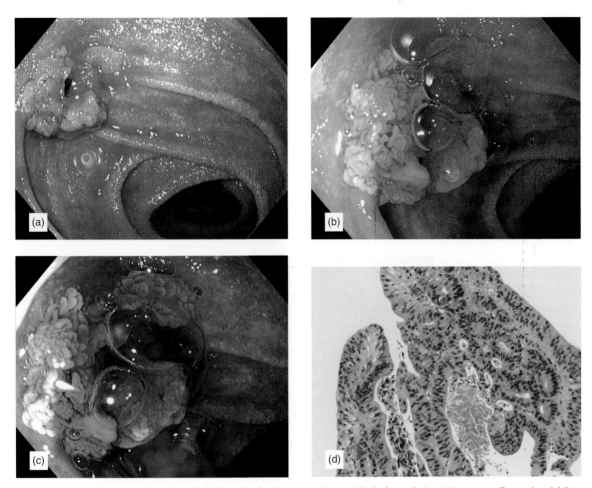

Figure 16.29 (a) Bile duct adenoma with high-grade dysplasia seen here with high-resolution WL (note yellow-colored bile). (b) Close-up high-resolution WL image of bile duct adenoma with high-grade dysplasia (note yellow-colored bile). (c) Close-up image of bile duct adenoma with high-grade dysplasia viewed with high-resolution NBI (note red-colored bile). (d) Histologic image of bile duct adenoma with high-grade dysplasia. (Mayo Clinic, Jacksonville.)

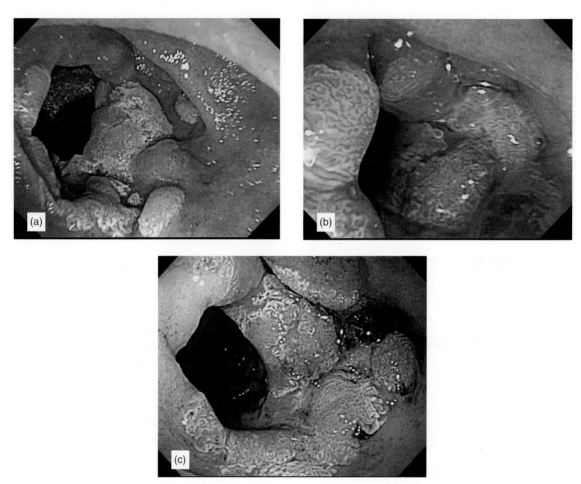

Figure 16.30 (a) WL view of duodenal adenoma. Note the white tufted appearance characteristic of adenomatous change in the duodenal mucosal. (b) WL near focus magnification of duodenal adenoma. (c) NBI view of duodenal adenoma. (Jonathan Cohen, NYU Langone School of Medicine).

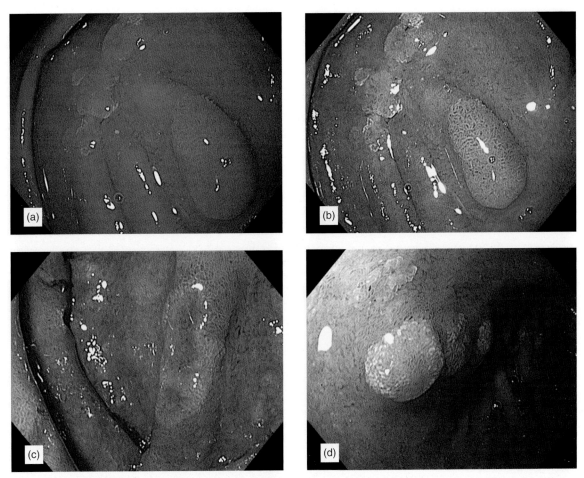

Figure 16.31 (a) WL H180 low-magnification view of familial adenomatous polyposis (FAP): duodenal lesions. (b) NBI image of FAP: duodenal lesions appear whitish on pink background. Better delineation and characterization than with WL. (c) Varying appearance of FAP: large gray–white lesion in the duodenum under NBI, low magnification. (d) FAP: several adenomas easily detected with NBI, here with a white appearance. Indigocarmine is not necessary for identification or assessment of borders. (Thierry Ponchon, Edouard Herriot Hospital.)

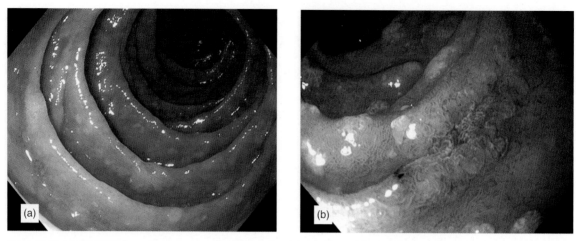

Figure 16.32 (a) WL H180 view of numerous small adenomas in D3 in a patient with FAP. (b) Magnification NBI view in this patient clearly defines the lesions as sessile adenomas. (James DiSario, University of Utah Health Sciences Center.)

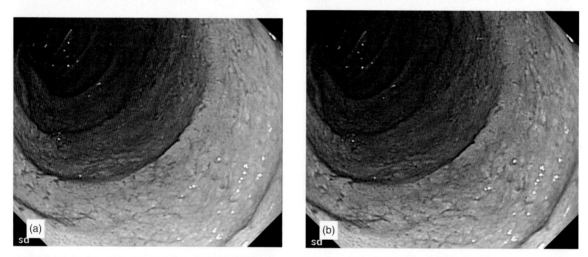

Figure 16.33 (a) Complete villous atrophy, WL H180 HRE low-magnification view. (b) Completely flattened villi seen on NBI low-magnification view. Histopathology confirmed endoscopic impression of total villous atrophy. (Jean-François Rey, Institut Arnault Tzanck.)

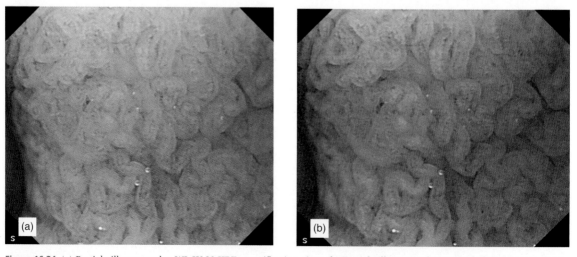

Figure 16.34 (a) Partial villous atrophy, WL H180 HRE magnification view. (b) Partial villous atrophy, magnified NBI image. (Jean-François Rey, Institut Arnault Tzanck.)

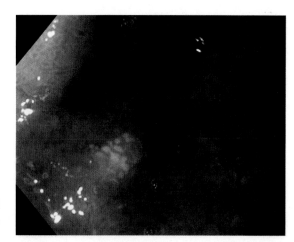

Figure 16.35 NBI H180 1.5× magnified view of jejunal lymphangiectasia in an efferent limb of a gastrojejunostomy. (Jonathan Cohen, NYU Langone School of Medicine.)

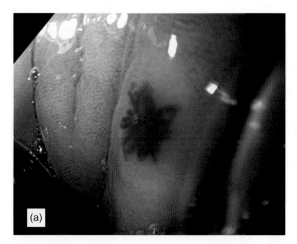

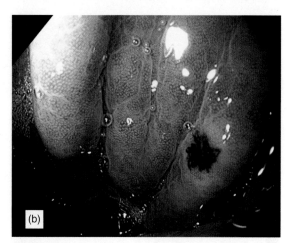

Figure 16.36 Arterio-vascular malformation (a) viewed with high-resolution WL H180. (b) viewed with high-resolution NBI. (Mayo Clinic, Jacksonville.)

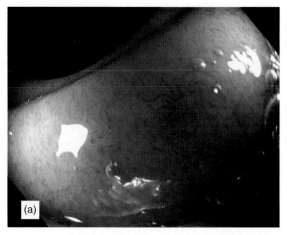

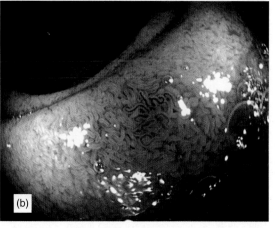

Figure 16.37 (a) Duodenal angioectasia with subtle appearance well appreciated using WL H180 HRE. (b) NBI view of the same lesion clearly enhances detection of this vascular abnormality. (Jean-François Rey, Institut Arnault Tzanck.)

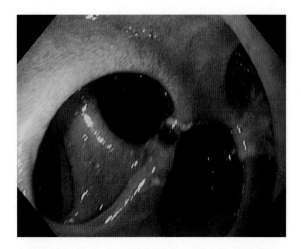

Figure 16.38 Multiple large duodenal diverticula, WL H180 low-magnification view. (Jean-François Rey, Institut Arnault Tzanck.)

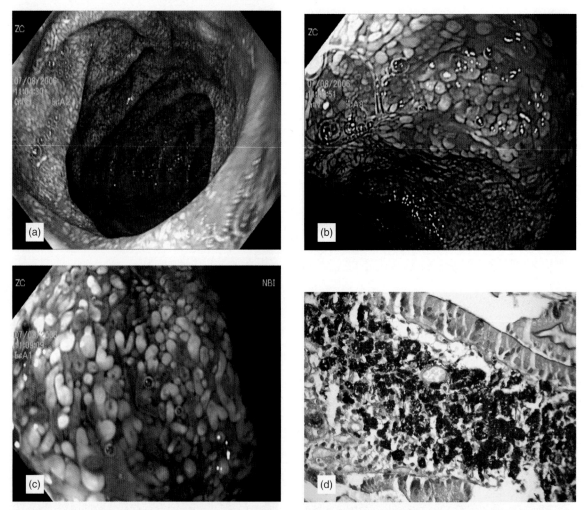

Figure 16.39 (a) Small bowel Whipple's disease with whitish plaque-like patches, WL H180 low-magnification view. (b) NBI view of small bowel Whipple's disease; the contrast highlights the whitish plaque-like patches. (c) NBI 1.5× magnification of small bowel Whipple's disease highlighting the whitish plaque-like patches. (d) Histologic image of Whipple's disease showing PAS-positive macrophages in lamina propria. (Guilherme Macedo, Hospital Sao Marcos.)

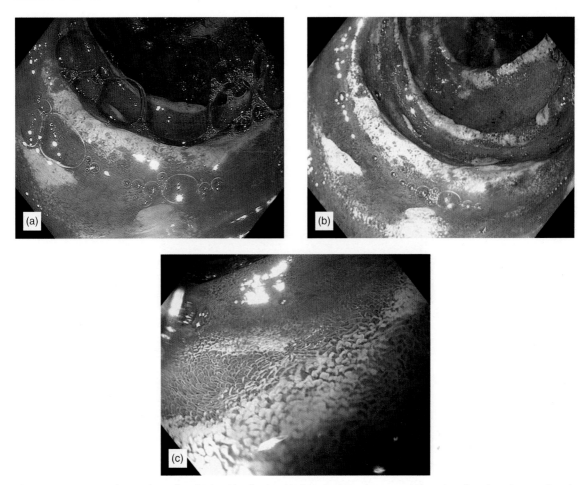

Figure 16.40 (a–c) Another etiology of multiple white duodenal lesions, in this case numerous large lymphangiectasias, seen here in WL H190 and NBI and NBI near focus views. (Jonathan Cohen, NYU Langone School of Medicine.)

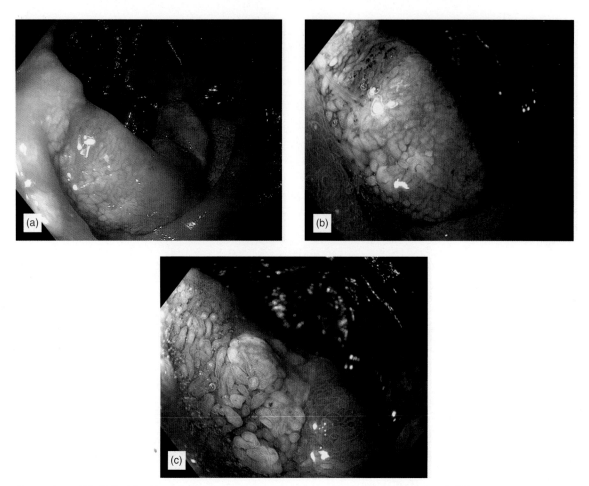

Figure 16.41 Thick fold with whitened villi raised suspicion for adenoma but biopsy diagnosed well-differentiated B-cell primary duodenal lymphoma: (a) WL H190, (b) NBI, and (c) NBI near-focus views. (Jonathan Cohen, NYU Langone School of Medicine.)

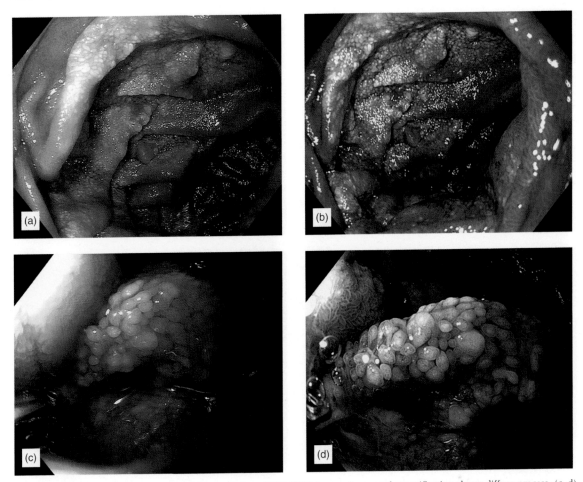

Figure 16.42 (a, b) Duodenal primary lymphoma, WL and NBI H190 images in normal magnification shows diffuse process. (c, d) Near-focus inspection of involved fold. (Jonathan Cohen, NYU Langone School of Medicine.)

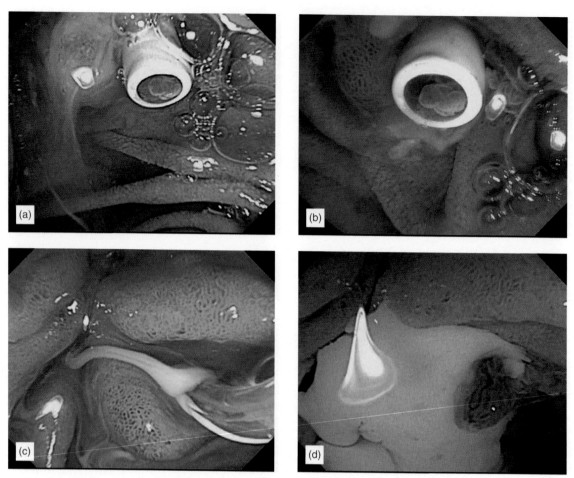

Figure 16.43 (a, b) Occluded bile duct stent and cholangitis WL and NBI view. (c–g) Stent removed with extrusion of pus followed metal biliary stent placement in this patient with locally advanced pancreatic cancer. (Jonathan Cohen, NYU Langone School of Medicine.)

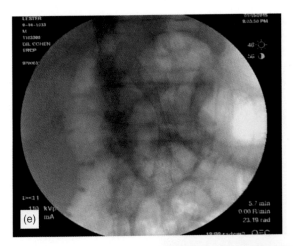

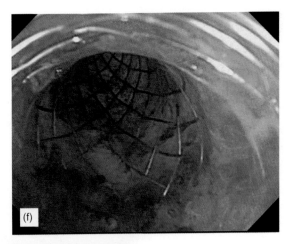

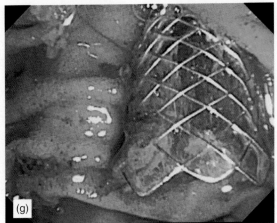

Figure 16.43 (Continued)

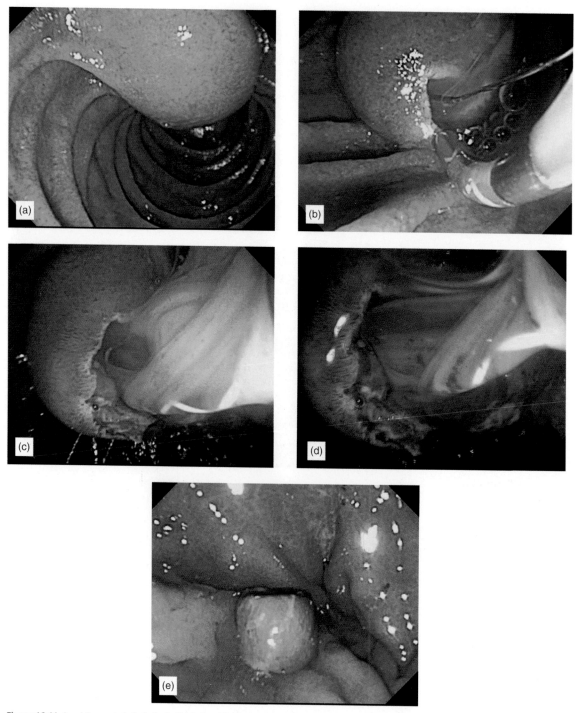

Figure 16.44 (a–e) Impacted choledocholithiasis with cholangitis and therapy. (Jonathan Cohen, NYU Langone School of Medicine.)

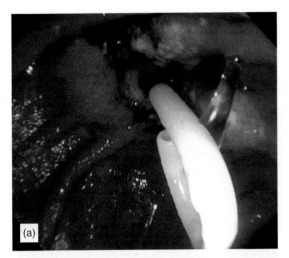 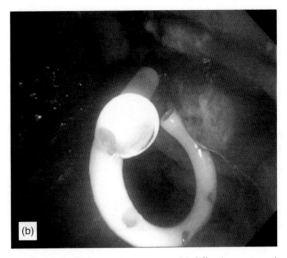

Figure 16.45 (a, b) Prophylactic 5 French pancreatic duct pigtail stent placed to prevent post-ERCP pancreatitis following pancreatic duct instrumentation. (Jonathan Cohen, NYU Langone School of Medicine.)

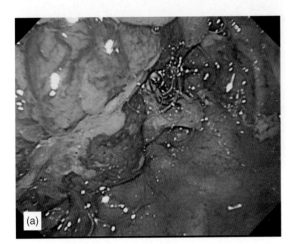 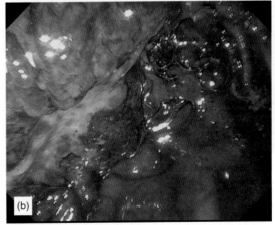

Figure 16.46 Occluded metal biliary stent in a patient with a gastrojejunostomy for duodenal obstruction from pancreatic cancer. (a, b) WL and NBI duodenoscope images of a mass growing into distal end of metal stent. (continued)

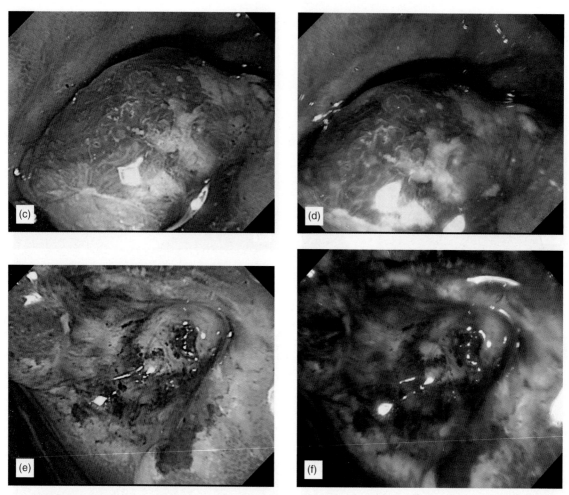

Figure 16.46 (Continued) (c, d) Mass obstructing the duodenum in the bulb. (e, f) Duodenal ulcerated mass in the afferent limb of a gastrojejunostomy anastomosis in patient with metastatic pancreatic cancer. (Jonathan Cohen, NYU Langone School of Medicine.)

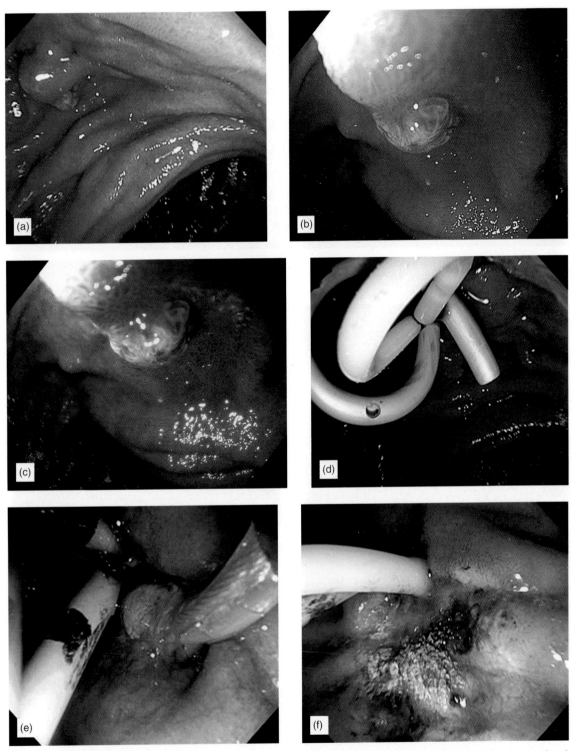

Figure 16.47 (a–f) WL and NBI images of ampullary adenoma before and after resection. Pancreatic and bile duct stents placed. (continued)

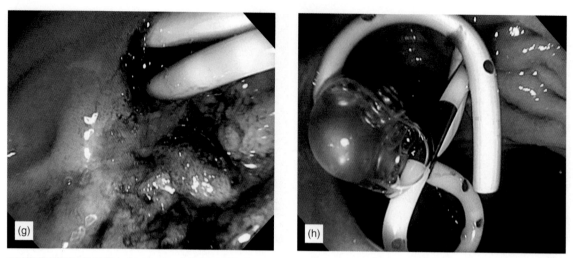

Figure 16.47 (Continued) (g, h) WL views of resection site showing cauterized borders and of dual biliary and pancreatic duct stents. (Jonathan Cohen, NYU Langone School of Medicine.)

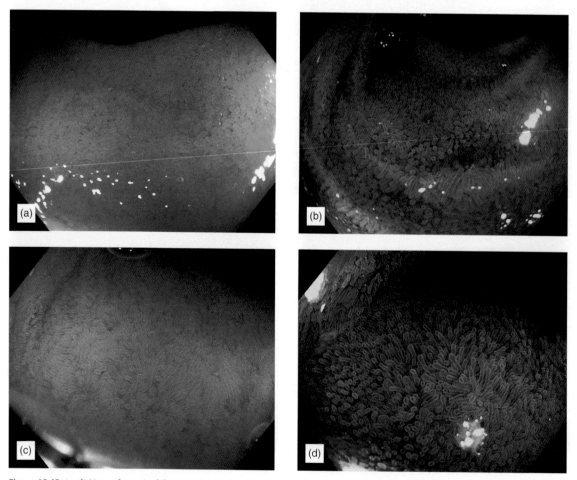

Figure 16.48 (a–d) Normal terminal ileum is shown in low magnification WL and NBI H190 and in near focus WL and NBI. (Jonathan Cohen, NYU Langone School of Medicine.)

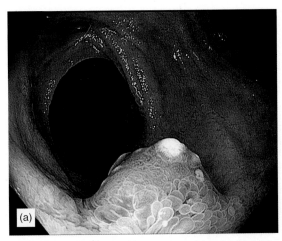
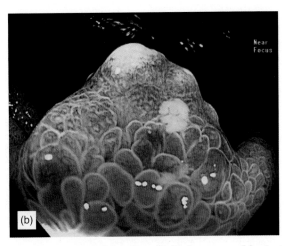

Figure 16.49 (a, b) WL low magnification H190 with methylene blue spray and NBI near focus views. Ileal inflammatory polyp just proximal to the ileocolonic anastomosis in a patient with inactive Crohn's ileocolitis after ileal resection. (Jonathan Cohen, NYU Langone School of Medicine.)

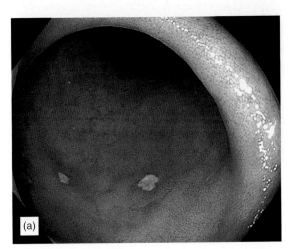
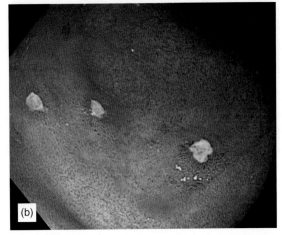

Figure 16.50 (a, b) WL and NBI H190 views of isolated small ileal erosions in otherwise normal mucosa with no clinical suspicion of Crohn's disease raises concern for non-IBD etiology such as NSAID use. (Jonathan Cohen, NYU Langone School of Medicine.)

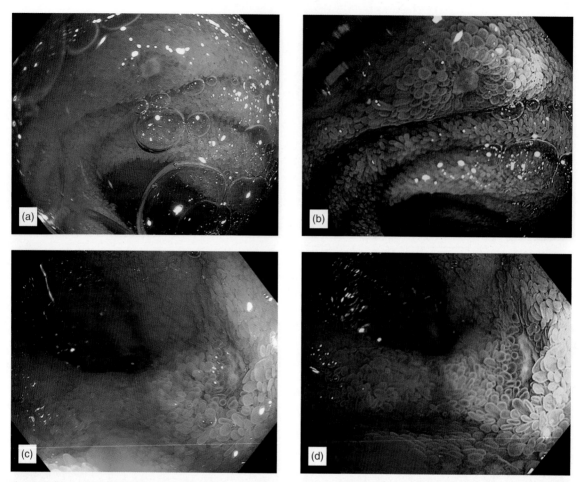

Figure 16.51 (a–d) Isolated ileal erosions of uncertain significance found incidentally on colonoscopy H190 WL and NBI low magnification views with normal surrounding ileal mucosa. Nonspecific ileitis on biopsy. (Jonathan Cohen, NYU Langone School of Medicine.)

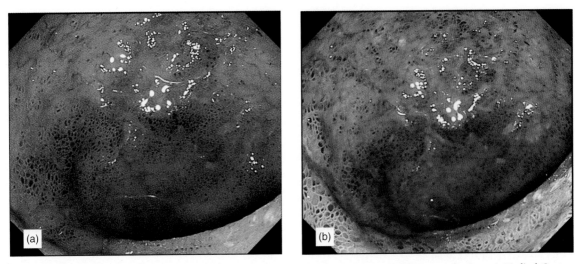

Figure 16.52 Ileitis in patient with active Crohn's disease, WL and NBI H190 views. (Krish Ragunath, Queen's Medical Centre, Nottingham.**)**

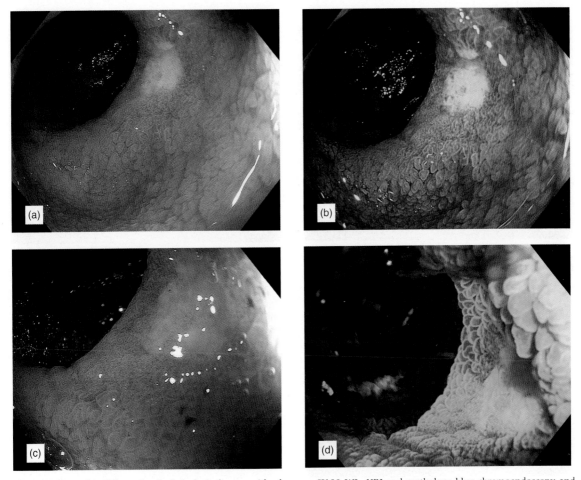

Figure 16.53 (a–d) Mildly active ileal Crohn's disease with ulcers on H190 WL, NBI and methylene blue chromoendoscopy and magnification view of larger ulcer with NBI. (Jonathan Cohen, NYU Langone School of Medicine.)

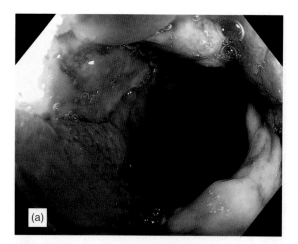

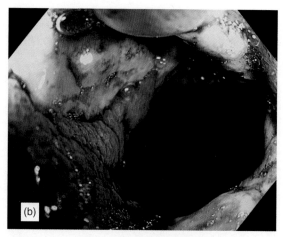

Figure 16.54 (a, b) Sizable Crohn's ulceration in terminal ileum in WL H190 with chromoendoscopy and NBI. (Jonathan Cohen, NYU Langone School of Medicine.)

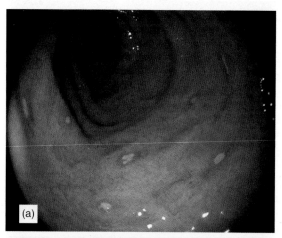

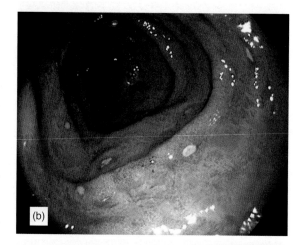

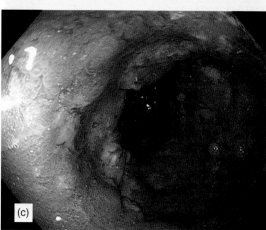

Figure 16.55 (a) WL H180 low-magnification image of multiple small ulcers of the distal ileum due to NSAIDs. Note the reddened borders of the punctate white lesions indicating that these are ulcerations. On NBI in (b), these appear as dark rings providing striking contrast to the erosions within. (b) NBI low-magnification image of distal ileal ulcers due to NSAIDs. (James DiSario, University of Utah Health Sciences Center). (c) WL view depicts multifocal abnormal ileal mucosa in Crohn's disease. This appearance is more diffuse than the punctate NSAID-associated ileal ulcers depicted in (a) and (b). The degree of mucosal irregularity stands in considerable contrast to the bumpy lymphoid tissue of the normal ileum (Figure 16.11). (Jean-François Rey, Institut Arnault Tzanck.)

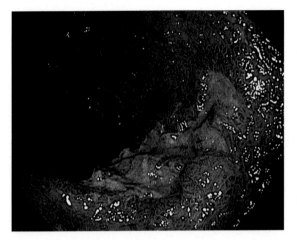

Figure 16.56 NBI H180 image clearly delineates a large ileal Crohn's ulcer along with diffuse inflammation of the surrounding tissue. (Jean-François Rey, Institut Arnault Tzanck.)

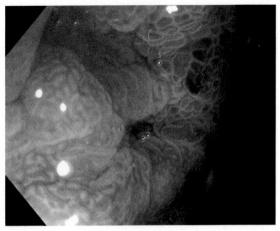

Figure 16.57 Aphthous ulcer in terminal ileum in Crohn's disease. The heaped-up epithelium surrounds a tiny ulcer. NBI H180 view. (Jerome Waye, Mount Sinai School of Medicine.)

ABBREVIATIONS

ERCP   endoscopic retrograde cholangiopancreatography
FAP   familial adenomatous polyposis
HDTV   high-definition TV
HRE   high-resolution endoscopy
NBI   narrowband imaging
NSAID   nonsteroidal anti-inflammatory drug
PAS   periodic acid–Schiff
WL   white light

 Video clips to accompany this book can be found in the online material at www.wiley.com/go/cohen/NBI

17 Colon atlas

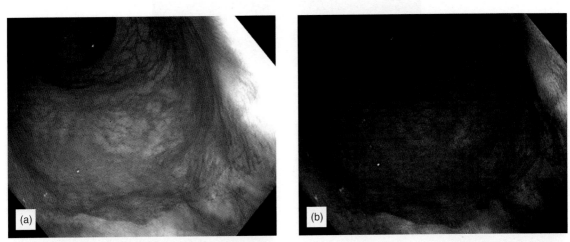

Figure 17.1 (a) WL H180 HRE low-magnification view of normal rectum with clear demarcation of the dentate line. (b) Similar view of normal rectum seen here in low-magnification NBI. (Jonathan Cohen, NYU Langone School of Medicine.)

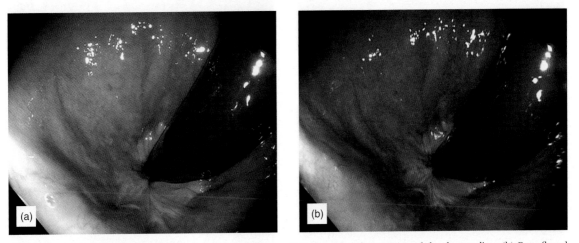

Figure 17.2 (a) Retroflexed H180 WL view of a normal rectum. Note the sharp demarcation of the dentate line. (b) Retroflexed NBI view of a normal rectum. Note the sharp demarcation of the dentate line. (James DiSario, University of Utah Health Sciences Center.)

Comprehensive Atlas of High-Resolution Endoscopy and Narrowband Imaging, Second Edition. Edited by Jonathan Cohen.
© 2017 John Wiley & Sons, Ltd. Published 2017 by John Wiley & Sons, Ltd.
Companion website: www.wiley.com/go/cohen/NBI

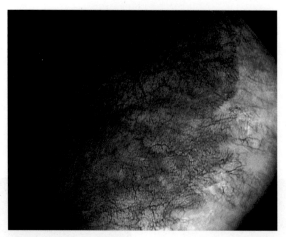

Figure 17.3 NBI view clearly demarcating dentate line. (Jonathan Cohen, NYU Langone School of Medicine.)

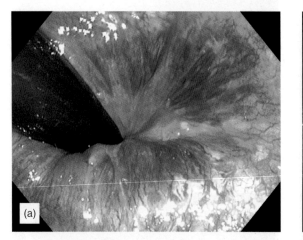

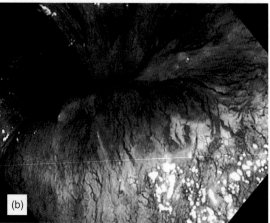

Figure 17.4 (a) WL H180 retroflex view of distal rectum. (b) NBI H180 rectal retroflex view highlights prominent vascular pattern. (Jonathan Cohen, NYU Langone School of Medicine.)

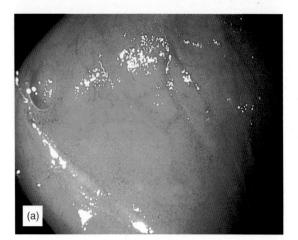

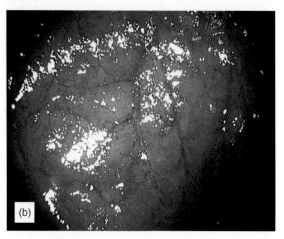

Figure 17.5 (a) WL H180 view of normal colon. (b) NBI non-magnified view of normal colon demonstrates vascular pattern poorly seen on WL view (a). (Jonathan Cohen, NYU Langone School of Medicine.)

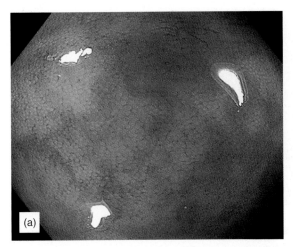
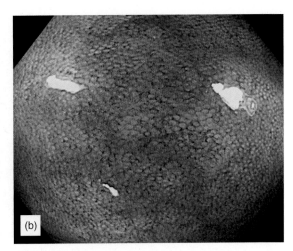

Figure 17.6 (a, b) Normal colon, WL and NBI H190 near-focus examination of the mucosal and vessel pattern. Deeper larger vessels appear bluish-green and the more superficial capillaries lining the normal pits appear brown and allow excellent inspection of the pit pattern. (Jonathan Cohen, NYU Langone School of Medicine.)

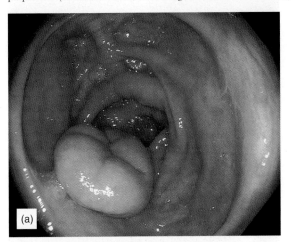
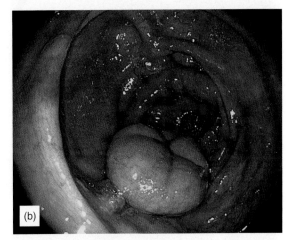

Figure 17.7 (a, b) Lipomatous enlarged ileocecal valve at first gives impression of mass; WL and NBI H190 views. (Jonathan Cohen, NYU Langone School of Medicine.)

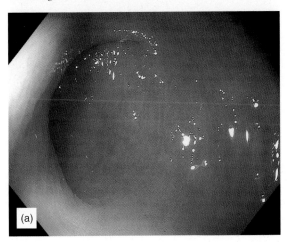
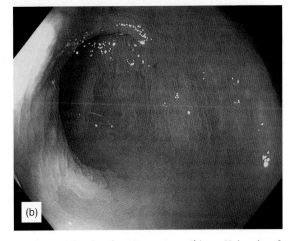

Figure 17.8 (a, b) Normal WL and NBI H190 view of the cecum normal appendiceal orifice. (James Lau, Chinese University of Hong Kong.)

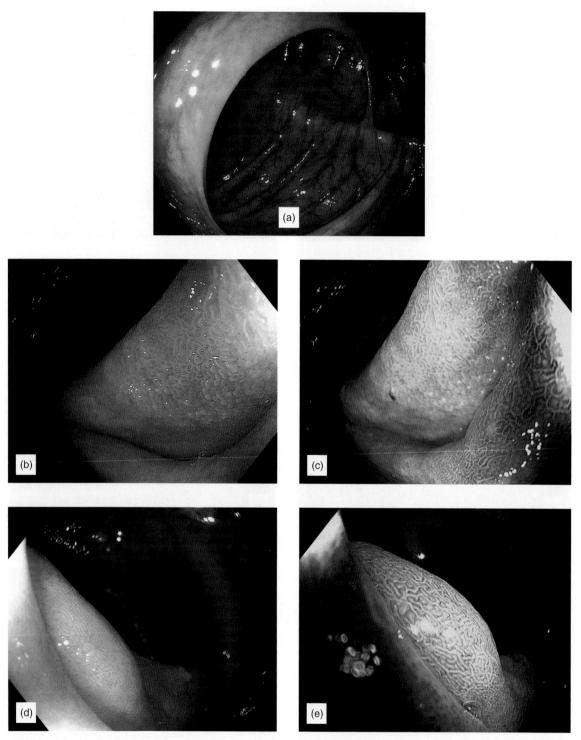

Figure 17.9 (a) WL view of ileocecal valve on approach to cecum. (b–e) WL and NBI views of transitional mucosa with regular flat villous pattern. (Jonathan Cohen, NYU Langone School of Medicine.)

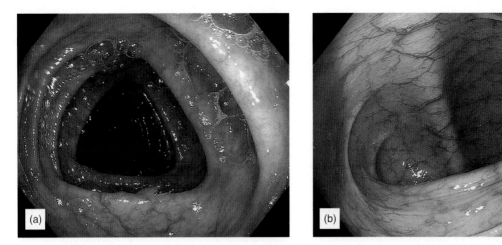

Figure 17.10 Normal transverse colon (a) and sharp angulation at splenic flexure (b) WL H190. (Jonathan Cohen, NYU Langone School of Medicine.)

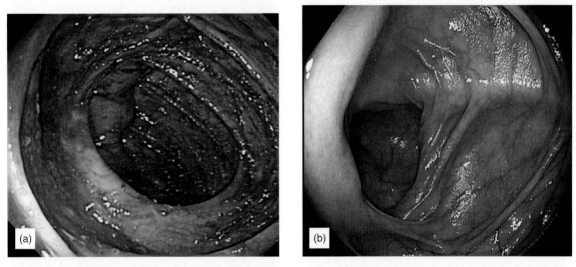

Figure 17.11 (a) Fair preparation not adequate to detect polyps <5 mm or flat serrated polyps and take advantage of imaging advances for detection and diagnosis of polyps. Unless sufficiently cleaned with irrigation during the examination, a sub-par preparation should prompt repeat examination within the year. (b) WL H180 image of the ileocecal valve with excellent preparation. (Jonathan Cohen, NYU Langone School of Medicine.)

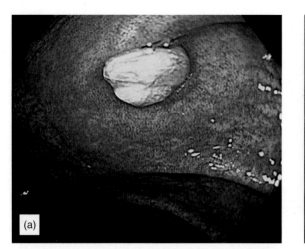
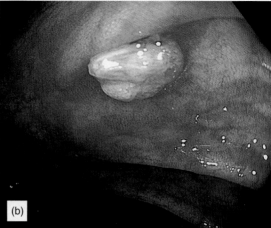

Figure 17.12 (a, b) Residual stool on NBI might be mistaken for a sessile polyp until clearly identified on WL H190 view. (Jonathan Cohen, NYU Langone School of Medicine.)

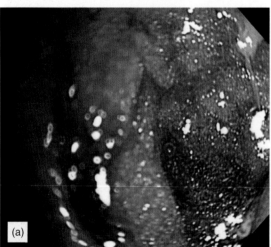
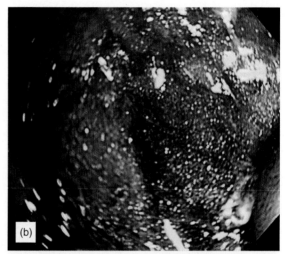

Figure 17.13 (a) Post-polypectomy from ileocecal valve, submucosal fat viewed under WL H180. (b) NBI image has no advantage in viewing submucosal fat. (Gregory Haber, Lenox Hill Hospital.)

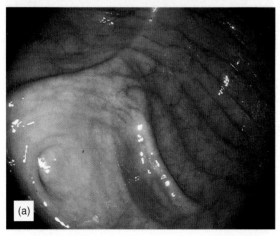
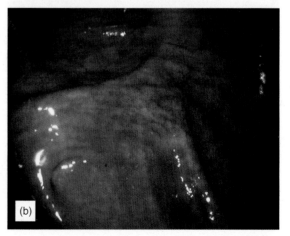

Figure 17.14 (a) Normal appendiceal orifice viewed with WL H180 HRE. (b) Normal appendiceal orifice viewed with NBI light. (James DiSario, University of Utah Health Sciences Center.)

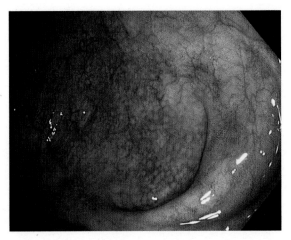

Figure 17.15 Non-magnified view of normal appendiceal orifice with prominent lymphoid tissue highlighted with NBI H180. (Jonathan Cohen, NYU Langone School of Medicine.)

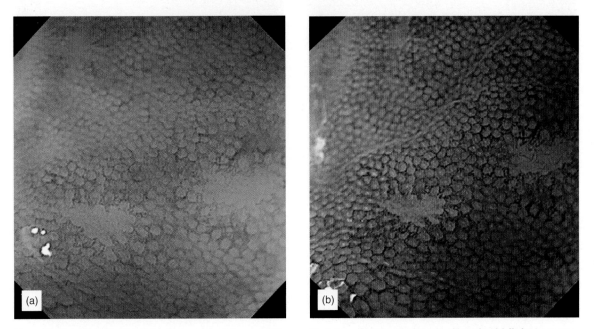

Figure 17.16 (a) Lymphoid follicles in cecum seen here on WL magnified view. (b) Magnified image of lymphoid follicles in cecum. Note honeycomb capillary plexuses around pits in normal mucosa seen well with NBI. (James East, St Mark's Hospital.)

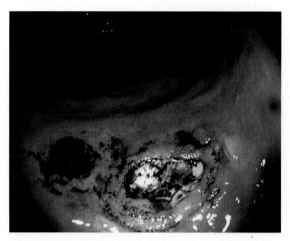

Figure 17.17 NBI H180 image post biopsy. (James DiSario, University of Utah Health Sciences Center.)

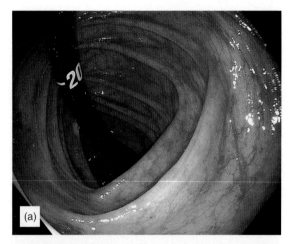

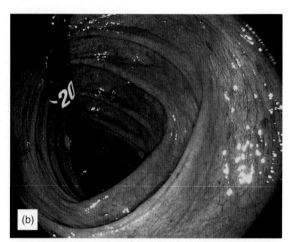

Figure 17.18 (a) Retroflexion WL view of one patient and (b) retroflexion NBI H190 view of another with normal right colon on surveillance examination. (Jonathan Cohen, NYU Langone School of Medicine.)

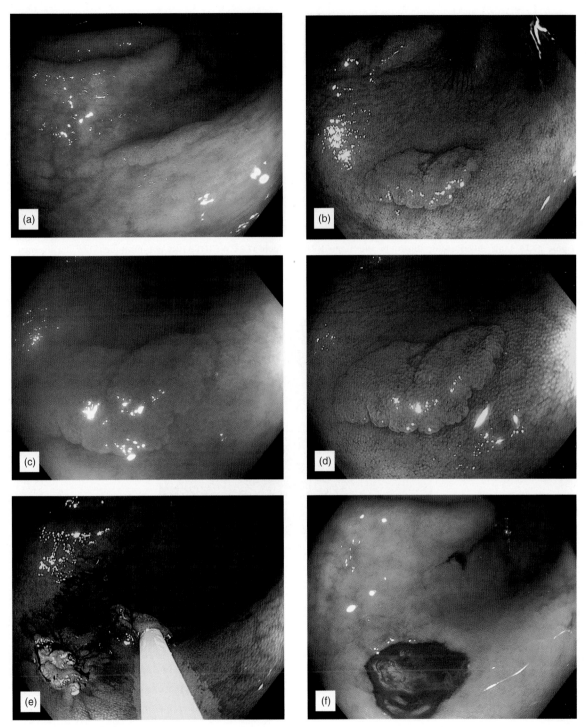

Figure 17.19 (a–f) Retroflexion in cecum: WL and NBI H190 views reveal 10-mm flat adenoma that was the only lesion in this 52-year-old male patient on screening examination. (Jonathan Cohen, NYU Langone School of Medicine.)

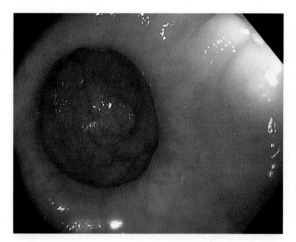

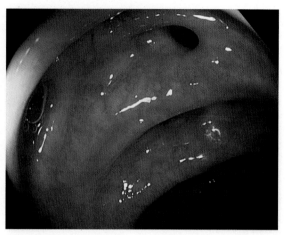

Figure 17.20 Large diverticulum shown in WL H180 HRE view. (Jonathan Cohen, NYU Langone School of Medicine.)

Figure 17.21 WL H180 HRE non-magnified view of a diverticulum. (Jonathan Cohen, NYU Langone School of Medicine.)

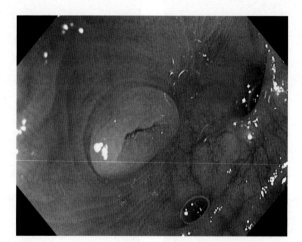

Figure 17.22 Everted diverticulum with NBI H180 image confirming normal colon pit pattern to avoid mistaken identification as a polyp. (Jonathan Cohen, NYU Langone School of Medicine.)

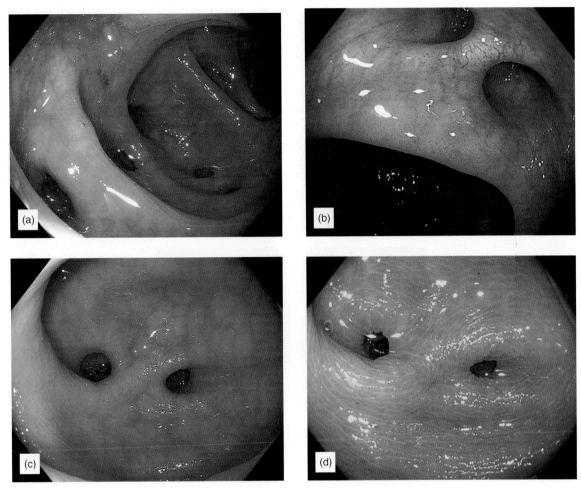

Figure 17.23 (a–d) Images of colonic diverticula H190 WL and NBI views (Jonathan Cohen, NYU Langone School of Medicine.)

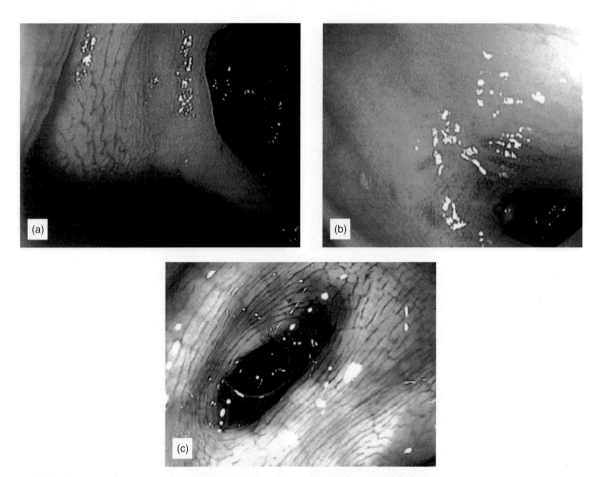

Figure 17.24 (a) WLE H180 view of active arterial bleeding from a diverticulum at 9 o'clock, during urgent colonoscopy. (b) Non-bleeding visible vessel at the neck of a diverticulum, a major stigma of gastrointestinal hemorrhage. (c) Adherent clot in a diverticulum, another major stigma. (Dennis Jensen, David Geffen School of Medicine at UCLA.)

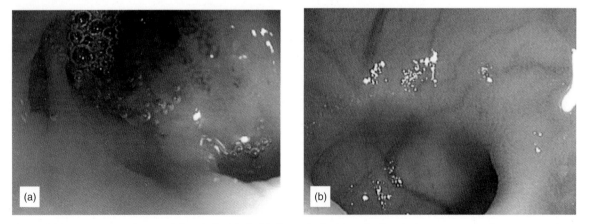

Figure 17.25 WL H180 HRE images of diverticula. (a) Flat black spot in the base of a diverticulum on urgent colonoscopy, a minor stigma of diverticular hemorrhage. (b) Clean diverticulum with normal vessels running from the neck into the base; diagnosis on urgent colonoscopy only presumptive of diverticular bleed since no stigmata seen. (Dennis Jensen, David Geffen School of Medicine at UCLA.)

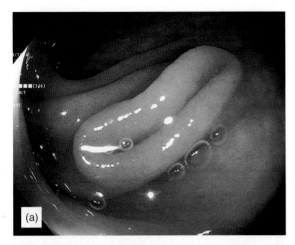 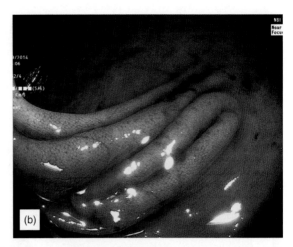

Figure 17.26 (a) An amorphous appearance on WL H190 view of this ridge-like protruberance with a depressed center. (b) With NBI and near focus, the normal pit pattern on the edges of this oblong ridge is clearly visible, and can be compared with the pattern on adjacent mucosal folds. This is a partially inverted diverticulum. (Jerome Waye, Mount Sinai School of Medicine.)

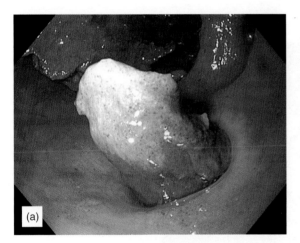 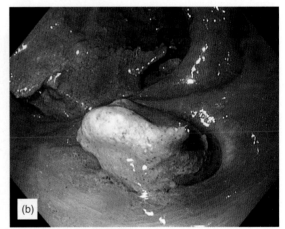

Figure 17.27 (a) Residual stool within diverticulum, WL H190 view. (b) NBI image of residual stool lodged in a diverticulum. Stool appears pink in NBI. (Jonathan Cohen, NYU Langone School of Medicine.)

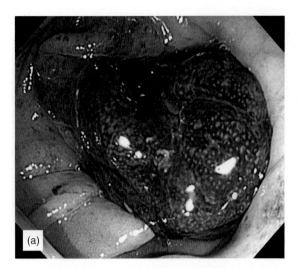 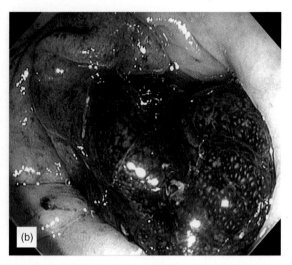

Figure 17.28 (a) Polypoid red fold of diverticular disease; note normal pit pattern. (b) Polypoid red fold of diverticular disease; note normal pit pattern on NBI H190 image. (Mount Sinai School of Medicine.)

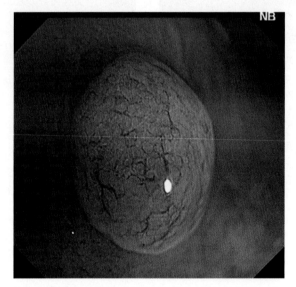

Figure 17.29 Magnified NBI H190 image of hyperplastic polyp showing fine vessels and type 2 pit pattern. (James East, St Mark's Hospital.)

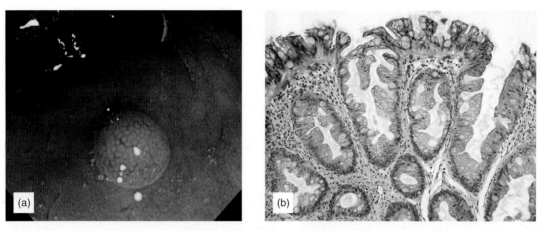

Figure 17.30 (a) Hyperplastic-appearing pit pattern on NBI non-magnified view of rectal polyp, Q180 non-high definition scope which still has NBI capability. (b) Hyperplastic polyp. Surface and gland epithelium, composed of tall cells with small basal nuclei and eosinophilic cytoplasm with mucin droplets, is thrown into papillary folds giving glands a serrated appearance. (Jonathan Cohen, NYU Langone School of Medicine.)

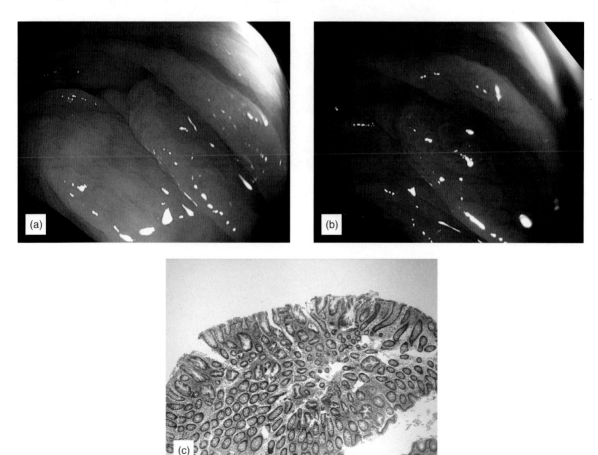

Figure 17.31 (a) Small hyperplastic polyp in the transverse colon in WL H180, low magnification. (b) NBI image of small hyperplastic transverse colon polyp, type 1 pits. (c) Small proximal colon hyperplastic polyp in low power. (Douglas K. Rex, Indiana University School of Medicine.)

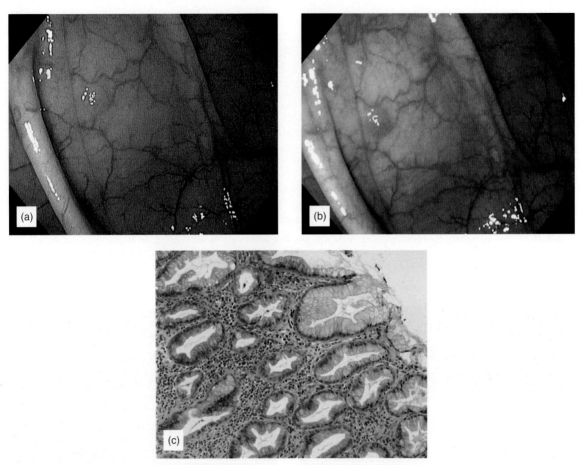

Figure 17.32 (a) WL H180 image fails to demonstrate a polyp. (b) NBI view reveals a tiny hyperplastic polyp seen only with NBI: red–brown in color. (c) Hyperplastic polyp. Gland lumens appear stellate in histologic section and are lined by bland mucinous epithelium. (Thierry Ponchon, Edouard Herriot Hospital.)

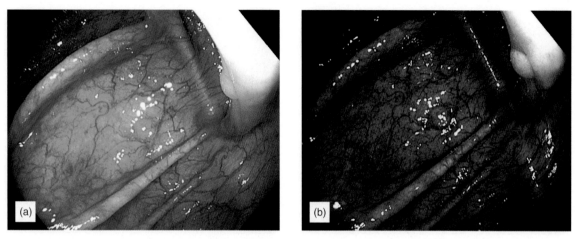

Figure 17.33 (a) Small polyp on fold in upper right of image barely visible even on high-resolution WL H180 view. (b) The same small polyp easily identified on NBI low-magnification view. (Jonathan Cohen, NYU Langone School of Medicine.)

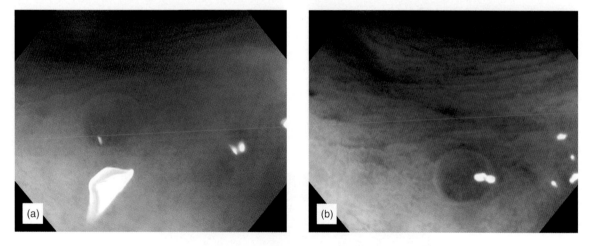

Figure 17.34 (a) Barely discernible 1-mm rectal polyp seen with WL H180. (b) Clearly discernible 1-mm rectal polyp seen with NBI light with the characteristic pitted appearance of a hyperplastic polyp. (James DiSario, University of Utah Health Sciences Center.)

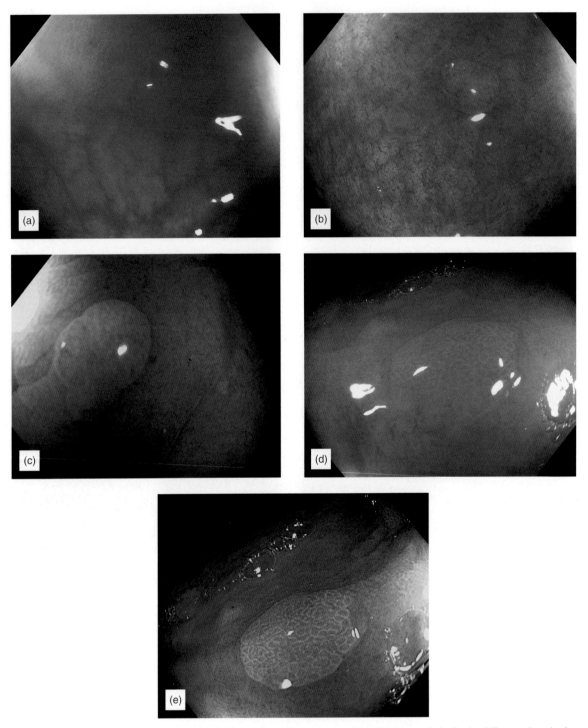

Figure 17.35 Hyperplastic polyps. (a, b) Typical bland vascular pattern on WL and NBI H190; note lack of color difference from background makes this polyp only detected on NBI view. (c) Small polyp NBI view shows round dark spots surrounded by white pattern. Note color of polyps similar to surrounding mucosa. (d, e) WL and NBI near focus identify the round dark spot pattern characteristic of hyperplastic polyps. (Jonathan Cohen, NYU Langone School of Medicine.)

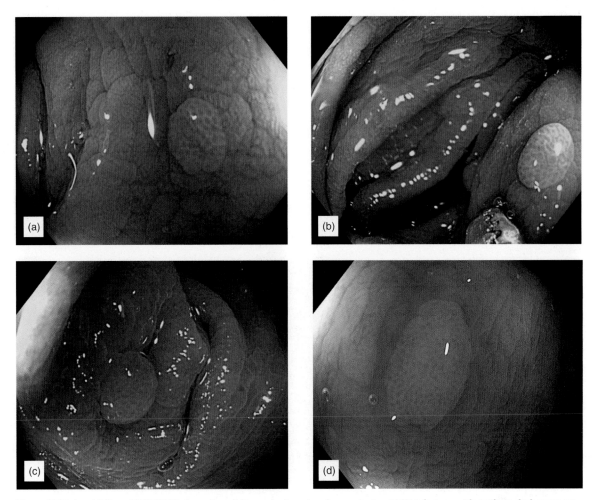

Figure 17.36 (a–g) WL and NBI H190 view of small hyperplastic polyp demonstrating NICE 1 feature with uniform dark spots surrounded by white borders. (Jonathan Cohen, NYU Langone School of Medicine.) (continued)

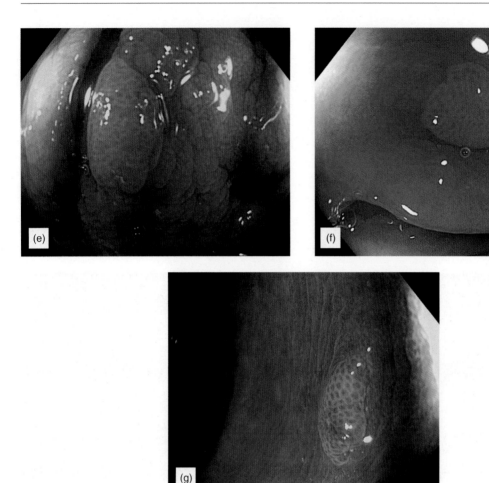

Figure 17.36 (Continued)

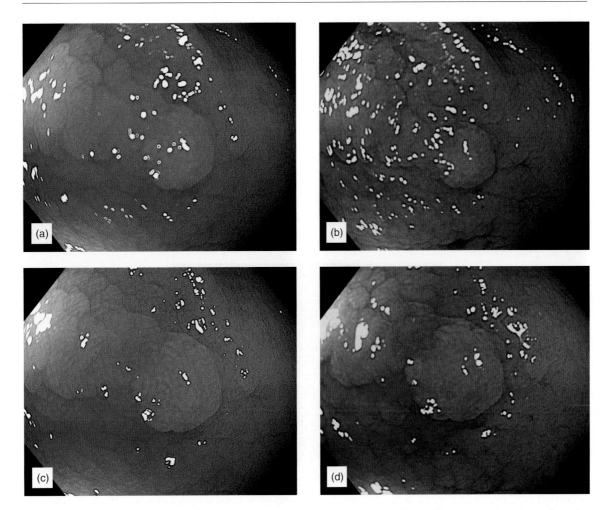

Figure 17.37 (a–d) This small polyp is suspicious for being a hyperplastic polyp on normal magnification NBI H190 view with a color similar to the background, yet is not possible to discern the mucosal and vascular patterns (a). (b, c) WL and NBI near focus views show the uniform distribution of black round dots surrounded by white, characteristic for hyperplastic polyps. (Jonathan Cohen, NYU Langone School of Medicine.)

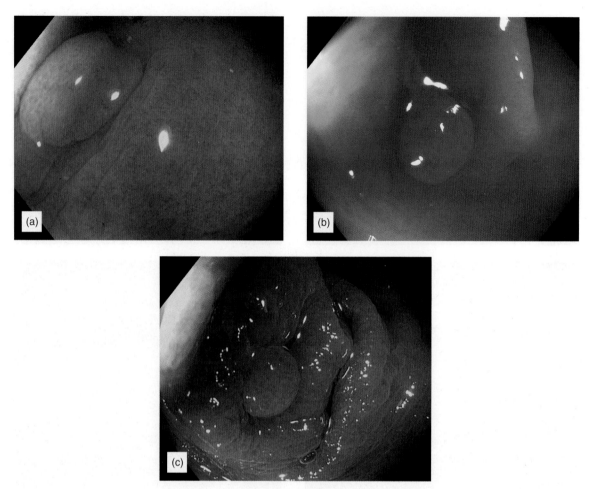

Figure 17.38 (a–c) Hyperplastic polyps with NICE 1 features on WL and NBI H190 views. Note round pattern with uniform dark spots with white background, and similar color of polyp and surrounding mucosa. (Jonathan Cohen, NYU Langone School of Medicine.)

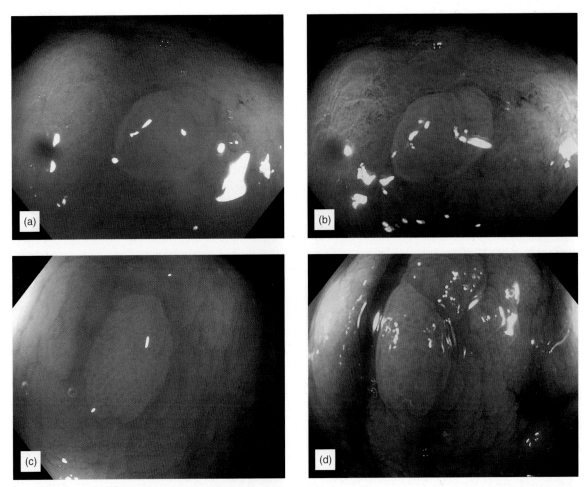

Figure 17.39 (a, b) Hyperplastic polyp with bland pattern with minimal to no visible vessels on polyp. (c, d) Hyperplastic polyp with round pattern on top half and bland pattern on lower half. WL and NBI H190 low magnification views. (Jonathan Cohen, NYU Langone School of Medicine.)

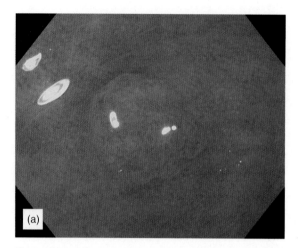

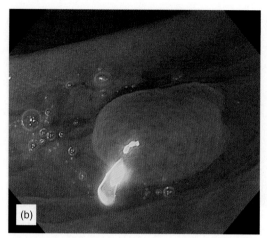

Figure 17.40 (a, b) H190 NBI images of hyperplastic NICE 1 polyp. Note Sano type 1 vessel pattern and similar color of polyp to surrounding normal mucosa. (James Lau, Chinese University of Hong Kong.)

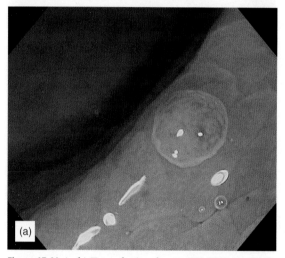

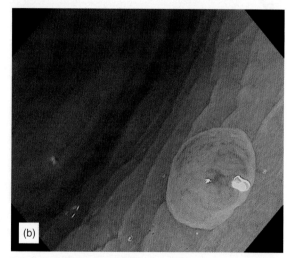

Figure 17.41 (a, b) Hyperplastic polyp on NBI H190 view in low and high magnification with bland mucosal pattern. (James Lau, Chinese University of Hong Kong.)

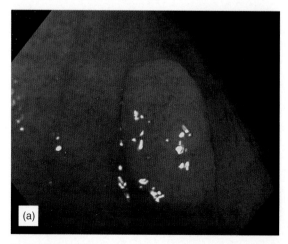

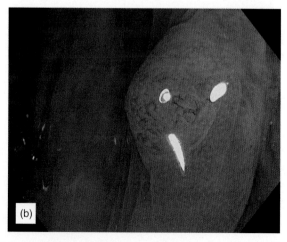

Figure 17.42 (a, b) Two polyps with mixed areas of NICE 1 and NICE 2 characteristics H190 NBI views. Any uncertainty in an optical diagnosis program necessitates histopathologic analysis as a low confidence lesion. (James Lau, Chinese University of Hong Kong.)

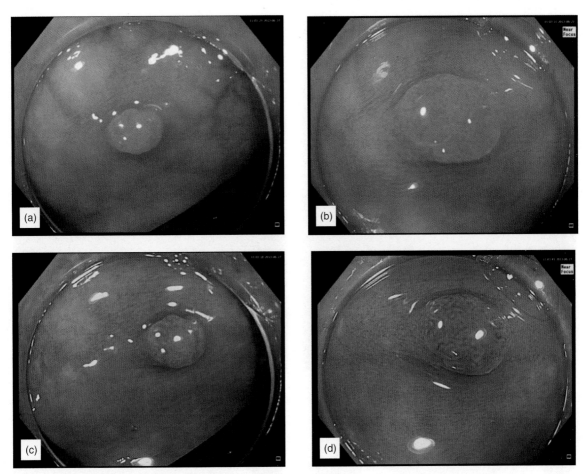

Figure 17.43 Tubular adenoma of colon. (a) H190 WL endoscopy reveals a sessile polyp measuring approximately 4 mm; after resection, pathology reveals the polyp to be a tubular adenoma. (b) WL near-focus view of the same polyp. (c) H190 NBI reveals a tubulo-gyrus surface pattern of the polyp consistent with an adenomatous colon polyp. (d) NBI near-focus view of the same polyp allows for better characterization of the polyp surface pattern. (Neil Gupta, Loyola University Health System.)

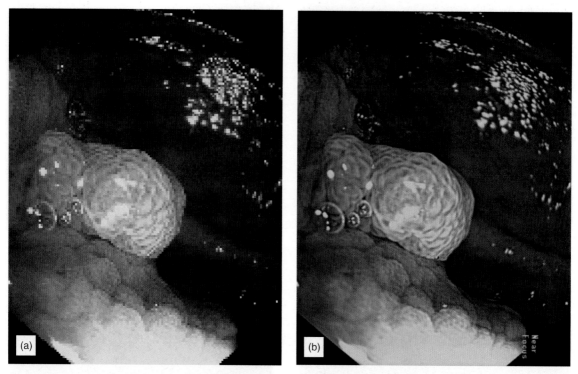

Figure 17.44 Near-focus H190 image of sessile adenoma: (a) low-resolution image storage (66 kb) and (b) high-resolution tiff format (843 kb) of the same polyp. Optical biopsy will require high-resolution photodocumentation and storage to confirm findings. (Jonathan Cohen, NYU Langone School of Medicine.)

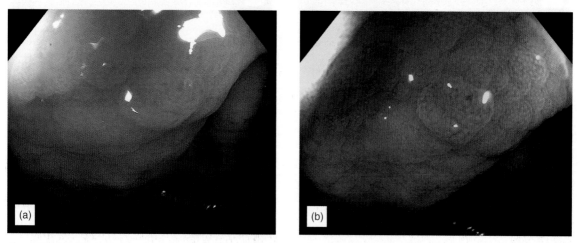

Figure 17.45 (a, b) Diminutive adenoma on WL and NBI H190 views. White dots surrounded by dark lines supports optical diagnosis of adenoma by NICE criteria. (Jonathan Cohen, NYU Langone School of Medicine.)

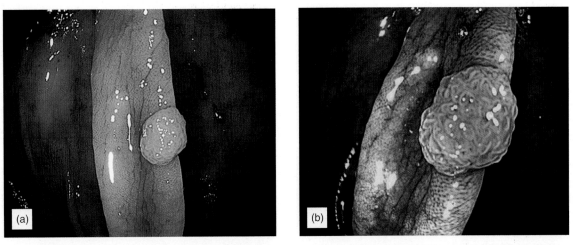

Figure 17.46 (a, b) Small tubular adenoma on WL and NBI H190 near-focus views. (Jonathan Cohen, NYU Langone School of Medicine.)

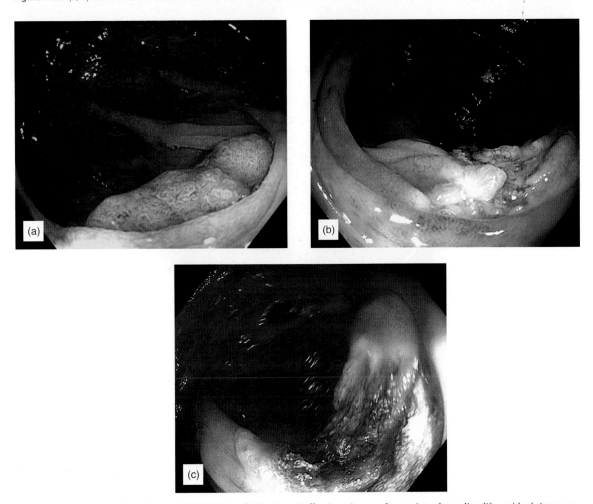

Figure 17.47 (a–c) Large flat adenoma NBI H190 and WL views. Following piecemeal resection after saline lift, residual tissue can be removed via avulsion with hot biopsy forceps. Argon plasma coagulation (APC) fulguration of the entire base is used to reduce residual adenoma at the site. (Jonathan Cohen, NYU Langone School of Medicine.)

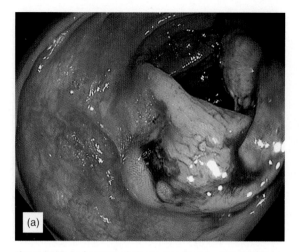 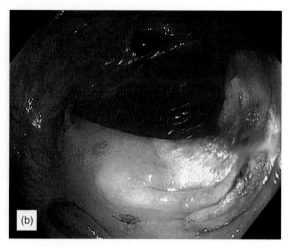

Figure 17.48 (a, b) Optimal placement of tattoo mark. Tattoos are seen better under WL H190 and not NBI. Note placement proximal and distal to APC-fulgurated base of resected sessile polyp, at least 3 cm away from the lesion. (Jonathan Cohen, NYU Langone School of Medicine.)

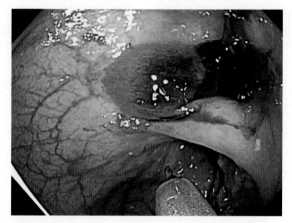

Figure 17.49 Ink tattoo in colon seen well in these images only on WL H190 view. (Jonathan Cohen, NYU Langone School of Medicine.)

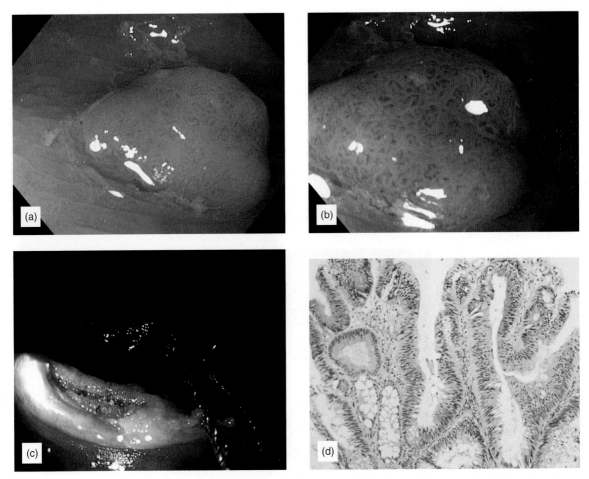

Figure 17.50 (a) WL H180 view of sessile polyp. (b) NBI image of adenoma; note high clusters of brown vessels. (c) Post-polypectomy inspection of polyp border NBI H180 view; normal pit pattern confirms complete resection. (d) Tubulovillous adenoma with low-grade dysplasia. Glands and villi are lined by mucin-depleted cells with enlarged stratified hyperchromatic nuclei that contrast with entrapped normal glands (bottom left). (Jonathan Cohen, NYU Langone School of Medicine.)

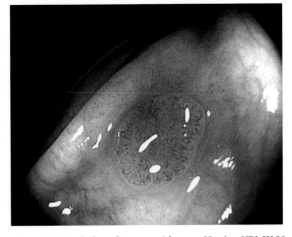

Figure 17.51 Tubular adenoma with type 3L pits. NBI H180 low-magnification view. Note also the well-demarcated margins (Douglas K. Rex, Indiana University School of Medicine.)

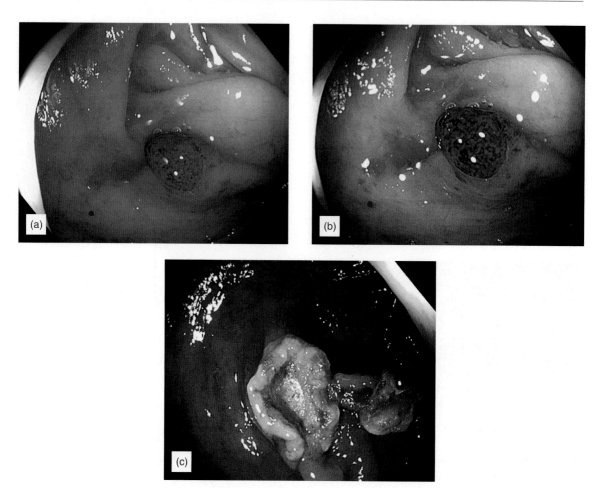

Figure 17.52 (a) WL H180 HRE suggests adenoma vs. inflammatory polyp in this patient with a history of malignant melanoma. (b) NBI magnification view of this small polyp provides extremely precise determination of its adenomatous pit pattern and vascularity, and pathology confirmed it to be a tubular adenoma. (c) NBI image following polypectomy clearly indicates complete removal of polyp tissue. (Jonathan Cohen, NYU Langone School of Medicine.)

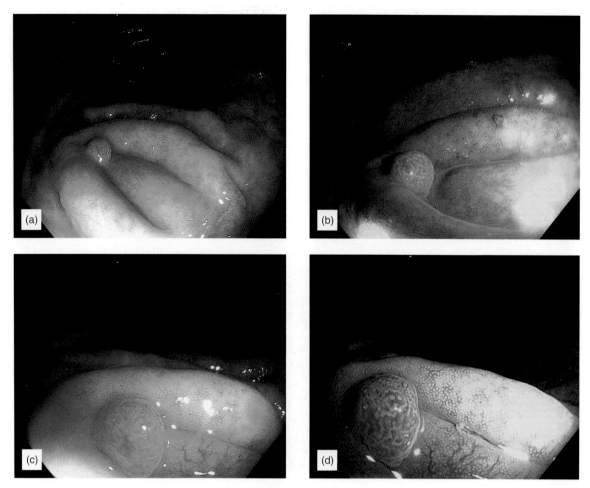

Figure 17.53 (a–d) WL and NBI H190 images of adenoma on the rim of the appendiceal orifice, normal and magnification near focus views. (Jonathan Cohen, NYU Langone School of Medicine.

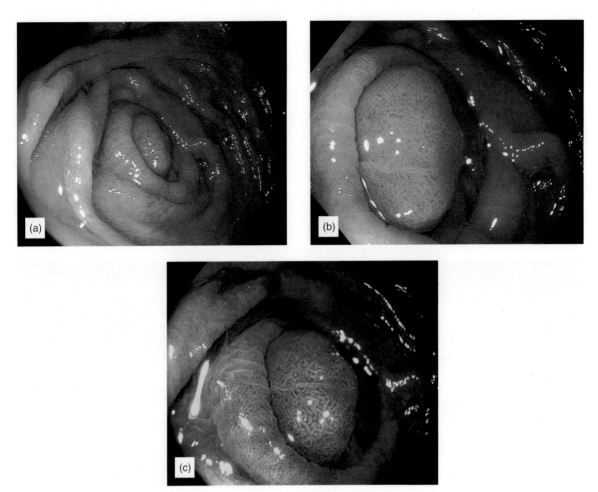

Figure 17.54 (a–c) Adenoma completely within the appendiceal orifice, WL and NBI H190 images. (Jonathan Cohen, NYU Langone School of Medicine.)

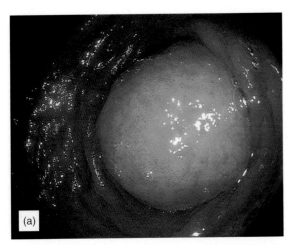 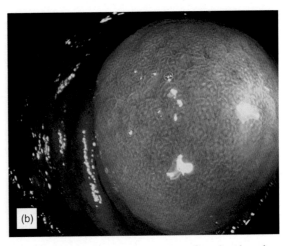

Figure 17.55 (a, b) Submucosal serous peri-appendiceal 2-cm cyst in WL and NBI H190 views. Diagnosis confirmed with probe-based endoscopic ultrasound. Near-focus NBI clearly shows normal mucosal pit pattern. (Jonathan Cohen, NYU Langone School of Medicine.)

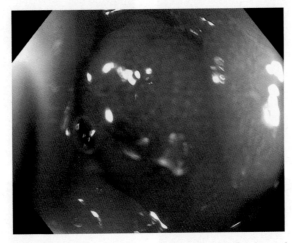

Figure 17.56 Acute inflammation in appendiceal orifice detected on colonoscopy in patient who presented with intermittent abdominal pain over 3 weeks WL H190 view. (Jonathan Cohen, NYU Langone School of Medicine.)

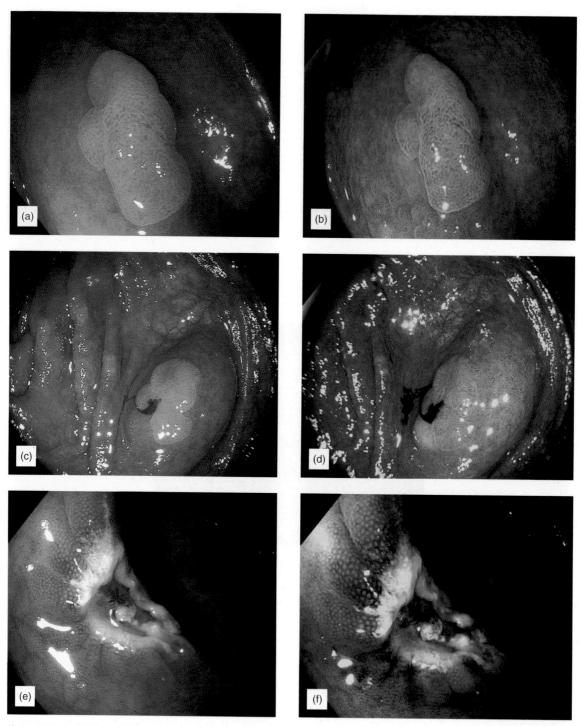

Figure 17.57 (a–f) WL and NBI H190 views of irregular border sessile adenoma, saline lift, and post-endoscopic mucosal resection (EMR) demonstration of normal surrounding pits confirming complete resection. (Jonathan Cohen, NYU Langone School of Medicine.)

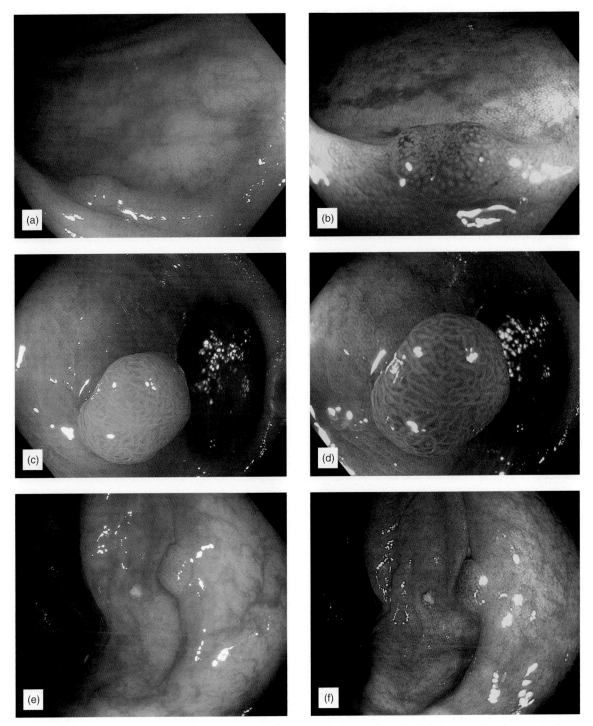

Figure 17.58 (a–j) NICE 2 adenomas in WL, NBI low magnification, and NBI near focus (b, d, j) demonstrating the gyrus pattern. (Jonathan Cohen, NYU Langone School of Medicine.) (continued)

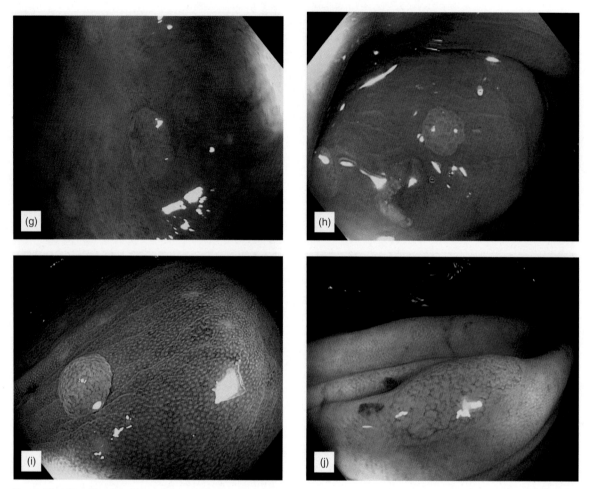

Figure 17.58 (Continued)

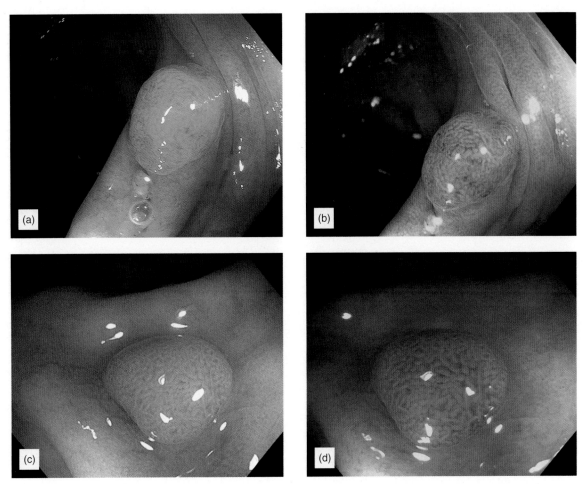

Figure 17.59 (a–d) WL and NBI H190 images of NICE 2 tubular adenomas. (Jonathan Cohen, NYU Langone School of Medicine.)

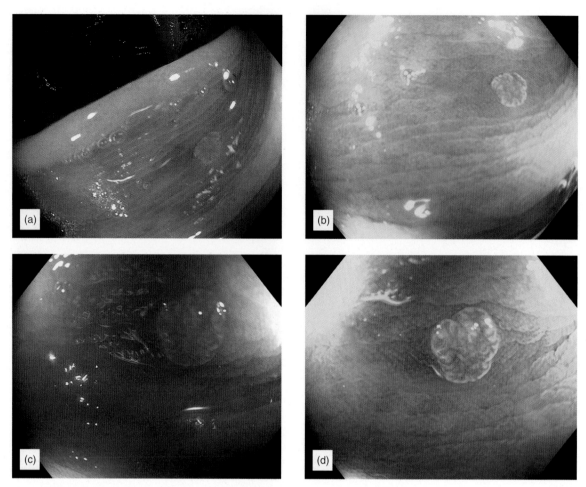

Figure 17.60 (a–d) Diagnosis of diminutive tubular adenoma by NICE criteria can be made with more confidence using magnification WL H190 and NBI with near focus. (Jonathan Cohen, NYU Langone School of Medicine.)

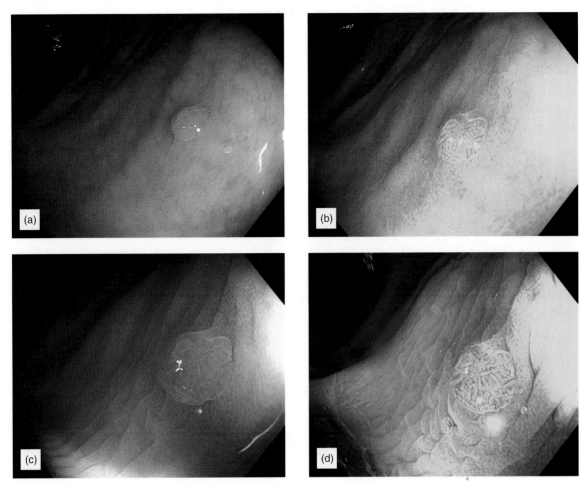

Figure 17.61 Diminutive tubular adenoma with characteristic findings discernible on WL H190 and NBI low-magnification views in this case (a, b) without requiring near focus (c, d). (Jonathan Cohen, NYU Langone School of Medicine.)

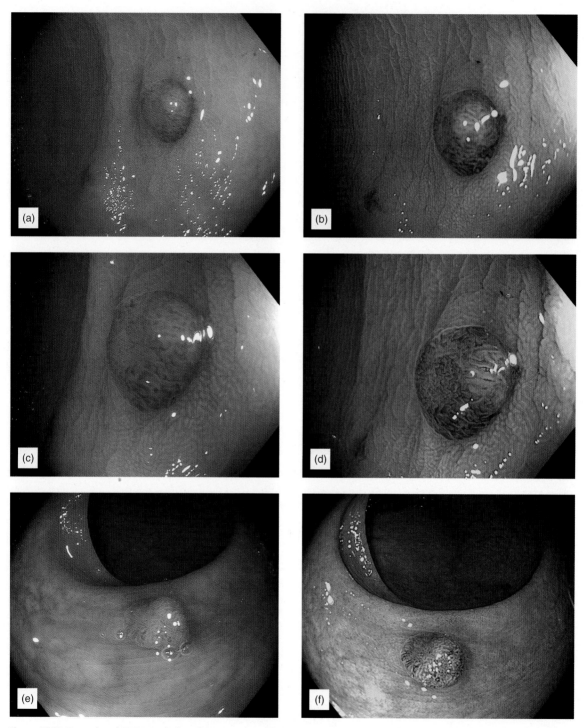

Figure 17.62 Examples of NICE 2 tubular adenomas amenable for optical diagnosis: (a–d) WL low-magnification and near-focus. (e–h) another small adenoma meeting NICE 2 criteria in WL and NBI in unmagnified and magnified views. (i-l) A third set of images which allow for high confidence recognition as adenoma. Note the slight central dimple on NBI with concentrated vessels characteristic of small NICE 2 tubular adenomas, the so-called "valley sign." (Jonathan Cohen, NYU Langone School of Medicine.)

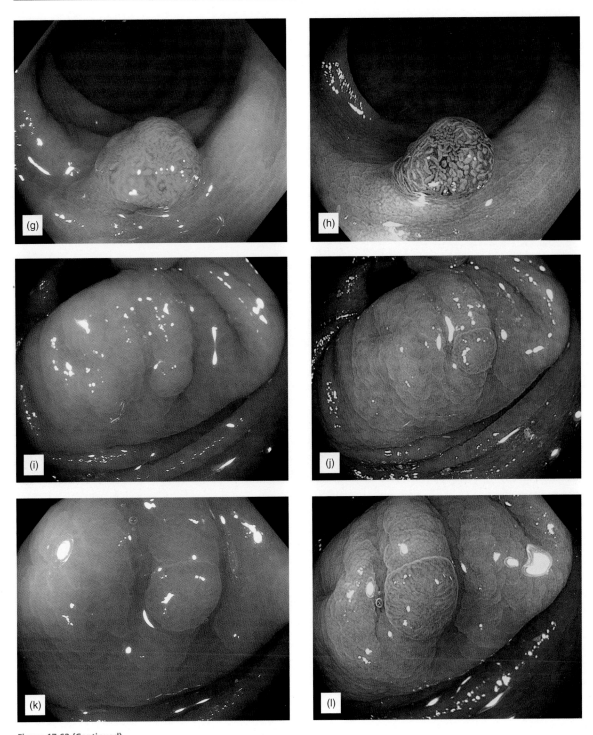

Figure 17.62 (Continued)

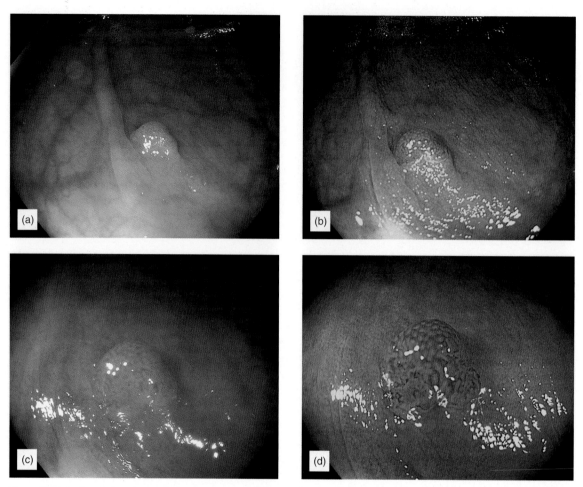

Figure 17.63 (a–d) Tubular adenoma NICE 2 polyps on WL and NBI H190 views. Top of polyp shows typical white round dots surrounded by dark line pattern, while lower half of polyp has typical gyrus and Sano type 2 vessels. (Jonathan Cohen, NYU Langone School of Medicine.)

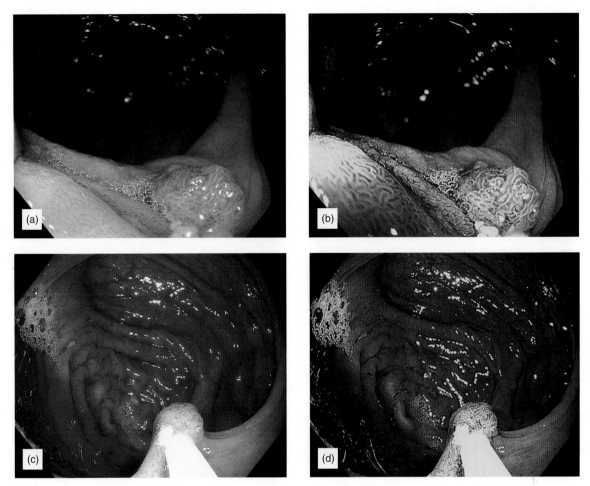

Figure 17.64 (a–d) Adenoma on ileocecal valve readily apparent in WL and NBI H190 near focus views with villous pit pattern. (Jonathan Cohen, NYU Langone School of Medicine.)

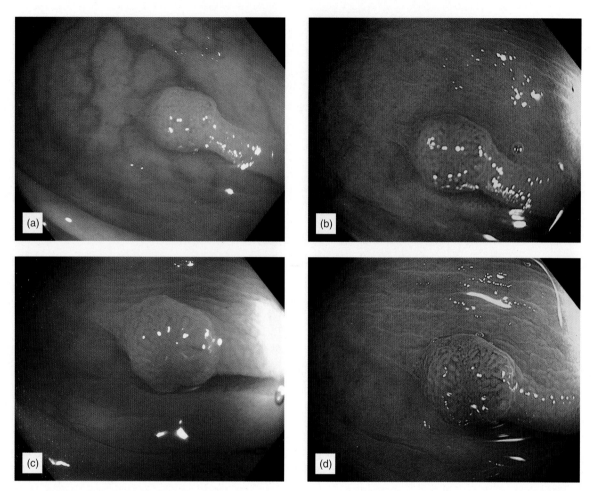

Figure 17.65 (a–d) NICE 2 sessile adenoma on WL and NBI low-magnification and near-focus views. Images (d) and (f) illustrate the valley sign of minute central depression with increased density vessels often seen in tubular adenomas. (Jonathan Cohen, NYU Langone School of Medicine.)

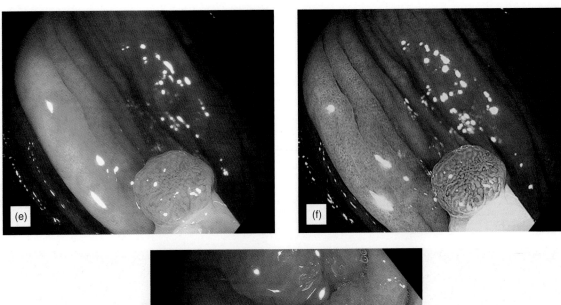

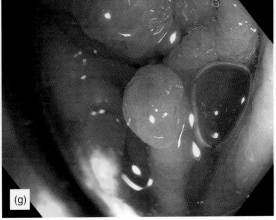

Figure 17.65 (Continued)

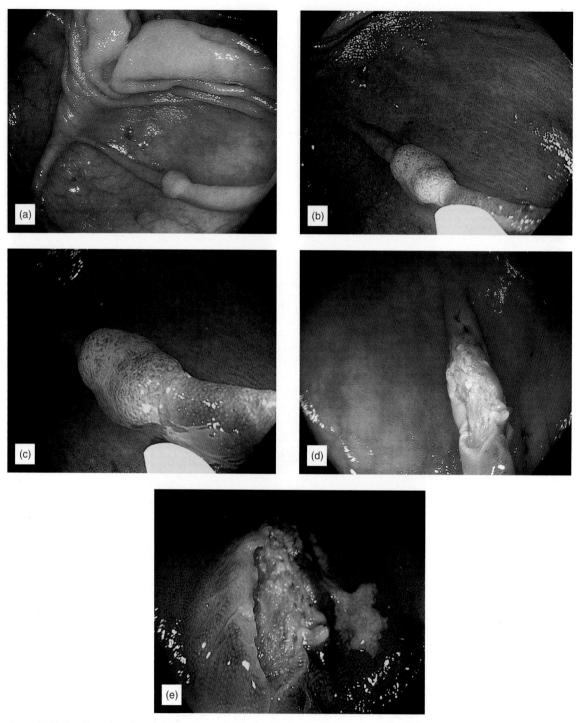

Figure 17.66 Small sessile right-sided adenoma on a fold near the ileocecal valve on (a, b) WL and NBI H190 low-magnification view and (c) NBI high-magnification view. (d, e) Post-resection WL and NBI views with demonstration of normal pits at the margin. (Jonathan Cohen, NYU Langone School of Medicine.)

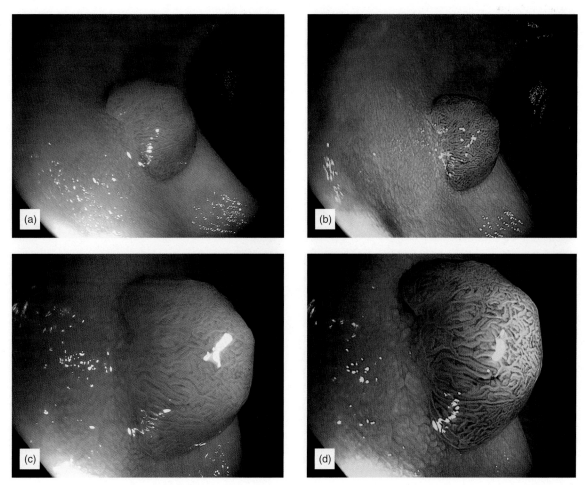

Figure 17.67 (a–d) Near-focus WL and NBI H190 views both demonstrate 3L pit patterns and fit NICE 2 criteria for adenoma. (Jonathan Cohen, NYU Langone School of Medicine.)

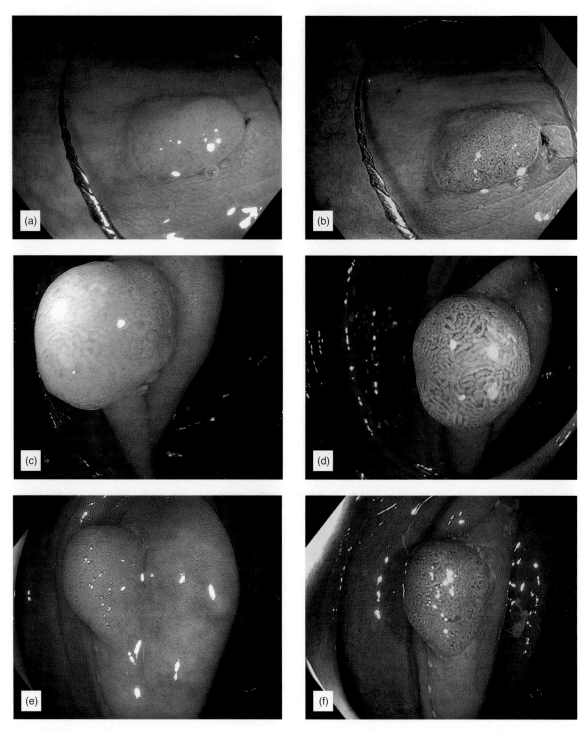

Figure 17.68 (a–i) Multiple WL and NBI H190 images of small tubular adenomas with NICE 2 features. (Jonathan Cohen, NYU Langone School of Medicine.)

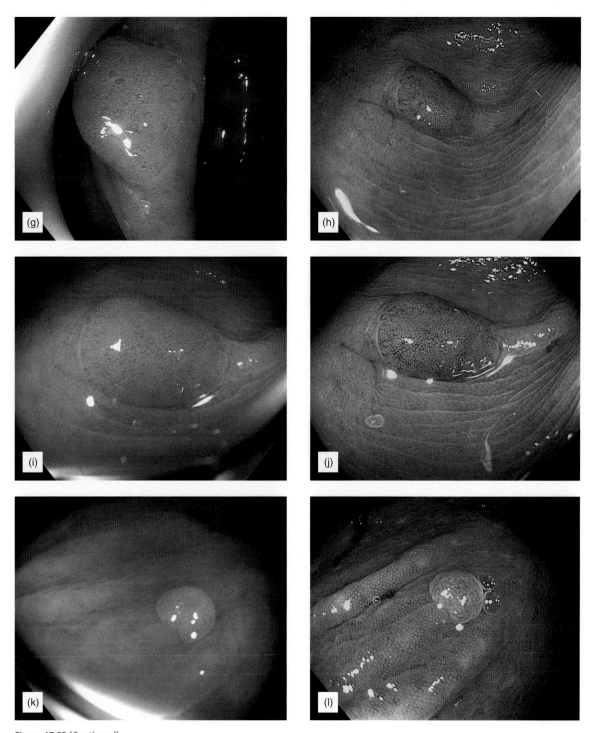

Figure 17.68 (Continued)

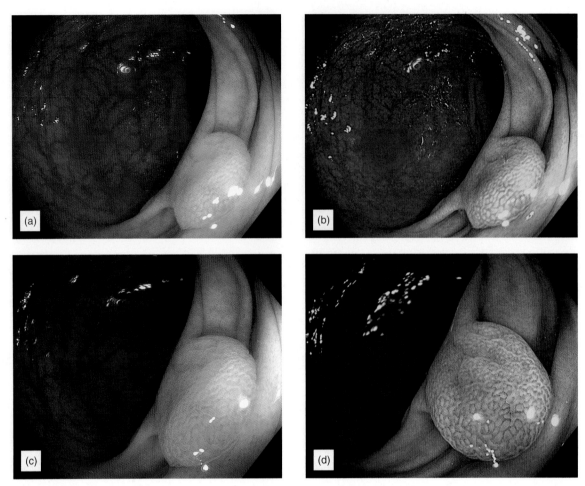

Figure 17.69 (a–d) Sessile tubular adenoma with central dimple in low and high magnification WL and NBI H190 with NICE 2 features clearly demonstrated. (Jonathan Cohen, NYU Langone School of Medicine.)

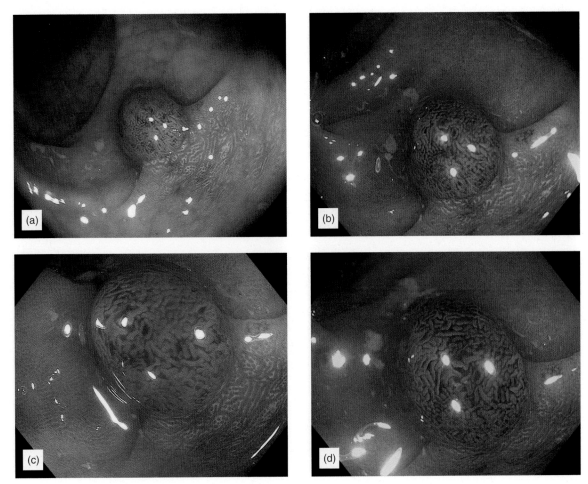

Figure 17.70 (a–d) Sessile tubular adenoma in low and high magnification WL and NBI H190 with NICE 2 features clearly demonstrated. (Jonathan Cohen, NYU Langone School of Medicine.)

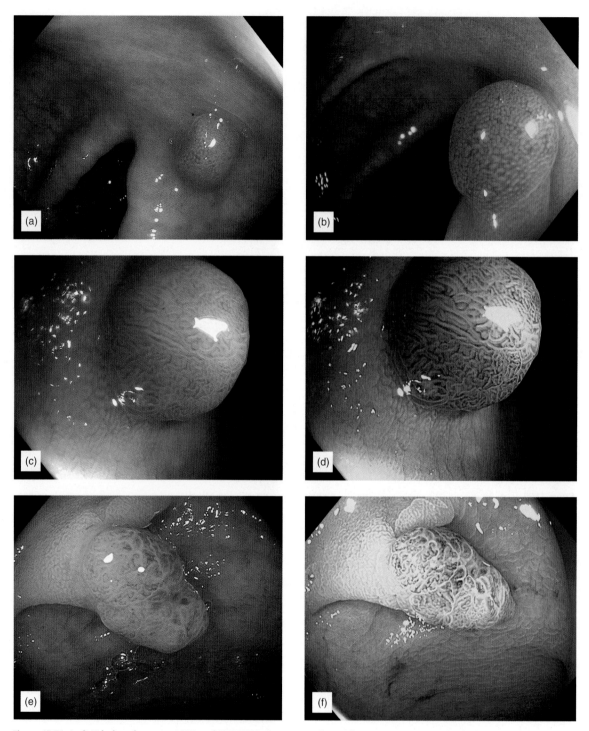

Figure 17.71 (a–f) Tubular adenoma on WL and NBI H190 views. (Jonathan Cohen, NYU Langone School of Medicine.)

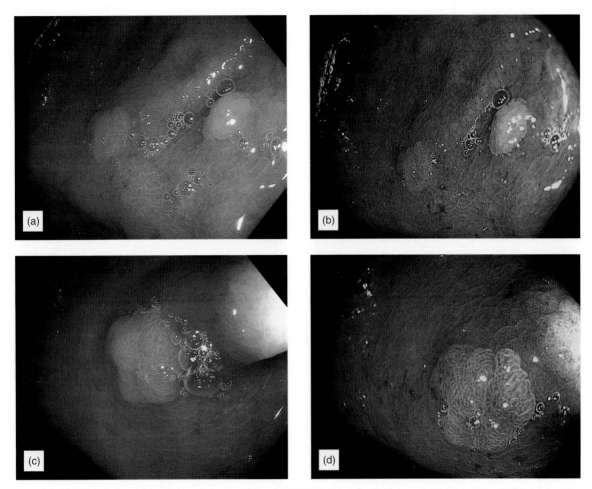

Figure 17.72 (a, b) A pair of flat tubular adenomas, WL and NBI H190 views. (c, d) High-magnification WL and NBI views of the polyp on the left of the pair. (Jonathan Cohen, NYU Langone School of Medicine.)

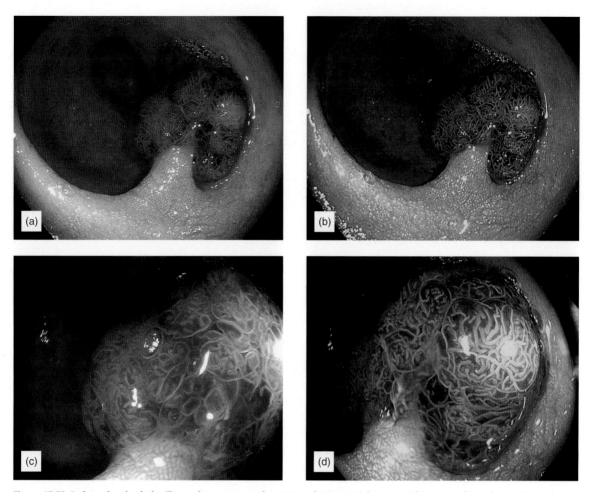

Figure 17.73 Pedunculated tubulovillous adenomatous polyp, WL and NBI H190 low magnification (a, b) and near-focus of adenoma (c, d).

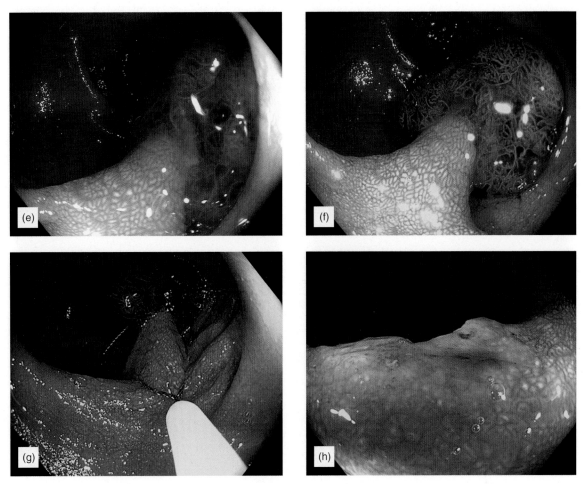

Figure 17.73 (Continued) (e, f) WL and NBI close-up inspection of stalk. (g) NBI of snare encircling base of stalk to ensure wide margin. (h) Normal pits at base of resected stalk. (Jonathan Cohen, NYU Langone School of Medicine.)

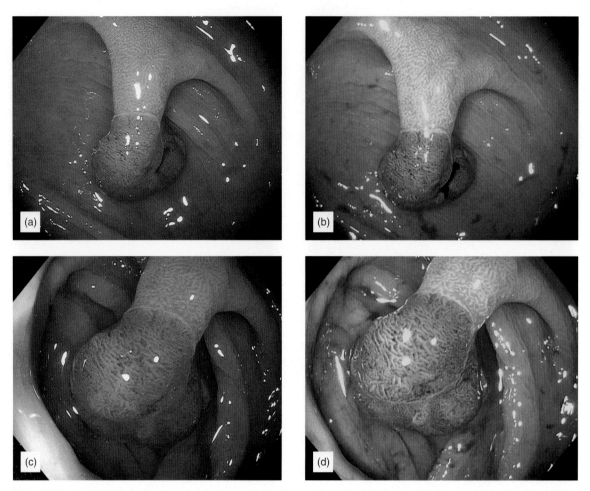

Figure 17.74 (a–g) This bilobed pedunculated adenoma with a long stalk is shown in low and high magnification in WL and NBI H190 pre and post resection. A clip is used to prevent bleeding from the wide stalk post resection. (Jonathan Cohen, NYU Langone School of Medicine.)

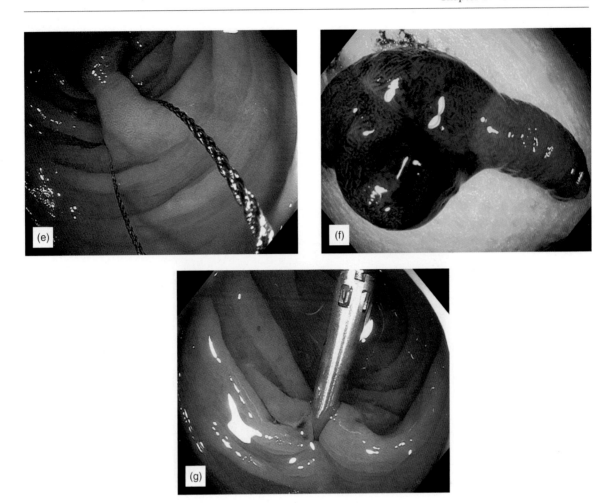

Figure 17.74 (Continued)

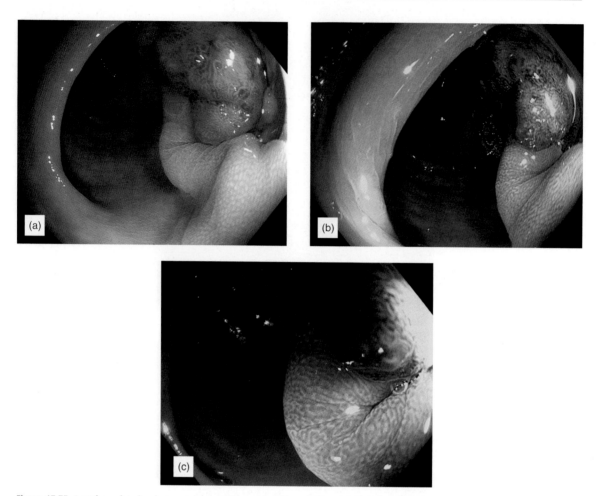

Figure 17.75 A pedunculated polyp on a long stalk seen in WL and NBI H190 low magnification (a, b) and near focus NBI view (c) of the stalk to direct polypectomy with sufficient negative margin. (Jonathan Cohen, NYU Langone School of Medicine.)

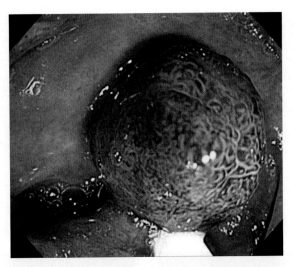

Figure 17.76 Sessile tubulovillous adenoma NBI H180 images demonstrate vessel pattern clearly. Stark color demarcation changes with surrounding mucosa, Sano 2 vessel patterns and surface pit patterns are all illustrated. (Jonathan Cohen, NYU Langone School of Medicine.)

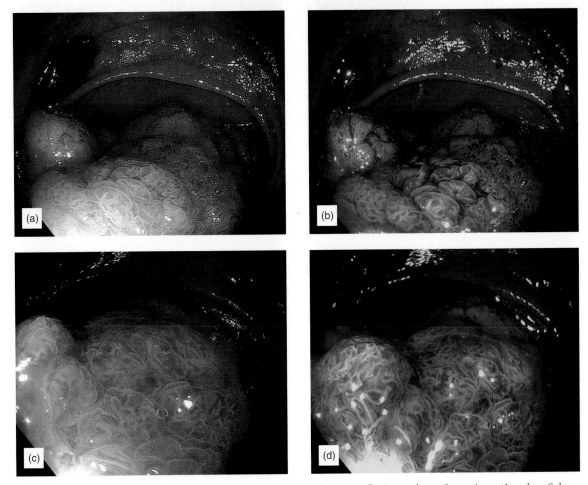

Figure 17.77 (a–h) Sessile tubulovillous adenoma WL and NBI H190 low magnification and near focus views. (Jonathan Cohen, NYU Langone School of Medicine.) (continued)

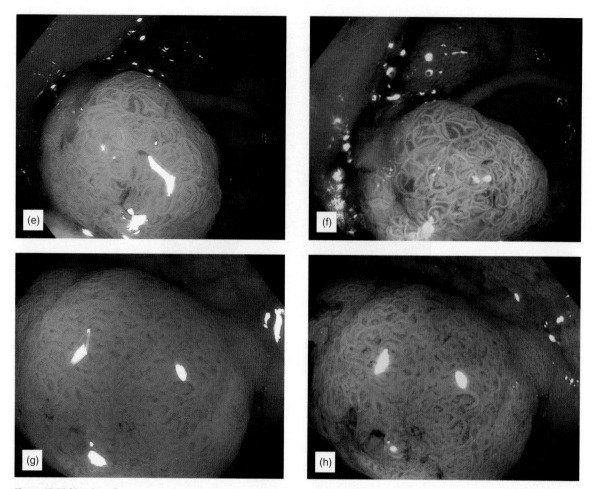

Figure 17.77 (Continued)

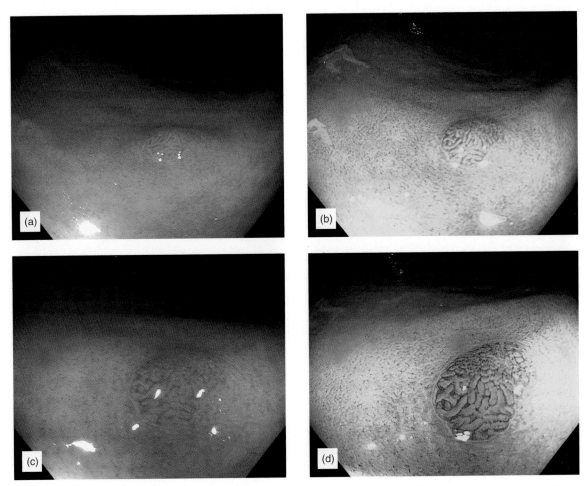

Figure 17.78 (a–d) Tiny flat rectal NICE 2 tubular adenoma on WL and NBI H190 low-magnification and near-focus views. (Jonathan Cohen, NYU Langone School of Medicine.)

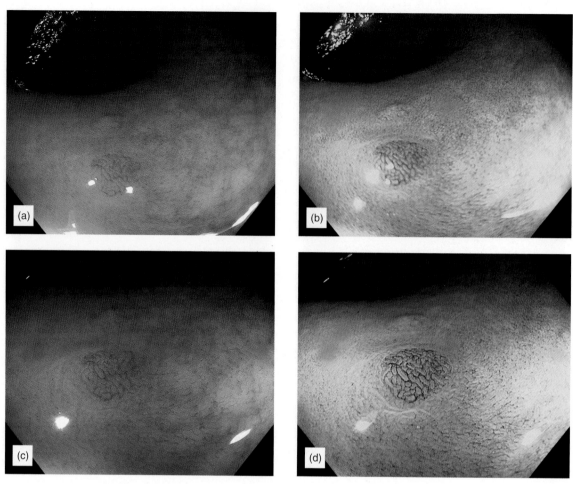

Figure 17.79 (a–d) Completely flat distal rectal NICE 2 adenoma on low-and high-magnification WL and NBI H190 views. (Jonathan Cohen, NYU Langone School of Medicine.)

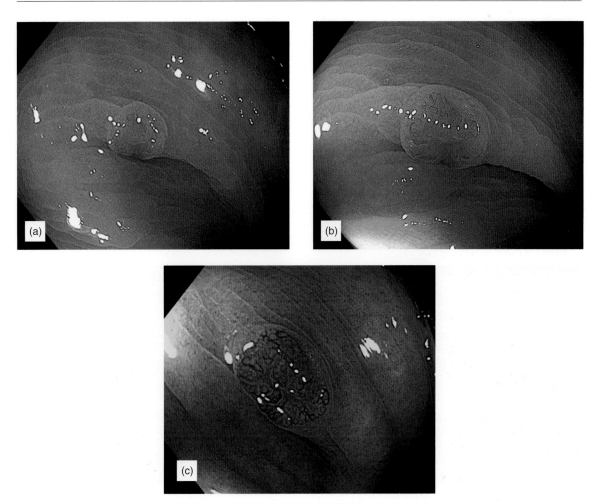

Figure 17.80 Tiny adenoma difficult to characterize on low-magnification WL H190 (a) but Sano type 2 vessels and NICE 2 characteristics seen well on WL and NBI near-focus views (b, c). (Jonathan Cohen, NYU Langone School of Medicine.)

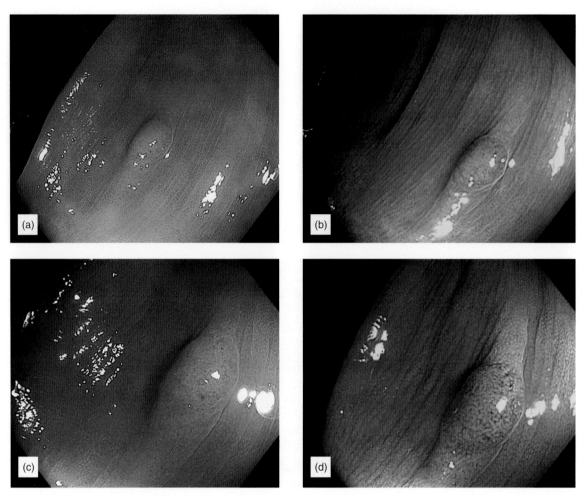

Figure 17.81 (a–d) Flat NICE 2 tubular adenoma on WL and NBI H190 views, with and without magnification. (Jonathan Cohen, NYU Langone School of Medicine.)

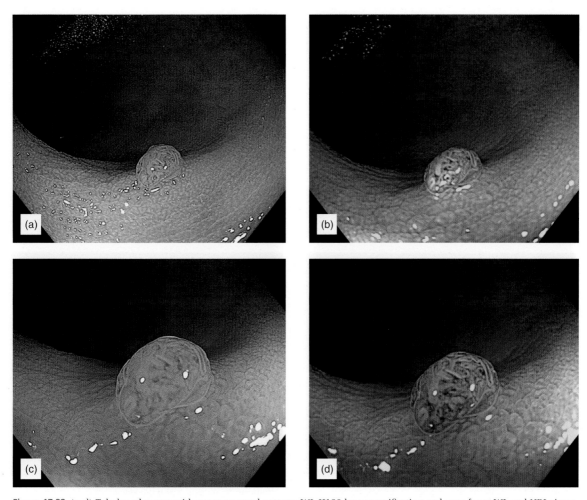

Figure 17.82 (a–d) Tubular adenoma with gyrus mucosal pattern: WL H190 low-magnification and near-focus WL and NBI views. (Jonathan Cohen, NYU Langone School of Medicine.)

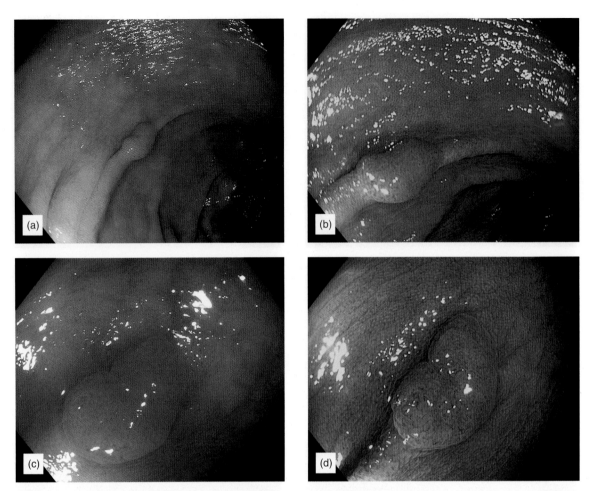

Figure 17.83 (a–d) Recurrent adenomatous polyp near ileocolonic anastomosis on WL and NBI H190 views. NICE 2 feature identified on near-focus NBI image. (Jonathan Cohen, NYU Langone School of Medicine.)

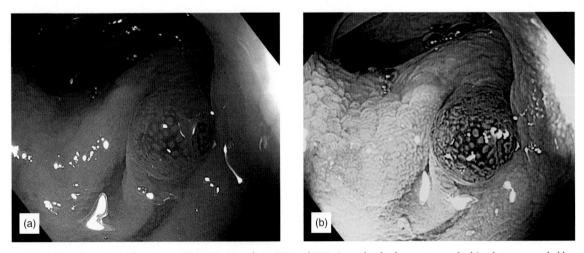

Figure 17.84 (a, b) NICE 2 adenoma on H190 WL. Near-focus WL and NBI views clearly show pattern of white dots surrounded by dark vessels. (Jonathan Cohen, NYU Langone School of Medicine.)

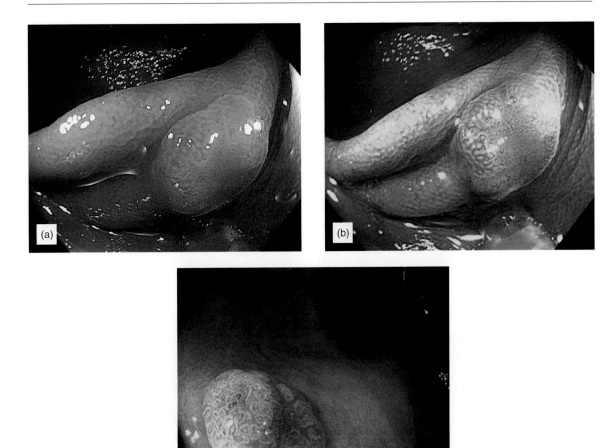

Figure 17.85 (a, b) Sessile tubular adenoma on WL and NBI views. While the broad central depression and change in vessel pattern raises some concerns for higher-grade dysplasia to prompt consideration of submucosal lift, histology here revealed tubular adenoma only. The area of depression is broader than the tiny "valley sign" often seen in tubular adenomas and accordingly this polyp would not be a good candidate for the resect and discard strategies described in Chapter 10, similar to those polyps for which a confident distinction of hyperplastic vs. adenoma can be made. (c) Similar sessile adenoma with central depression on NBI raises similar concerns but not diagnostic of advanced histology. This polyp also has a nodular appearance raising the possibility that it is a serrated sessile adenoma. Histologic analysis is advised for any lesions in which high grade dysplasia is at all suspected or in which the operator is not confident of the diagnosis. (Jonathan Cohen, NYU Langone School of Medicine.)

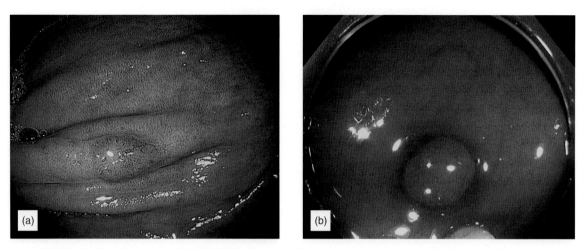

Figure 17.86 (a, b) Flat adenomas in NBI H190 light, low magnification. Pink rim of trace residual stool facilitates detection. (Jonathan Cohen, NYU Langone School of Medicine.)

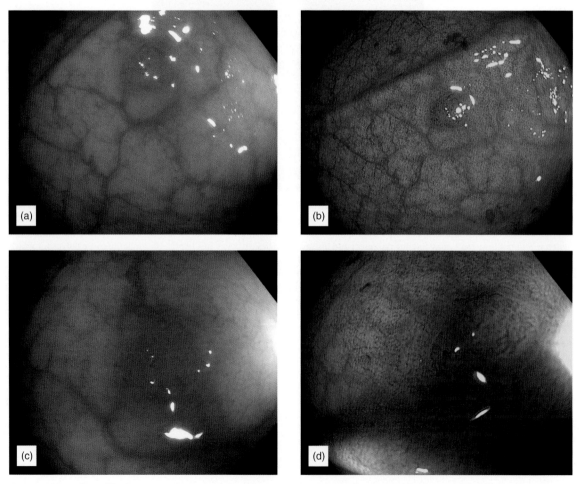

Figure 17.87 (a–d) Small adenoma evident on WL by abrupt end of blood vessel; NBI image shows stark color contrast with surrounding mucosa. NICE 2 features seen better on near focus NBI H190. (Jonathan Cohen, NYU Langone School of Medicine.)

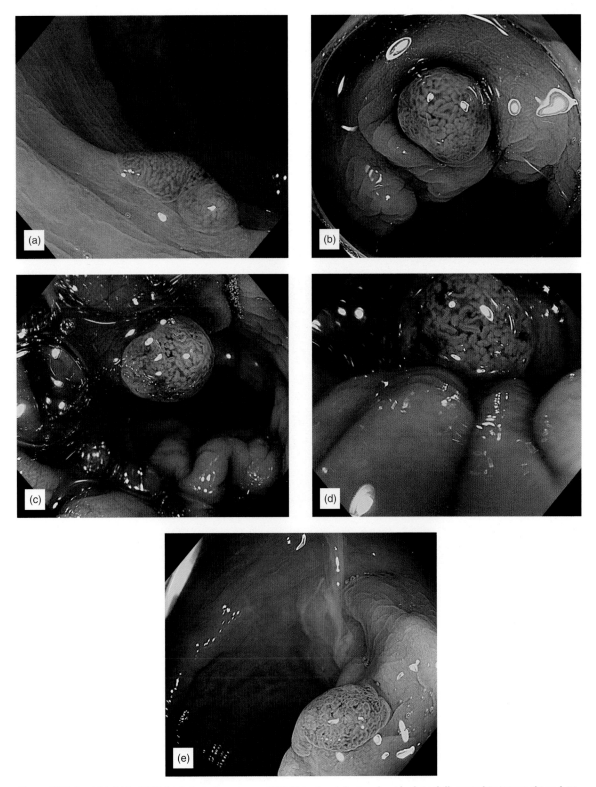

Figure 17.88 (a–e) Multiple NICE 2 tubular adenomas on NBI. Note the pink rim of residual stool illustrated in images (b) and (c). (James Lau, Chinese University of Hong Kong.)

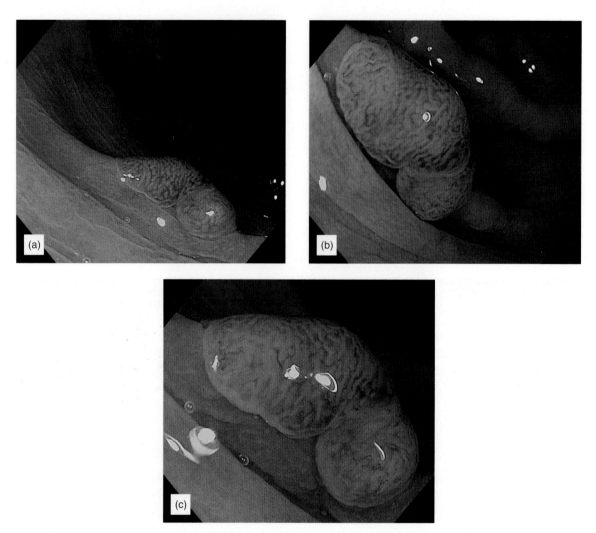

Figure 17.89 (a–c) Sessile tubular adenoma NBI H190 low and higher magnification views. (James Lau, Chinese University of Hong Kong.)

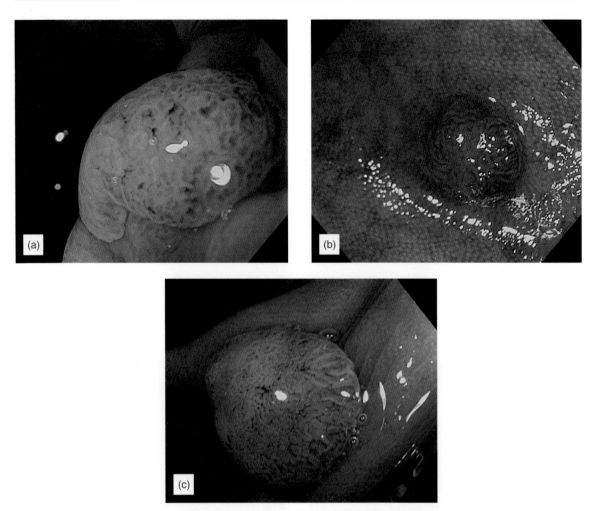

Figure 17.90 (a–c) NBI H190 images of NICE 2 tubular adenomas. (James Lau, Chinese University of Hong Kong.)

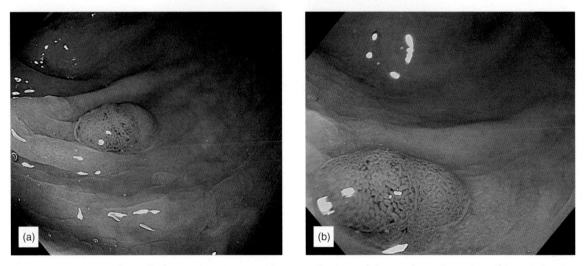

Figure 17.91 NICE 2 sessile small adenoma in NBI H190 (a) low magnification and (b) near focus. (James Lau, Chinese University of Hong Kong.)

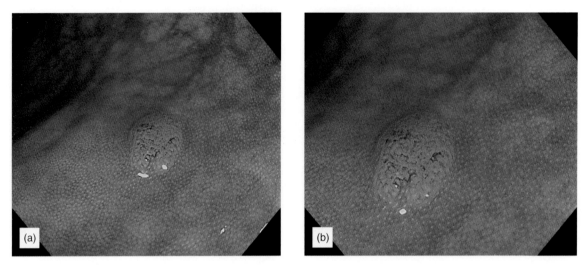

Figure 17.92 (a, b) NBI H190 low- and high-magnification views show a few lacy vessels and generally dark spots surrounded by white in a NICE 1 pattern suggesting hyperplastic change. (James Lau, Chinese University of Hong Kong.)

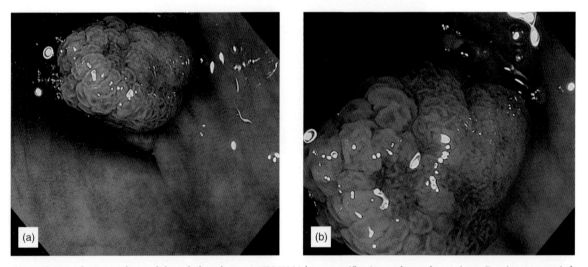

Figure 17.93 (a, b) Somewhat nodular tubular adenoma. NBI H190 low magnification and near focus views. Despite some varied surface topography with nodularity suggestive of serrated changes, the vessel and mucosal pattern shows no worrisome feature and pathology confirmed low-grade dysplasia. (James Lau, Chinese University of Hong Kong.)

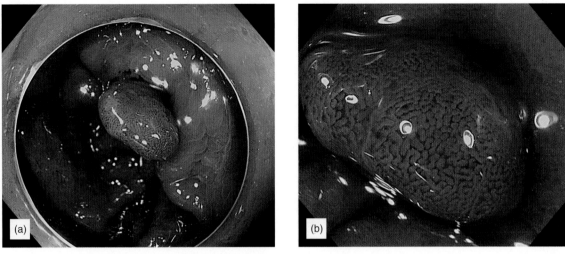

Figure 17.94 (a) NBI H190 low magnification view of sessile NICE 2 adenoma. (b) Near focus NBI view of large sessile tubular adenoma. (James Lau, Chinese University of Hong Kong.)

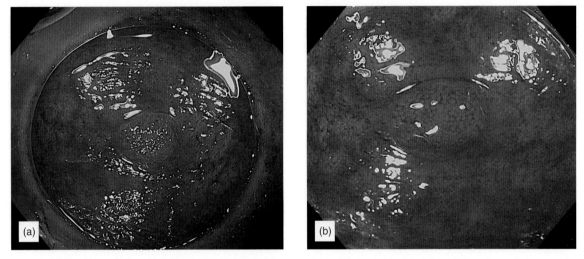

Figure 17.95 (a) Tiny tubular adenoma seen on low-magnification NBI H190 view. Note the abrupt ending of vessels interrupted by polyp margin, which helps to detect this subtle lesion. (b) High-magnification NBI identifies this as an adenoma by virtue of the white dot pattern surrounded by thin but dark vessels. (James Lau, Chinese University of Hong Kong.)

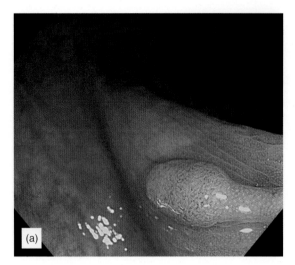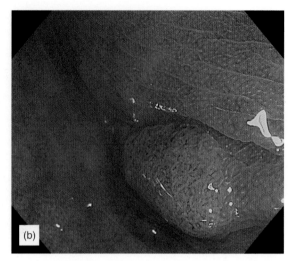

Figure 17.96 (a, b) Flat tubular adenoma on fold, NBI H190 low- and high-magnification views. Note the sharp transition from tubulo-gyrus NICE 2 mucosal pattern on the right of the polyp to normal Kudo type 1 pits to mark the lateral polyp border. (James Lau, Chinese University of Hong Kong.)

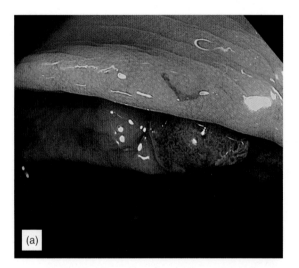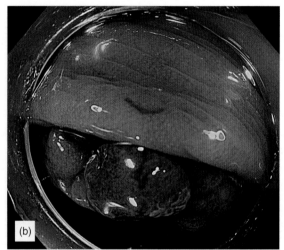

Figure 17.97 (a, b) NBI H190 low- and high-magnification views of NBI adenoma between two folds. (James Lau, Chinese University of Hong Kong.)

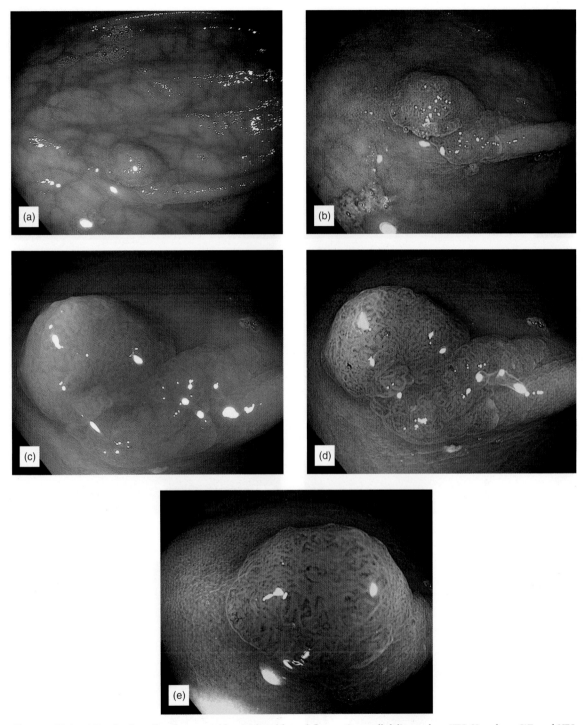

Figure 17.98 (a–e) Proximal sessile adenoma with raised and lateral flat portion well delineated on NBI. Near-focus WL and NBI H190 views show NICE 2 gyrus pattern and Sano type 2 vessels; saline lift; and post resection showing normal pits surrounding polypectomy. (Jonathan Cohen, NYU Langone School of Medicine.)

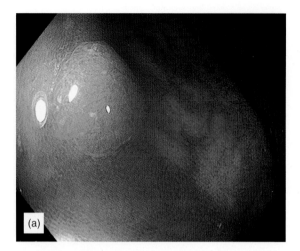
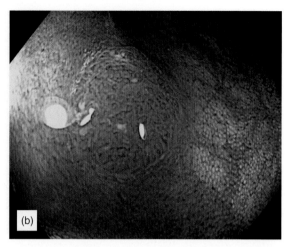

Figure 17.99 (a, b) Hepatic flexure sessile adenoma on WL and NBI H190 near-focus views. (Jonathan Cohen, NYU Langone School of Medicine.)

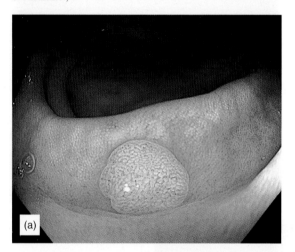
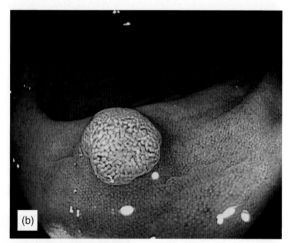

Figure 17.100 (a, b) Flat cecal adenoma on WL and NBI H190 views clearly show NICE 2 features. (Jonathan Cohen, NYU Langone School of Medicine.)

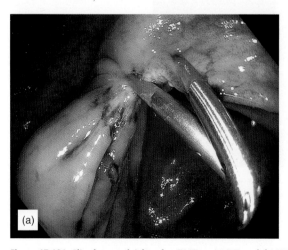
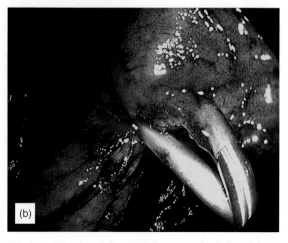

Figure 17.101 Clip closure of right colon EMR on (a) WL and (b) NBI H190 views. (Jonathan Cohen, NYU Langone School of Medicine.)

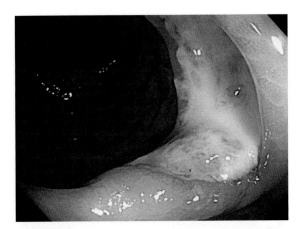

Figure 17.102 Ulceration in colon at base of recent large piece-meal mucosal resection WL H190 low magnification. (Jonathan Cohen, NYU Langone School of Medicine.)

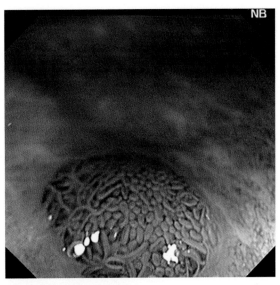

Figure 17.103 Magnified NBI H190 image of a 3-mm mildly dysplastic tubular adenoma with type 3L pit pattern (James East, St Mark's Hospital.)

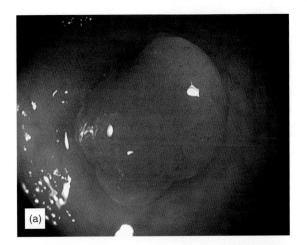

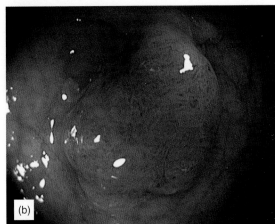

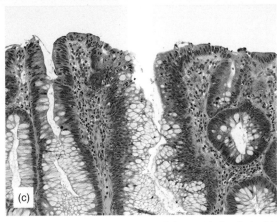

Figure 17.104 (a) WL H180 view of sigmoid colon tubular adenoma with low-grade dysplasia. (b) NBI image of sigmoid colon tubular adenoma with low-grade dysplasia showing 3L pits. (c) Tubular adenoma with low-grade dysplasia, high-power view. (Douglas K. Rex, Indiana University School of Medicine.)

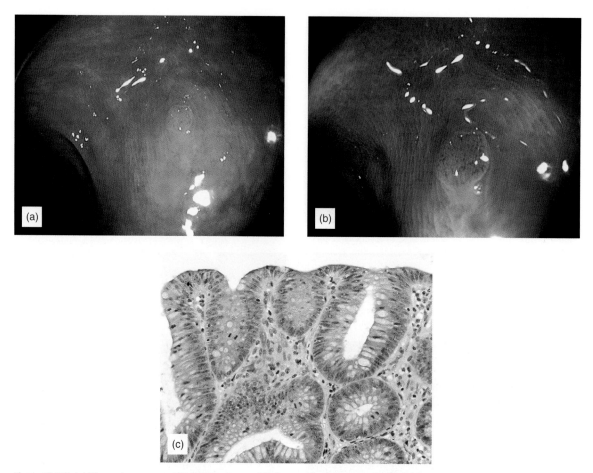

Figure 17.105 (a) Tiny polyp seen on WL H180 non-magnified view. (b) Adenoma pattern and well-demarcated borders evident on low-magnification NBI view. (c) Tubular adenoma with low-grade dysplasia. Epithelial cells of the glands and surface are crowded with enlarged, stratified hyperchromatic nuclei and an increased nuclear/cytoplasmic ratio. (Jonathan Cohen, NYU Langone School of Medicine.)

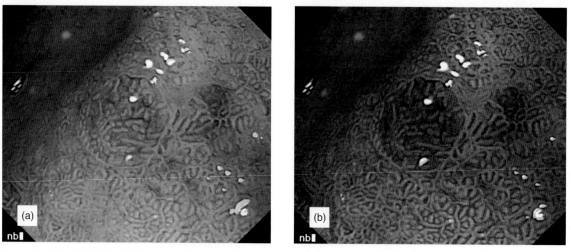

Figure 17.106 (a) WL H180 HRE low magnification of flat adenoma. (b) NBI image of the same lesions. (Jean-François Rey, Institut Arnault Tzanck.)

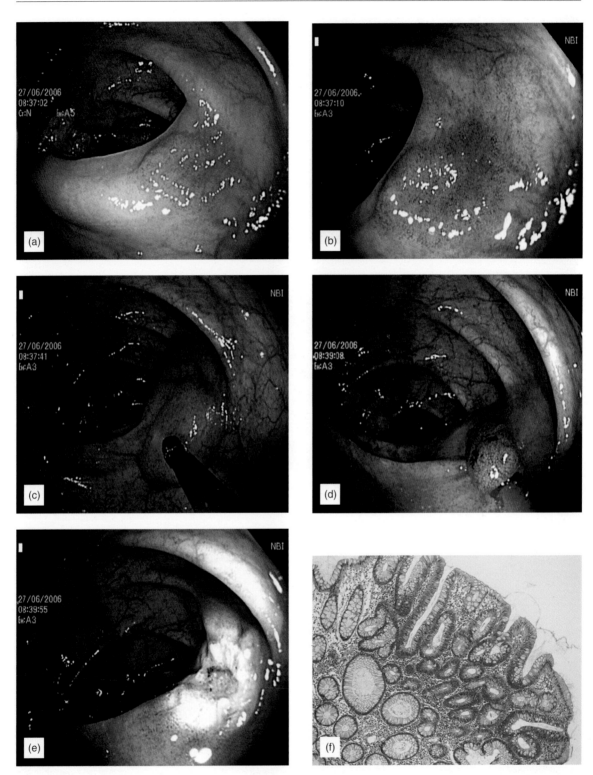

Figure 17.107 (a) Adenomatous polyp with low-grade dysplasia in sigmoid colon WL H180 view. (b) Low-grade dysplasia adenomatous polyp, with NBI highlighted borders. (c) Submucosal injection previous to polypectomy. (d) Polypectomy image with NBI. (e) Polypectomy resection base with surrounding normal pits. (f) Adenomatous polyp with low-grade dysplasia. (Guilherme Macedo, Hospital Sao Marcos.)

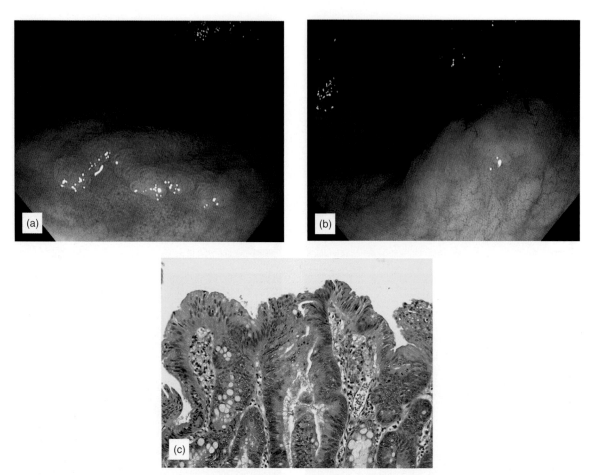

Figure 17.108 (a) Flat adenoma in cecum with NBI H180 showing 3L pits. (b) WL HRE view of flat adenoma in the cecum after submucosal injection with saline and methylene blue. (c) Portion of tubulovillous adenoma in high power. (Douglas K. Rex, Indiana University School of Medicine.)

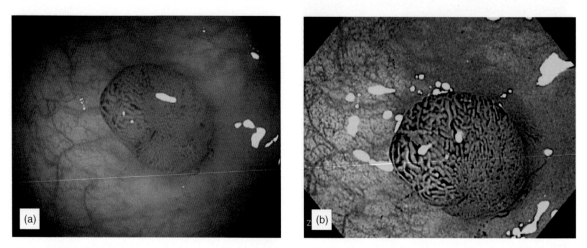

Figure 17.109 (a) WL H180 low-magnification view of colonic polyp. (b) NBI view of colonic adenoma with 1.5′ magnification. Pit pattern and vessel pattern consistent with pathologic diagnosis of tubulovillous adenoma. (Jean-François Rey, Institut Arnault Tzanck.)

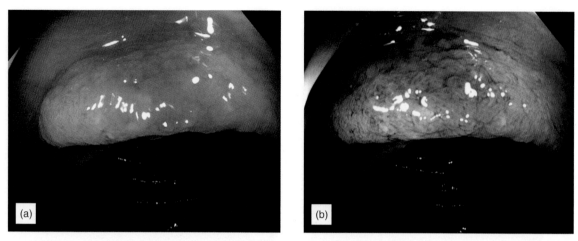

Figure 17.110 (a) WL H180 HRE low-magnification view of villous adenoma on a fold. (b) NBI light view of a villous adenoma. Note the typical villiform and sulcated surface appearance (James DiSario, University of Utah Health Sciences Center.)

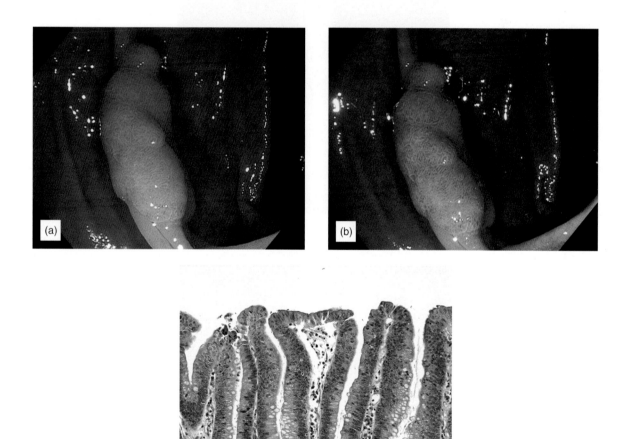

Figure 17.111 (a) WL image of tubulovillous adenoma in transverse colon with focal high-grade dysplasia. (b) NBI H180 image of tubulovillous adenoma in the transverse colon with focal high-grade dysplasia and type 3L and 4 pits. (c) Tubulovillous adenoma in transverse colon with focal high-grade dysplasia in high power. (Douglas K. Rex, Indiana University School of Medicine.)

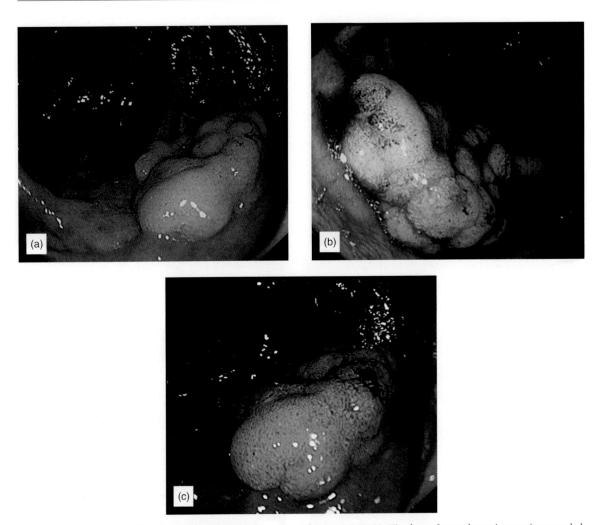

Figure 17.112 (a) Large sessile colon polyp seen here in low-magnification WL H180. Histology after endoscopic resection revealed a tubulovillous adenoma with free resection margins. (b) Chromoendoscopy with methylene blue nicely reveals the borders of the lesion in preparation for polypectomy. (c) Low-magnification NBI view of the polyp also provides excellent demarcation of the border comparable to chromoendoscopy. (University of Amsterdam.)

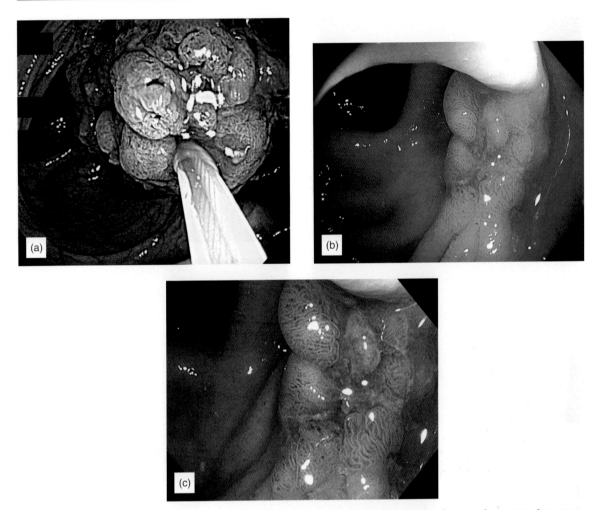

Figure 17.113 (a) Non-HRE WL view of a giant tubulovillous colon adenoma undergoing piecemeal snare polypectomy after tattoo-ing. Note the difference in resolution with the subsequent H180 HRE images taken for the follow-up examination. (b) WL HRE eas-ily identifies the site of scar and residual polyp 5 weeks following near complete piecemeal resection of 6-cm tubulovillous adenoma with APC fulguration. (c) NBI low-magnification view shows central scar and villous adenoma pit pattern in this residual lesion. Pathology confirmed residual tubulovillous adenoma. (Jonathan Cohen, NYU Langone School of Medicine.)

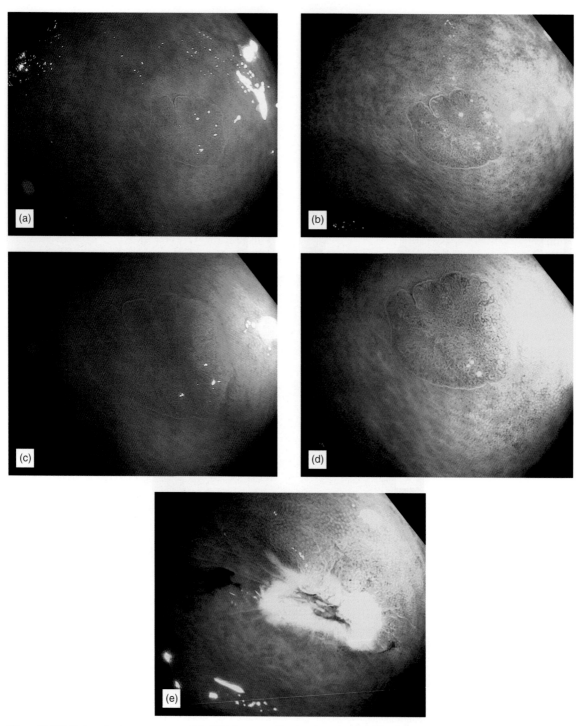

Figure 17.114 Flat cecal adenoma seen on WL H190 low magnification (a) only after identification on NBI (b). (c, d) Magnification WL and NBI views and (e) post resection. (Jonathan Cohen, NYU Langone School of Medicine.)

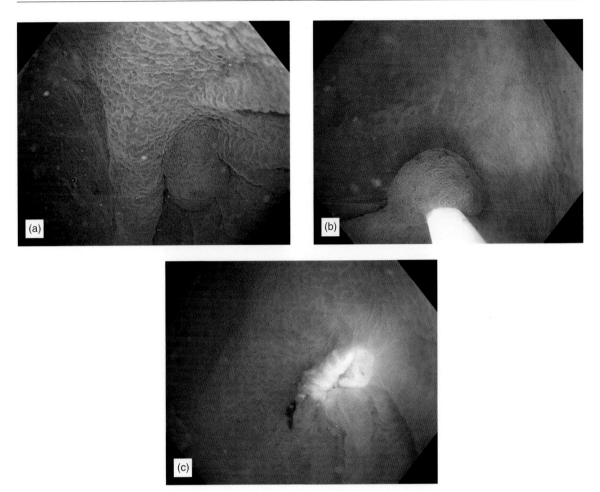

Figure 17.115 (a–c) Sessile adenoma in the cecum seen in NBI and in WL H190 under water to facilitate polypectomy without saline lift and subsequent underwater resection site. (Jonathan Cohen, NYU Langone School of Medicine.)

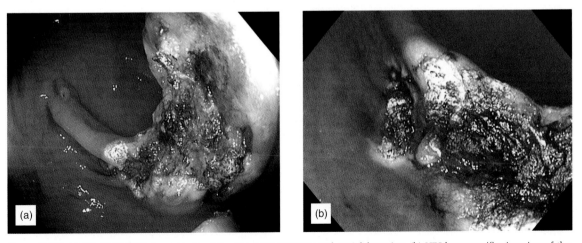

Figure 17.116 (a) WL H180 HRE view of lesion following snare resection and APC fulguration. (b) NBI low-magnification view of the lesion following snare resection and APC fulguration. No residual polypoid tissue is visualized. (Jonathan Cohen, NYU Langone School of Medicine.)

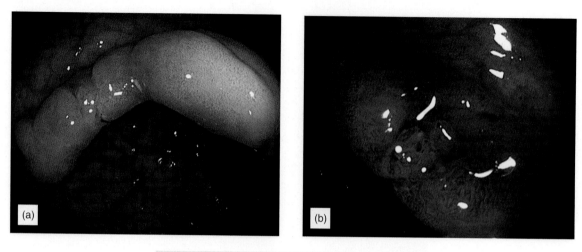

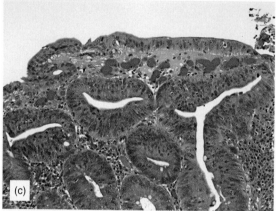

Figure 17.117 (a) WL H180 low-magnification image of tubular adenoma. (b) NBI image of tubular adenoma with high-grade dysplasia. (c) Tubular adenoma with high-grade dysplasia in high power. (Douglas K. Rex, Indiana University School of Medicine.)

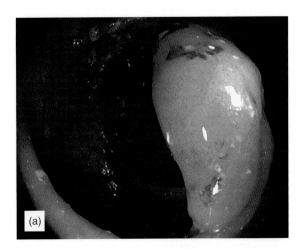

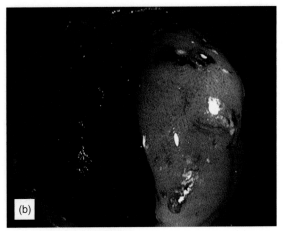

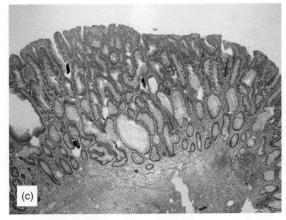

Figure 17.118 (a) WL H180 image of a tubulovillous adenoma with low-grade dysplasia in the transverse colon. (b) NBI image of tubulovillous adenoma in the transverse colon with low-grade dysplasia. Note type 3L and 4 pits. (c) Tubulovillous adenoma in low power. (Douglas K. Rex, Indiana University School of Medicine.)

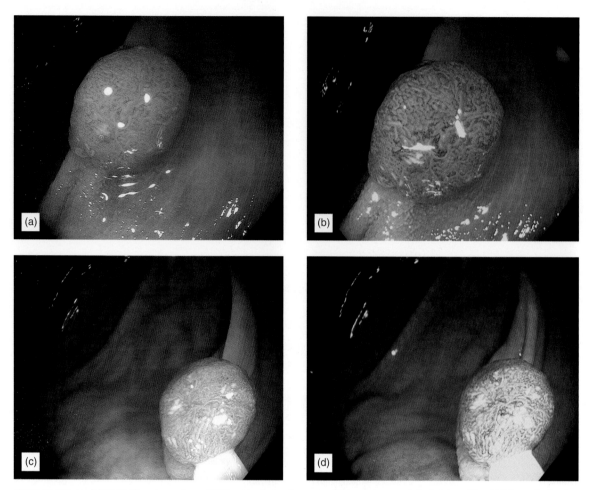

Figure 17.119 (a–d) WL H190 and near-focus NBI images show adenoma with irregular vessels indicative of focal high-grade dysplasia. Vessel pattern is accentuated when snare is closed around the polyp base. (Jonathan Cohen, NYU Langone School of Medicine.)

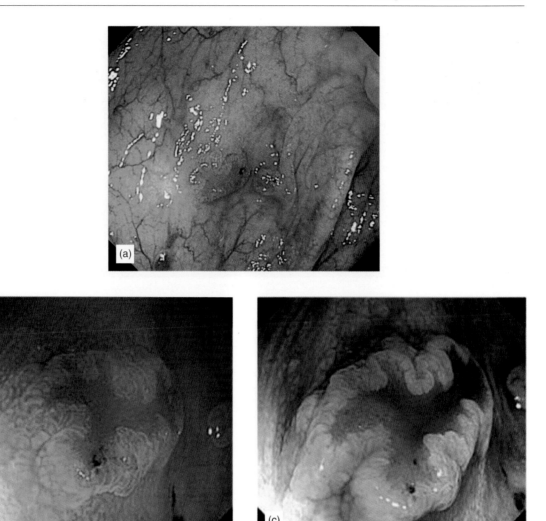

Figure 17.120 (a) Depressed type lesion (IIc+IIa) 9 mm in size, transverse colon. The lesion is identified by a tiny oozing during standard endoscopy. (b) Ordinary view, magnified showing central depression. (c) Indigocarmine dye spraying view. Pit pattern is not well recognized in either view. (continued)

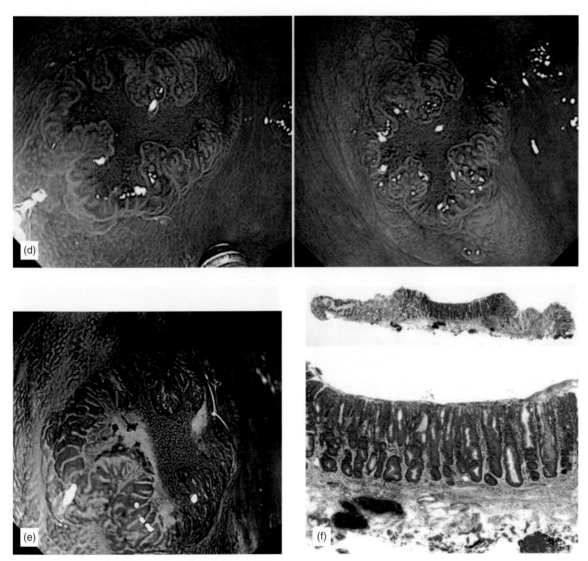

Figure 17.120 (Continued) (d) NBI colonoscopy with magnification. Kudo IIIs pit pattern is observed clearly without dye spraying. (e) Crystal violet staining. Kudo IIIs pit pattern is observed clearly same as NBI colonoscopy. (f) Pathologic findings: adenoma with high-grade dysplasia. (Copyright Yasushi Sano, Sano Hospital.)

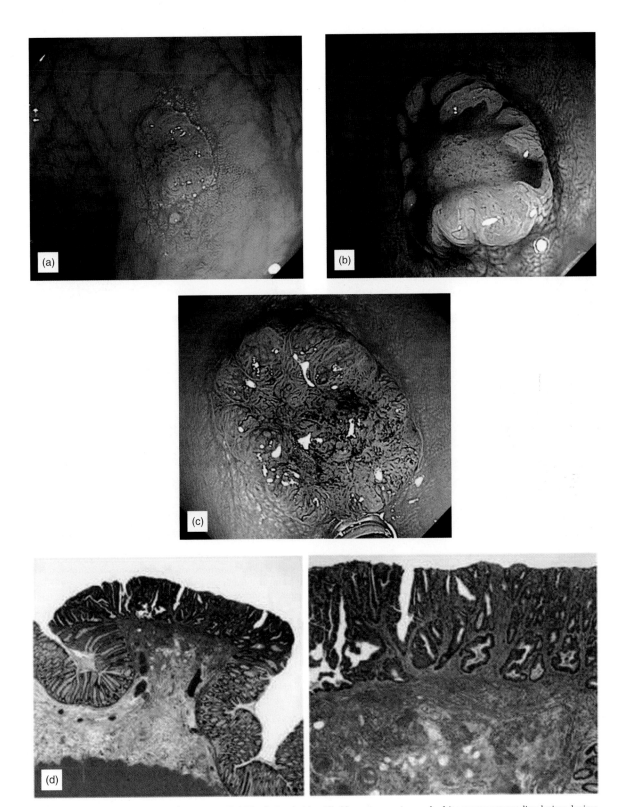

Figure 17.121 (a) Depressed type lesion (IIa+IIc.) The lesion is identified by a tiny oozing and white spots surrounding lesion during standard endoscopy. (b) Indigocarmine dye spraying view. Pit pattern is not well recognized due to dense mucus. (c) NBI colonoscopy with magnification. Sano capillary pattern type III is observed clearly without dye spraying. (d) Well-differentiated intramucosal adenocarcinoma without lymphatic, vascular or neural invasion. (Copyright Yasushi Sano, Sano Hospital.)

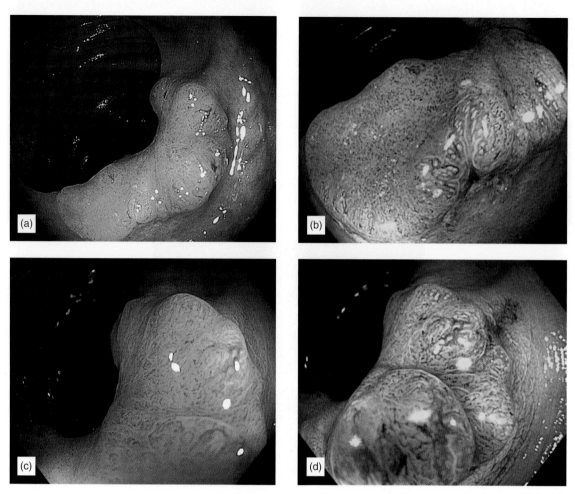

Figure 17.122 (a, b) WL and NBI H190 images of interval colon cancer in sessile right-sided polyp within 3 years of prior colonoscopy at outside institution. Central depression and ulceration and non-lifting point to the diagnosis. Missed lesions due to failure to reach the base of the cecum or sub-par preparation and incomplete polypectomy are leading possible causes. Special care is advised to inspect the back side of folds when resecting sessile polyps on folds and re-examine patients following piecemeal resection of large sessile polyps within a short interval. (c, d) WL and NBI near-focus views show highly irregular Sano type 3 vessels indicative of advanced histology. (Jonathan Cohen, NYU Langone School of Medicine.)

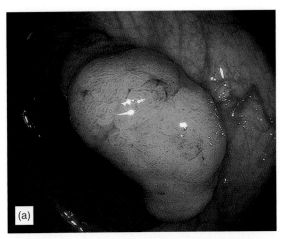
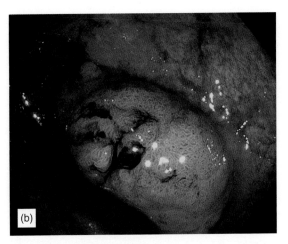

Figure 17.123 Larger sessile polyp right colon with smooth outer edge H180 WL and NBI low magnification views (a). Despite lack of advanced vessels, central depression or non-lifting, histopathology following complete piecemeal resection revealed invasive adenocarcinoma (b). (Jonathan Cohen, NYU Langone School of Medicine.)

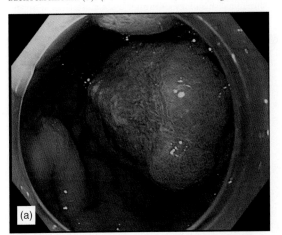
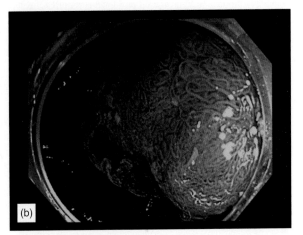

Figure 17.124 A 2-cm large rectal polyp with highly irregular vessels apparent on high-resolution WL view (a) and NBI H190 view (b), endoscopically suspicious for a polyp cancer. Pathology showed a moderately differentiated adenocarcinoma. (University of Amsterdam.)

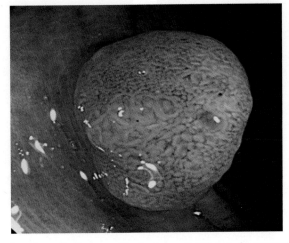

Figure 17.125 NBI H190 near focus view of a sessile adenoma with a focal area of highly irregular pattern of vessels and thick vessels indicating high-grade dysplasia. This finding warrants use of saline lift even in a polyp that might otherwise undergo simple snare resection. (Jonathan Cohen, NYU Langone School of Medicine.)

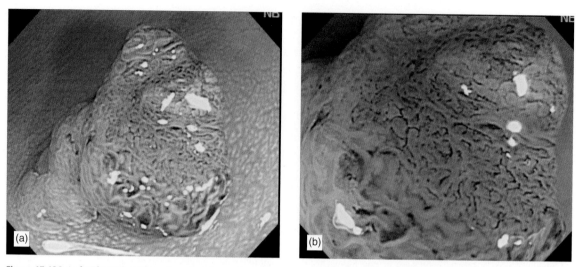

Figure 17.126 (a, b) This polyp shows Sano type 3 vessels and has a central depression, both alerting the endoscopist that this is likely a malignant polyp. Submucosal lift and EMR is required if resection is attempted. Histology confirmed as adenocarcinoma in situ. (Copyright Yasushi Sano, Sano Hospital.)

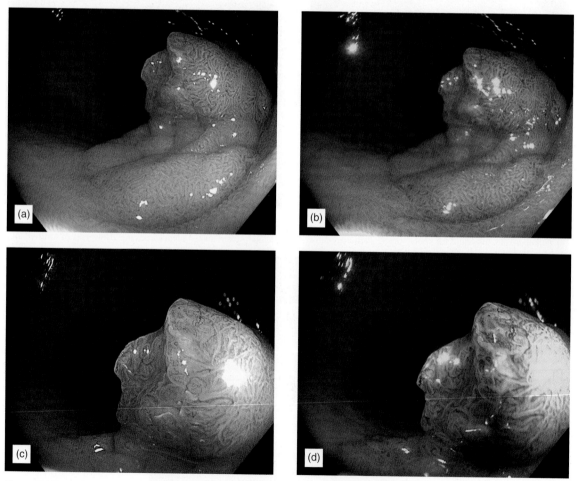

Figure 17.127 (a–d) Rectal tubulovillous adenoma WL and NBI H190 low magnification and then near focus views. Careful use of imaging delineates margins prior to resection. Near focus views (c, d) show highly irregular vessels and there is a central excavated area characteristic of at least high-grade dysplasia.

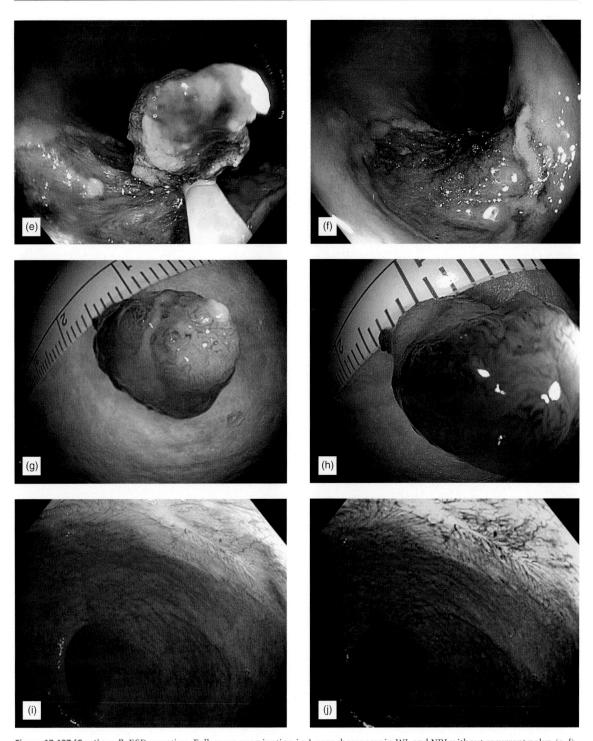

Figure 17.127 (Continued) ESD resection. Follow up examination in 1 year shows scar in WL and NBI without recurrent polyp (e, f). (g, h) WL and NBI near-focus examination of specimen identifies Sano type 3 vessels. (i, j) Follow-up 1 year without recurrence. (Jonathan Cohen, NYU Langone School of Medicine.)

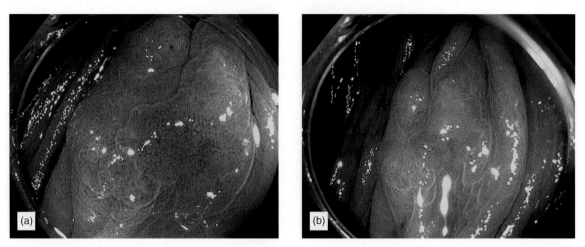

Figure 17.128 (a, b) Colon type IIa+IIc high-grade dysplasia. H190 NBI near focus (b) clearly shows adenomatous raised pattern with central depression, raising suspicion for high-grade dysplasia. (Michael Wallace, Mayo Clinic Jacksonville.)

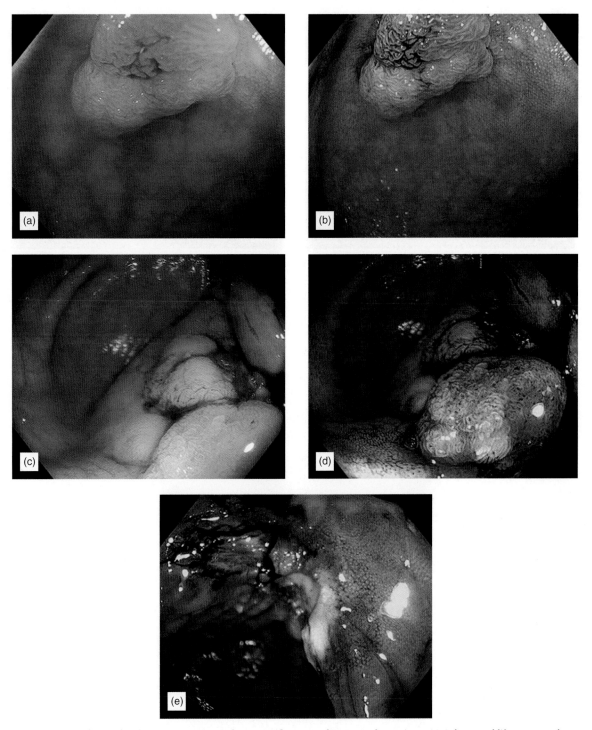

Figure 17.129 (a, b) Sessile adenoma on H190 WL low magnification and NBI near focus views. (c) Submucosal lift: WL notes borders well demarcated with just saline and methylene blue. (d) NBI low-magnification view. (e) Post-resection inspection of borders shows normal pit pattern. (Jonathan Cohen, NYU Langone School of Medicine.)

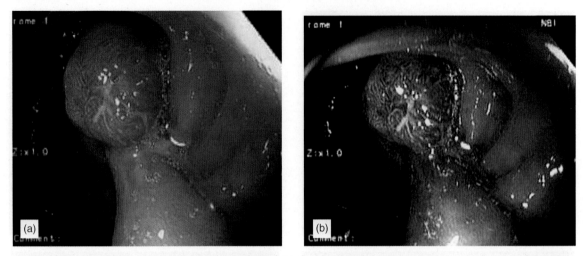

Figure 17.130 (a) WL H180 low-magnification view of pedunculated polyp. (b) NBI low magnification view of pedunculated polyp (Guido Costamagna, Catholic University of the Sacred Heart.)

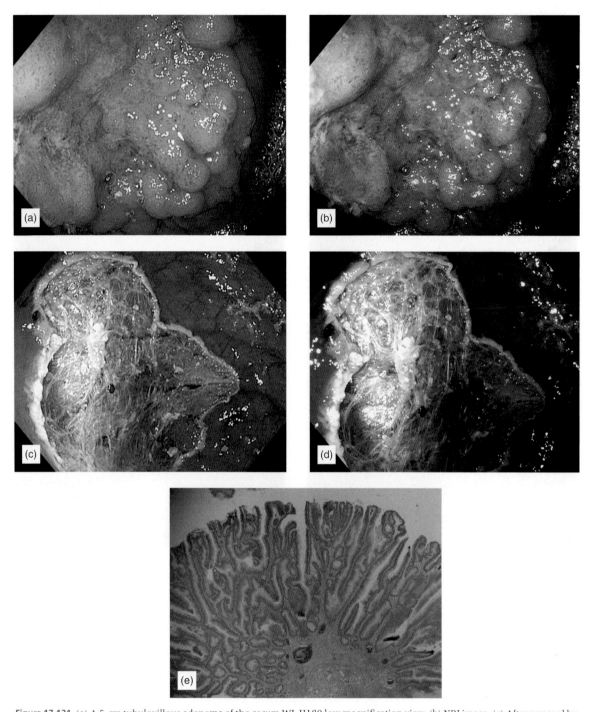

Figure 17.131 (a) A 5-cm tubulovillous adenoma of the cecum WL H180 low magnification view. (b) NBI image. (c) After removal by piecemeal polypectomy. (d) After removal by piecemeal polypectomy (NBI image). (e) Pathology. (Mount Sinai School of Medicine.)

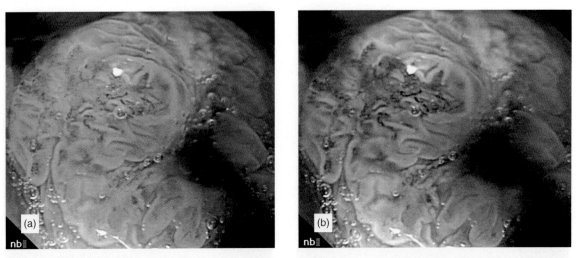

Figure 17.132 (a) Magnified WL H180 HRE view of colon adenocarcinoma. (b) NBI magnification view of intramucosal adenocarcinoma. Note the area of frank malignancy showing completely distorted pit pattern. (Jean-François Rey, Institut Arnault Tzanck.)

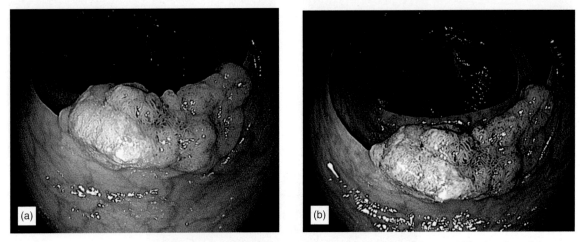

Figure 17.133 (a) WL H180 low-magnification view of a laterally spreading colon tumor. (b) NBI low-magnification view of the same lesion. (Jean-François Rey, Institut Arnault Tzanck.)

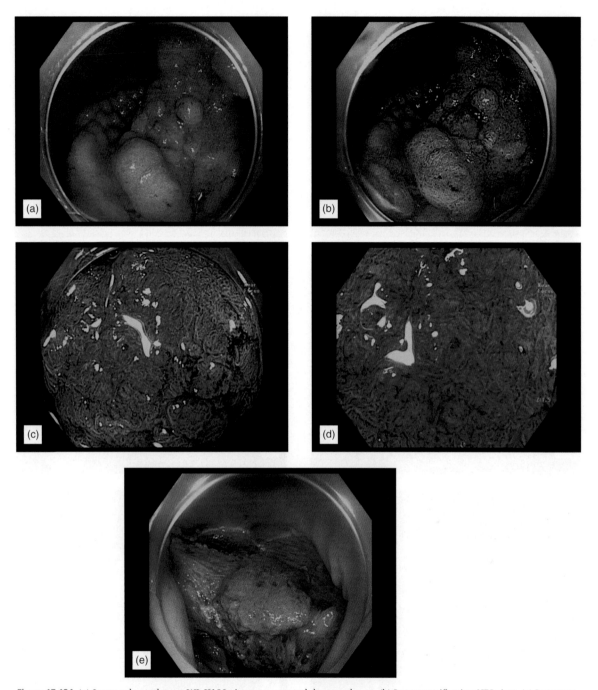

Figure 17.134 (a) Large colon polyp on WL H190 view; note central depressed area. (b) Low-magnification NBI view. (c) Low-magnification NBI inspection of depressed area. (d) Depressed area on high magnification shows an avascular pattern in keeping with suspected invasive cancer. (e) During the attempted wide piecemeal mucosal resection, the central depressed area fails to lift, further supporting the impression that this is an invasive cancer. (Rajvinder Singh, Lyell McEwin Hospital, Adelaide.)

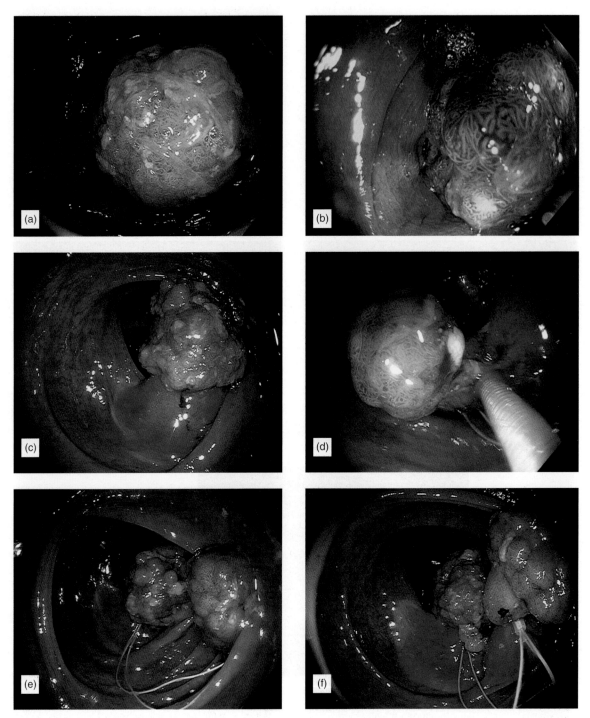

Figure 17.135 Large pedunculated adjacent adenomatous polyps with short and thick stalks. (a, b) WL and NBI H190 near focus demonstrates tubulovillous pattern. (c) Injection with saline and methylene blue together highlights adenoma margin and facilitates resection.

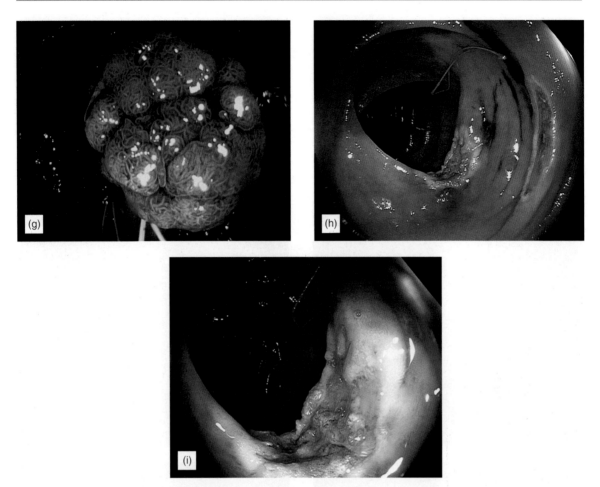

Figure 17.135 (Continued) (d–g) Detachable loops employed to reduce post-polypectomy bleeding given the wide stalk base. (h, i) Complete resection examination of bases and post-APC fulgaration of base. (Jonathan Cohen, NYU Langone School of Medicine.)

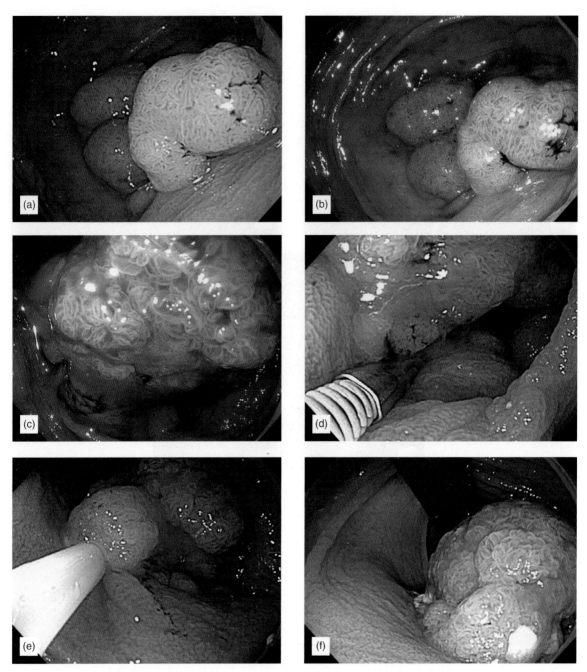

Figure 17.136 (a–k) H190 HRE WL and NBI imaging used to asses and clearly define the borders to assist in the piecemeal resection of this very large sessile mass-like tubulovillous adenoma at the splenic flexure. Injection and resection performed both anterograde and in retroflexion using a gastroscope with a 3 mm clear cap on the scope tip. A prominent vessel is identified and coagulated with using a grasper forceps and soft coagulation (g, h).

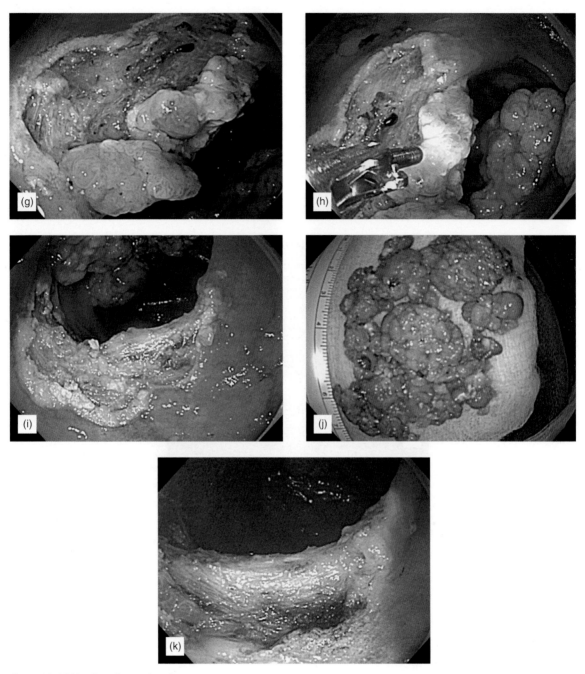

Figure 17.136 (Continued) (continued)

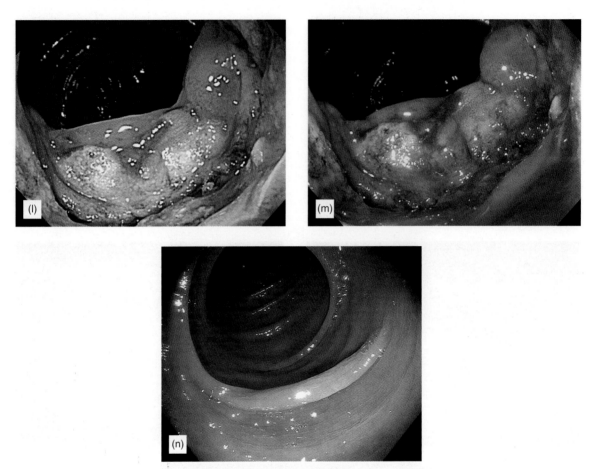

Figure 17.136 (Continued) (l, m) WL and NBI of retracted polyp base following resection and APC fulgaration around the margin. (n) WL image at 1 year follow up examination of the resection site shows tattoo mark and no residual or recurrent adenoma. (Jonathan Cohen, NYU Langone School of Medicine.)

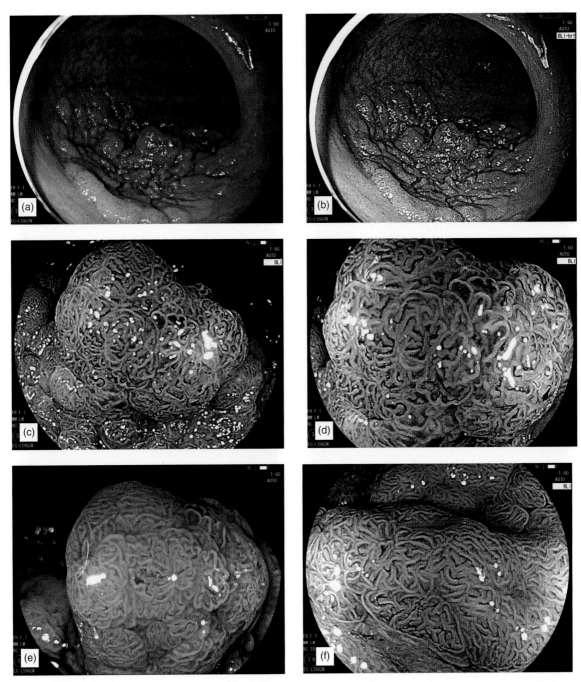

Figure 17.137 (a–h) WL and Fujinon blue laser imaging (BLI) of large lateral spreading tumor, granular type (LST-G) with normal and magnification view. The lesion was removed with endoscopic submucosal dissection (ESD) and the histopathology shown to correlate with the endoscopic optical diagnosis. (a) WL low magnification reveals a LST-G in the distal colon with a prominent raised area in the middle of the lesion. (b) Low magnification BLI image of the LST-G in the distal colon. (c) The raised portion of the LST-G is generally an area of concern for more invasive parts of the lesion. (d) High magnification BLI image from the central raised area identifies highly irregular vessels. (e) Chromoendoscopy is performed with magnification of the central nodule. (f) A more regular 3L pit pattern is seen corresponding to the more flat areas of the LST. (continued)

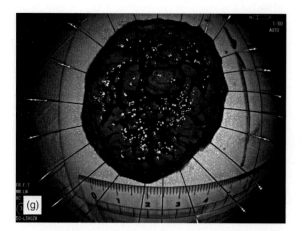

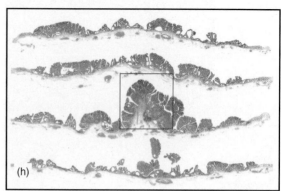

Figure 17.137 (Continued) (g) En bloc ESD specimen. (h) Histopathology reveals a laterally spreading adenoma with high grade dysplasia in the elevated central region where superficial submucosal invasion cannot be excluded. (Courtesy of Naohisa Yoshida, Kyoto Prefectural University of Medicine.)

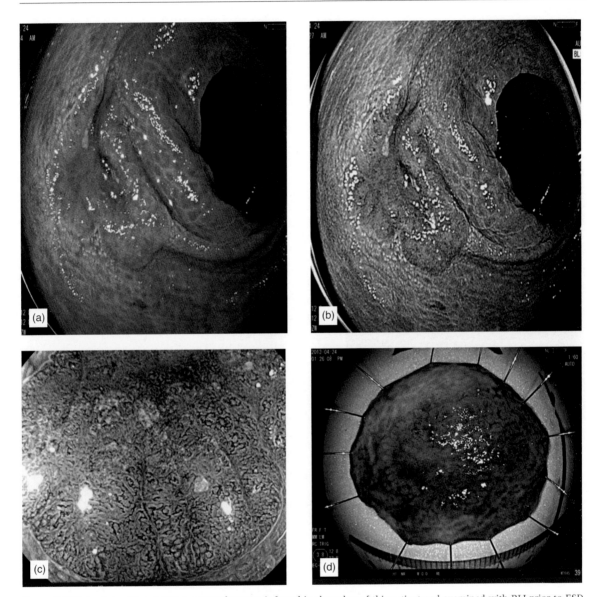

Figure 17.138 (a–e) An 18-mm LST, nongranular type, is found in the colon of this patient and examined with BLI prior to ESD. (a) WL, (b) FICE, and (c) BLI magnification views. (d) ESD specimen. (continued)

(e)

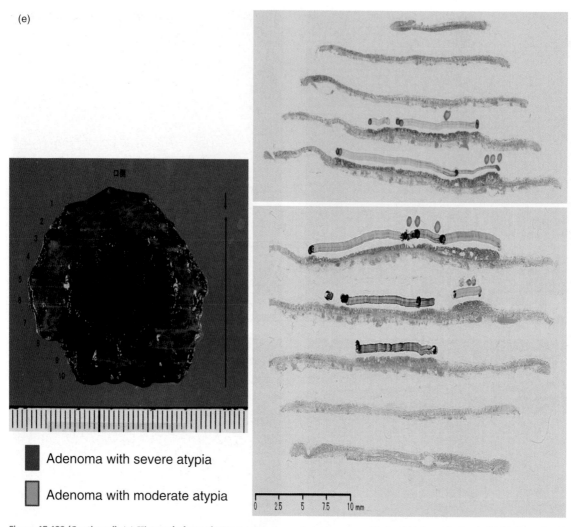

Adenoma with severe atypia

Adenoma with moderate atypia

Figure 17.138 (Continued) (e) Histopathology of ESD specimen revealed adenoma with focal high-grade dysplasia (high-grade adenoma, HM0, VM0). (Courtesy of Naohisa Yoshida, Kyoto Prefectural University of Medicine.)

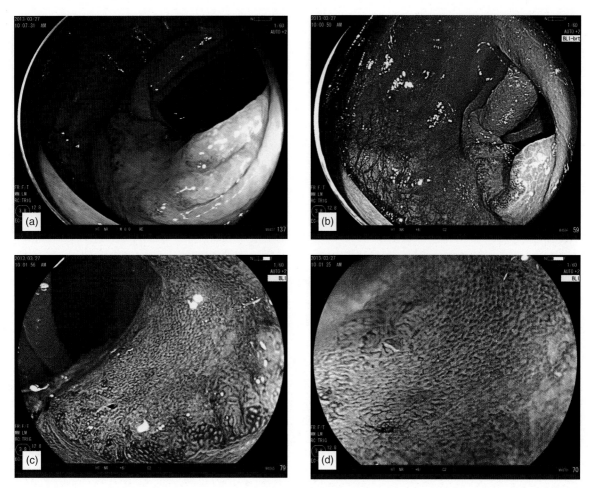

Figure 17.139 (a) WL view of LST, nongranular type, 0-IIa, 20 mm with central depression in the transverse colon. (b) BLI view. (c) Magnification of the depressed central region. (d) High magnification view. (continued)

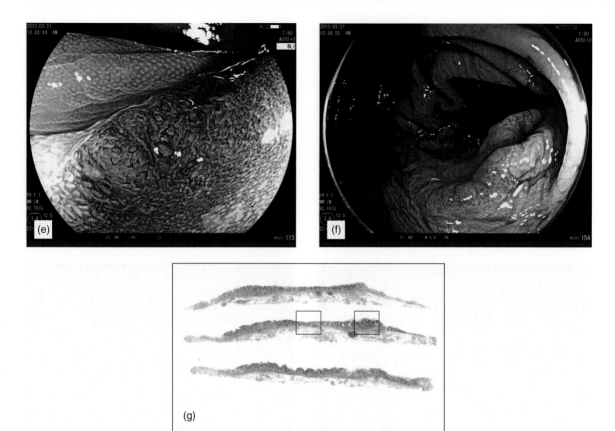

Figure 17.139 (Continued) (e) Magnification of the tumor lateral raised edge reveals highly abnormal vessels. (f) Chromoendoscopy is performed to inspect for signs of invasive cancer. (g) Histopathology reveals a lateral spreading adenoma with low and focal high grade dysplasia. (Courtesy of Naohisa Yoshida, Kyoto Prefectural University of Medicine.)

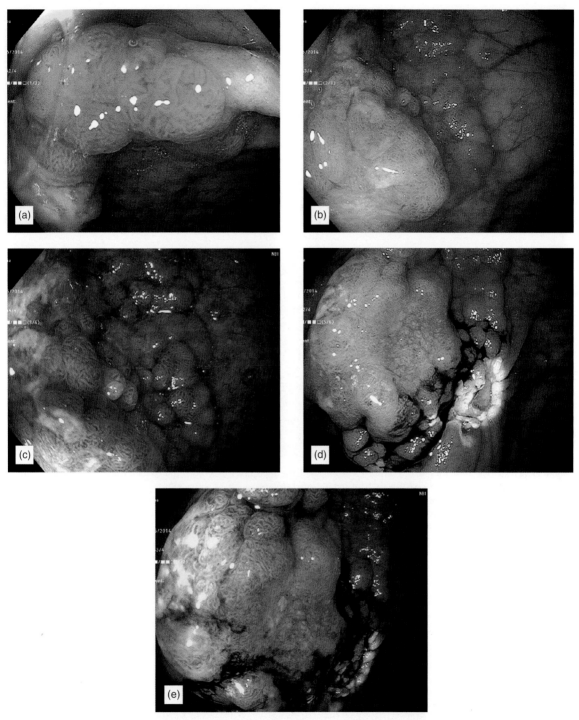

Figure 17.140 Malignant polyp in ascending colon. (a) A 3-cm sessile polyp in ascending colon WL H190 view. (b) Edge of polyp clearly demonstrated. (c) NBI demonstrates surface morphology of this portion of polyp. (d) This portion of polyp did not elevate with submucosal injection of saline. A close look revealed an indentation in the polyp with an amorphous appearance in that area. (e) NBI demonstrates a lack of usual adenomatous vascularity in the depressed area with a chaotic pattern in the center as compared to the surrounding adenoma. On biopsy this was an invasive carcinoma. (Jerome Waye, Mount Sinai School of Medicine.)

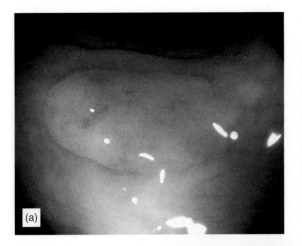

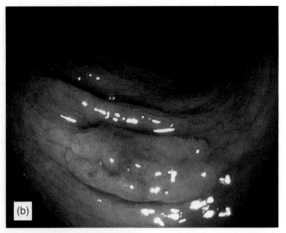

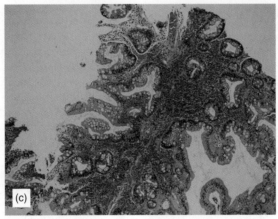

Figure 17.141 (a) Typical appearance of a serrated adenoma with the appearance of an accentuated fold. The architecture is indistinct on this WL H180 view, (b) seen with NBI light. The architecture is somewhat pitted with villiform components and is better defined than on the WL view. (c) Colonic mucosa with hyperplastic glands having a "sawtooth" appearance at the surface and dilation at the base with basal goblet cells. No dysplasia is seen. (James DiSario, University of Utah Health Sciences Center.)

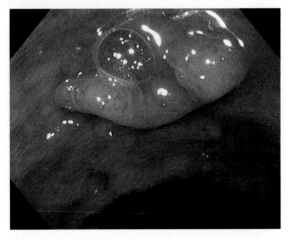

Figure 17.142 NBI H190 non-magnified view of a sessile polyp with a mixed surface vascular pattern, found on pathology to be a serrated polyp. (Jonathan Cohen, NYU Langone School of Medicine.)

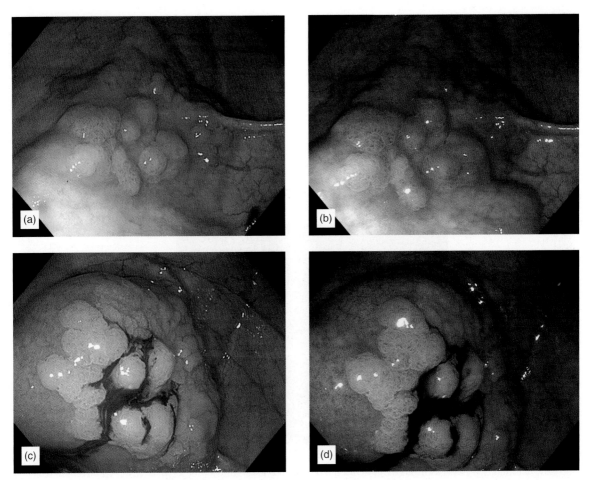

Figure 17.143 (a) Laterally spreading adenoma in cecum WL H180 view. (b) NBI low-magnification view. (c) Cecal adenoma elevated on pillow of saline from submucosal injection prior to piecemeal resection. (d) NBI view of the cecal adenoma following submucosal injection of saline. (continued)

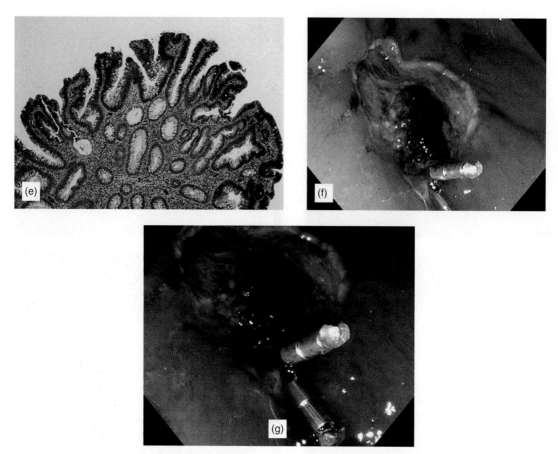

Figure 17.143 (Continued) (e) Laterally spreading adenoma in cecum (pathology). (f) Post-polypectomy site after APC and clips. Polypectomy done under WL. NBI used afterwards to rule out residual polyp. (g) NBI view of polyp site following piecemeal resection and APC with two clips for hemostasis; no residual polyp present. (Mount Sinai School of Medicine.)

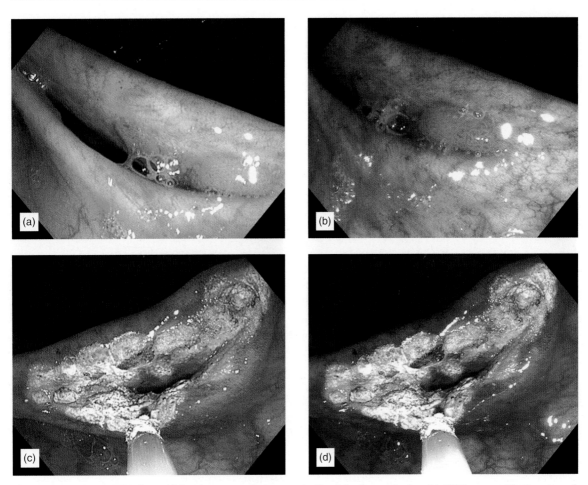

Figure 17.144 (a) WL H190 view with barely apparent polyps on the lip of the ileocecal valve. (b) NBI low-magnification view of two polyps on the lip of the ileocecal valve. (c) APC fulguration of polyps on lip of ileocecal valve. (d) NBI view of APC fulguration of polyps on ileocecal valve. (Mount Sinai School of Medicine.)

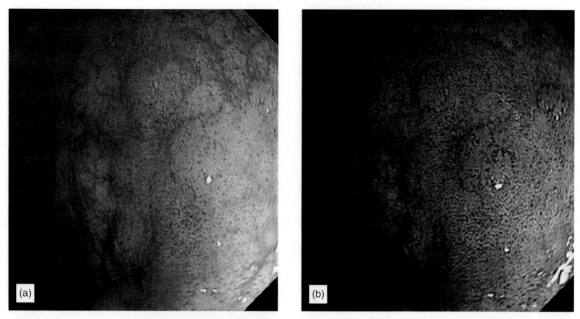

Figure 17.145 (a) Multiple rectal adenomas in familial adenomatous polyposis (FAP) H180 WL view. (b) Multiple adenomas in FAP. Note with NBI improved contrast for adenoma edges. (James East, St Mark's Hospital.)

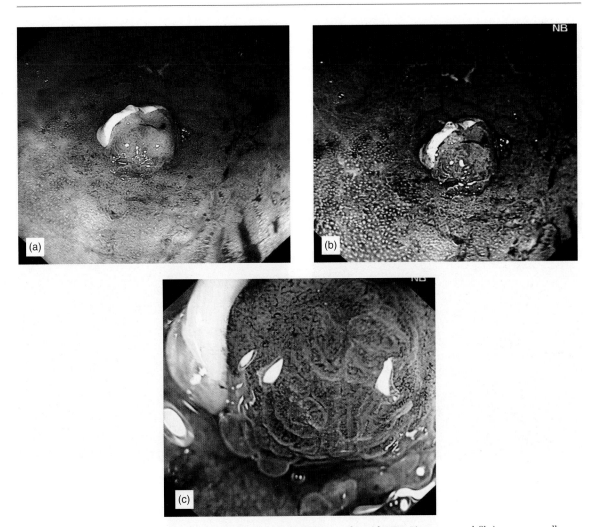

Figure 17.146 (a) Inflammatory polyp in ulcerative colitis with fibrin cap, (b) with NBI. Pit pattern and fibrin cap are well seen. (c) Magnification NBI view of inflammatory polyp in ulcerative colitis with pseudo type 4 pit pattern. However, histopathology reveals mainly granulation tissue. (James East, St Mark's Hospital.)

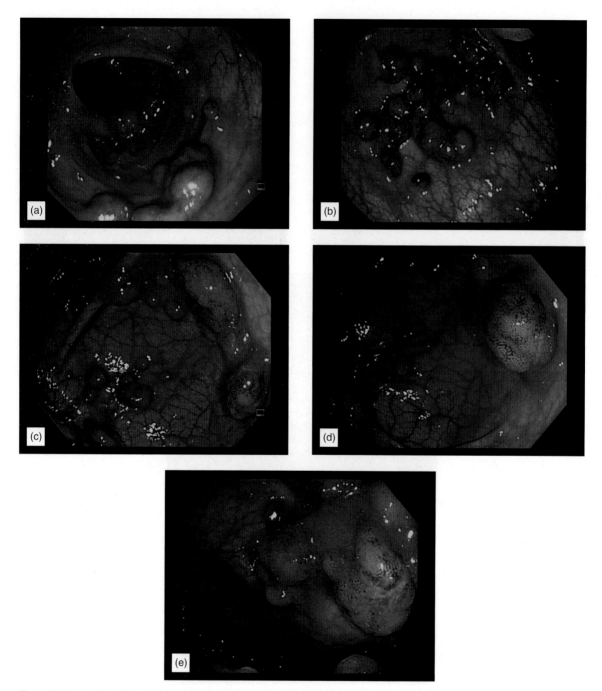

Figure 17.147 (a–e) An 18-year-old male patient with FAP (mutation in *APC* gene), paternally inherited. During first screening colonoscopy, around 200–300 adenomatous polyps were seen, increasing in size and number distally, with more than 20 polyps in the rectum H190 WL images. (University of Amsterdam.)

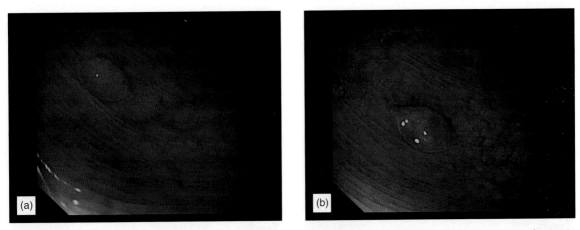

Figure 17.148 A 33-year-old male patient with hereditary nonpolyposis colorectal cancer (HNPCC, *MSH6* mutation.) In the proximal transverse colon, a 3-mm flat lesion is seen in (a) WL H190 and (b) NBI. Histology showed a tubular adenoma with low-grade dysplasia. (University of Amsterdam.).

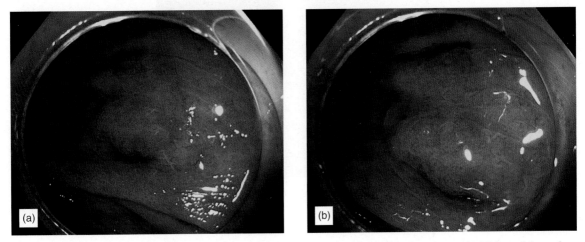

Figure 17.149 (a, b) Sessile serrated adenoma (SSA): NBI H190 low magnification and near focus images highlight nodular surface and waxy film with traces of residual fecal material. (Michael Wallace, Mayo Clinic Jacksonville.)

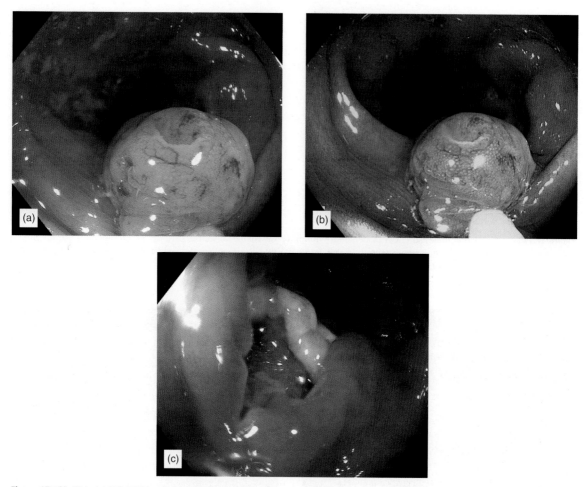

Figure 17.150 SSA: (a) WL H190 and (b) NBI views and (c) post EMR. (Jonathan Cohen, NYU Langone School of Medicine.)

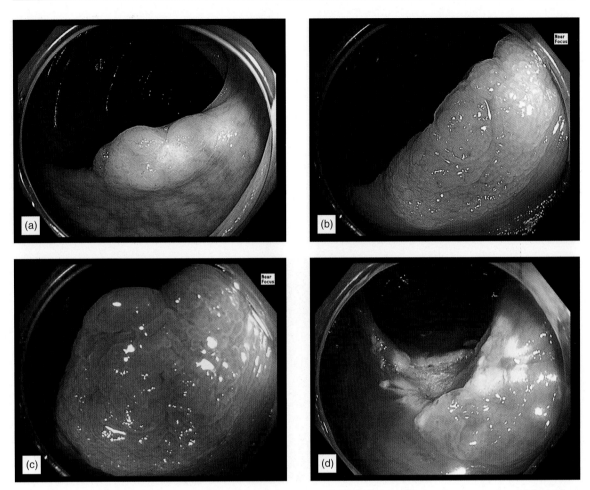

Figure 17.151 (a–c) H190 WL low magnification and near focus views and NBI high magnification demonstrate the nodular surface pattern typical of a serrated sessile adenoma. There is a bland vascular pattern. (d) Post saline injection assisted polypectomy. (Jonathan Cohen, NYU Langone School of Medicine.)

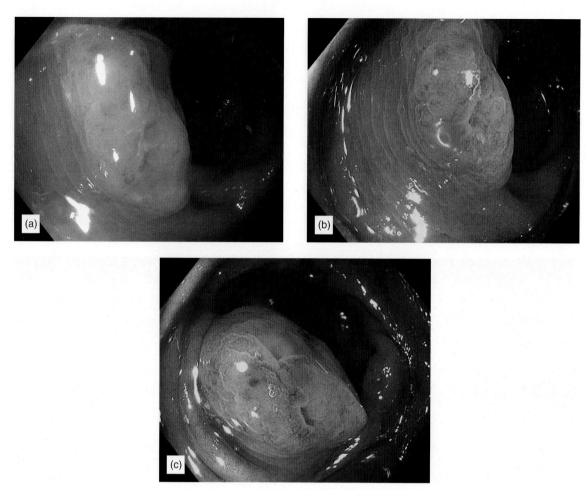

Figure 17.152 (a–c) SSA: nodular surface and mucoid cap on WL and NBI H190 views; NBI following injection accentuates features. (Jonathan Cohen, NYU Langone School of Medicine.)

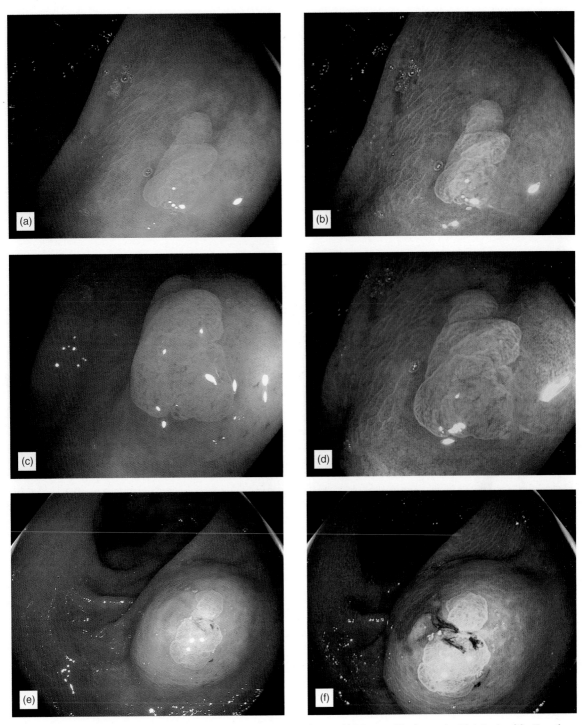

Figure 17.153 (a–f) Flat serrated sessile adenoma WL and NBI H190 low and high magnification and with injection lift. (Jonathan Cohen, NYU Langone School of Medicine.)

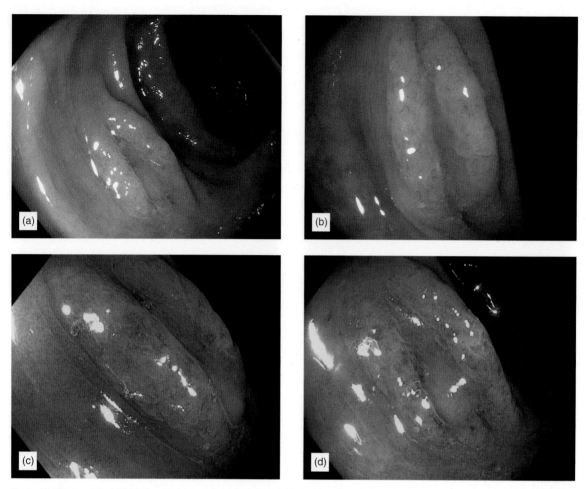

Figure 17.154 A residual SSA following biopsy alone is seen on folds in the right colon seen on WL and NBI H190 in both low magnification (a) and near focus WL and NBI (b, c). (d) Shows central scarring from the prior intervention between the two serrated portions of the lesion.

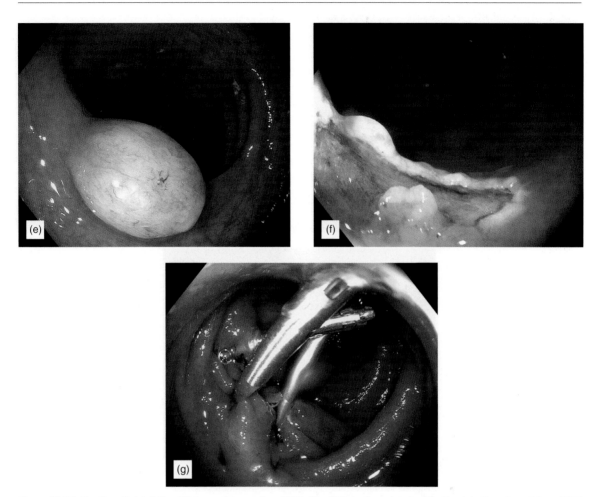

Figure 17.154 (Continued) (e) Saline lift is possible to allow EMR (f) which is then closed with clips (g). (Jonathan Cohen, NYU Langone School of Medicine.)

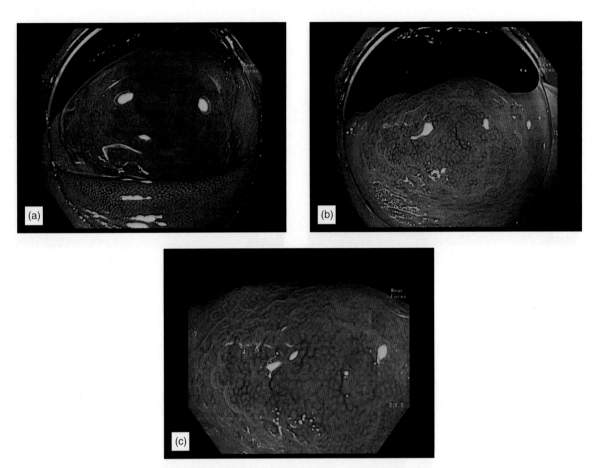

Figure 17.155 (a) Classic mucous cap atop SSA seen here in NBI H190 view. (b) Polyp following washing off of surface mucus and debris. (c) Near-focus NBI view illustrates several features of SSA, including cloud-like pits, round pits, and thin spidery vessels. (Rajvinder Singh, Lyell McEwin Hospital, Adelaide.)

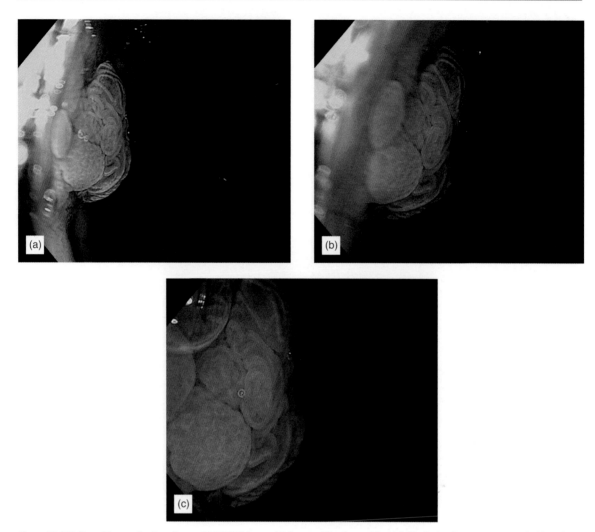

Figure 17.156 Rectal hyperplastic polyp on NBI H190 low to high magnification, with thick black circular spots surrounded by white. (James Lau, Chinese University of Hong Kong.)

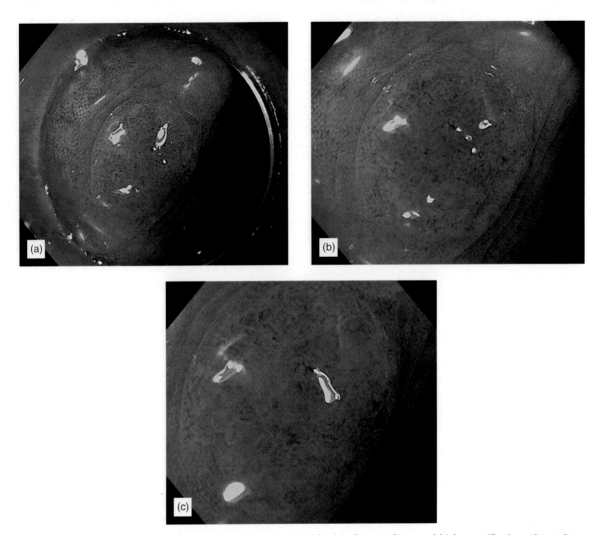

Figure 17.157 (a–c) Tiny low-grade dysplasia in adenoma in sigmoid colon: low, medium, and high magnification. (James Lau, Chinese University of Hong Kong.)

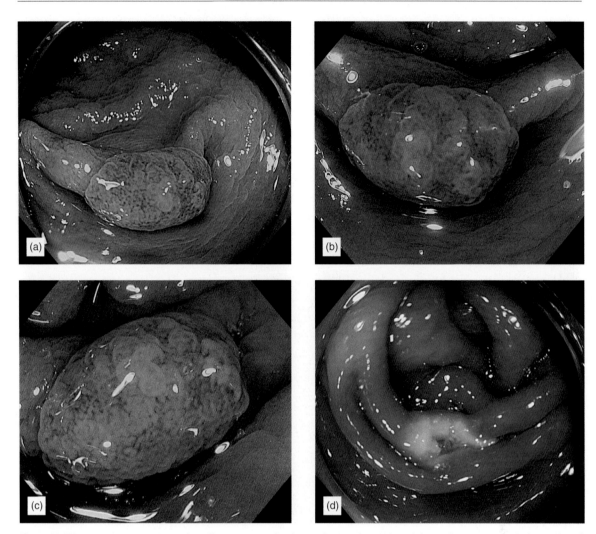

Figure 17.158 (a–c) NBI H190 views of small transverse colon hyperplastic polyp with nodular surface, raising optical question of serrated polyp in increasing magnification on Lucera NBI. (d) Post-polypectomy WL view. (James Lau, Chinese University of Hong Kong.)

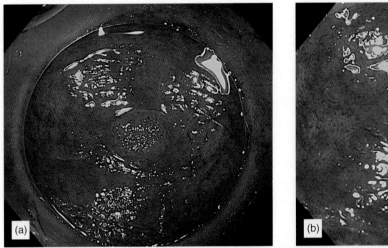

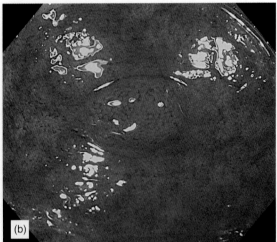

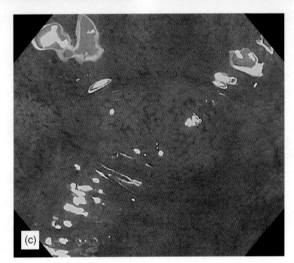

Figure 17.159 Diminutive flat adenoma seen in NBI H190 low (a), medium (b), and high (c) magnification demonstrating NICE 2 pattern of round white dots surrounded by dark vessels. (James Lau, Chinese University of Hong Kong.)

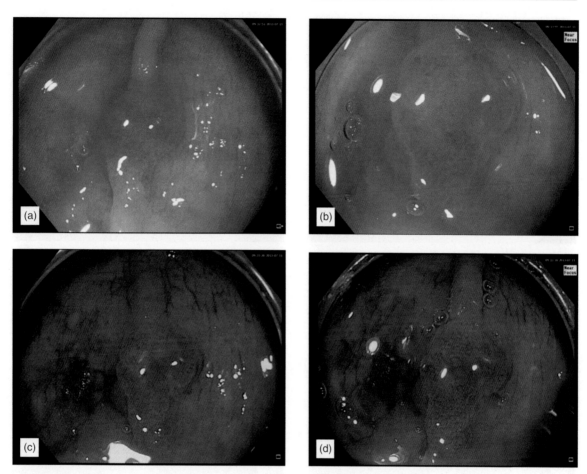

Figure 17.160 Traditional SSA of colon. (a) H190 WL endoscopy shows a flat (Paris IIa) colon polyp, here shown covered with a mucous cap. (b) After washing off the mucous cap, H190 WL near-focus view of the same polyp highlights some of the surface pattern as distinctly different from the surrounding normal colon mucosa. (c) H190 NBI of the same polyp highlights the exact borders of the polyp from the surrounding mucosa. (d) H190 NBI near-focus view of same polyp demonstrates the unique surface pattern that contains both tubulo-gyrus features and circular dot features. (Neil Gupta, Loyola University Health System.)

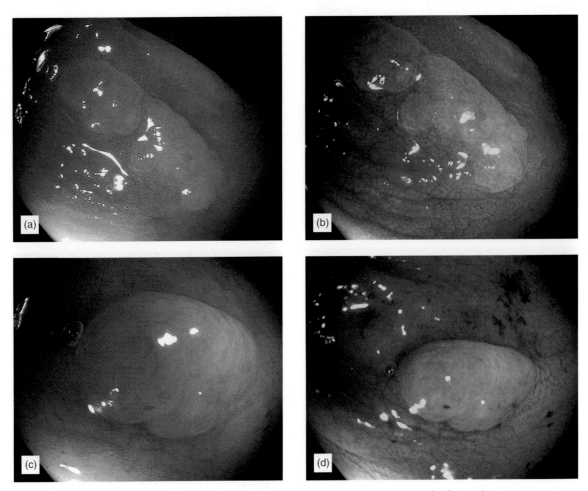

Figure 17.161 (a–d) Serrated polyp, WL and NBI H190 views. (Jonathan Cohen, NYU Langone School of Medicine.)

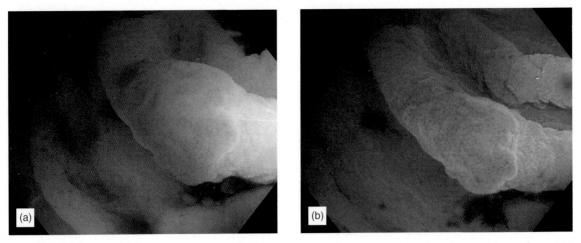

Figure 17.162 (a, b) Serrated flat polyp seen underwater in WL and NBI H190 low magnification views. (Jonathan Cohen, NYU Langone School of Medicine.)

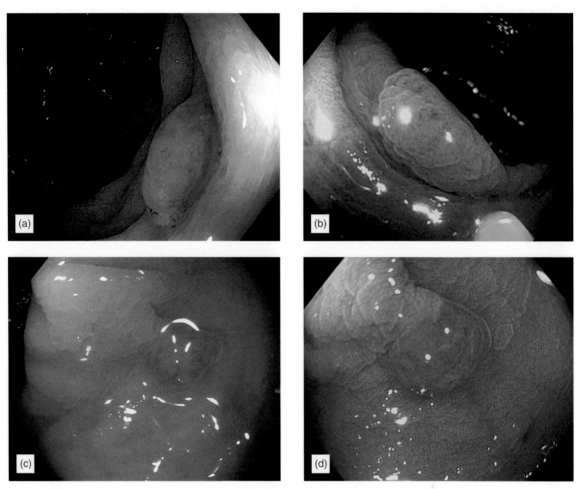

Figure 17.163 (a, b) Normal magnification WL and NBI H190 view of SSA; note the nodular surface and relatively bland vascular pattern. This small serrated polyp is shown in WL and NBI low magnification (c, d). (continued)

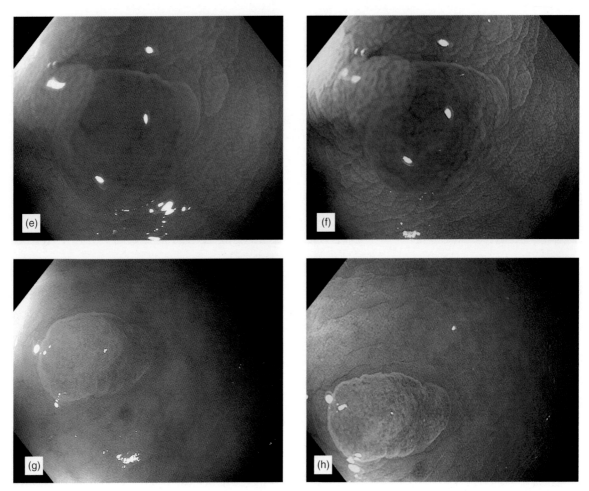

Figure 17.163 (Continued) (e, f) Small serrated polyp shown with near focus. (g, h) Sessile small SSA in WL and NBI H190 near focus view. (Jonathan Cohen, NYU Langone School of Medicine.)

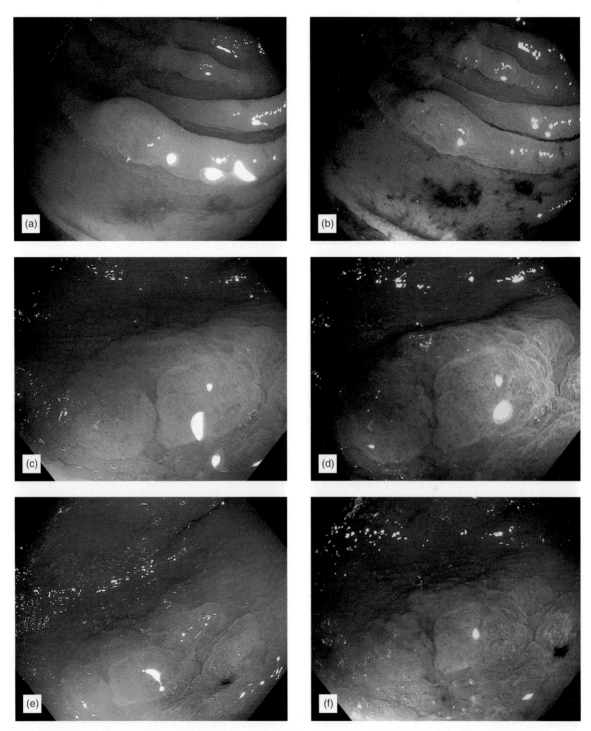

Figure 17.164 (a–f) More SSA polyps, WL and NBI H190 views. (Jonathan Cohen, NYU Langone School of Medicine.)

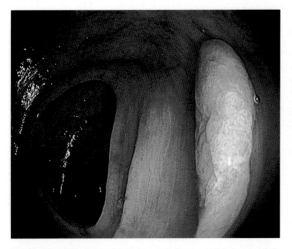

Figure 17.165 Suspected adenoma with serrated features, right colon, WL H190 view. (Jonathan Cohen, NYU Langone School of Medicine.)

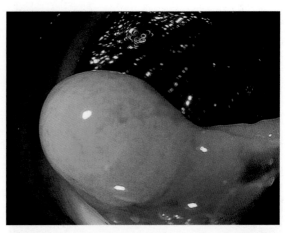

Figure 17.166 An 8-mm SSA with clear pearly mucoid surface appearance with largely bland mucosal pattern H190 WL view. (Jonathan Cohen, NYU Langone School of Medicine.)

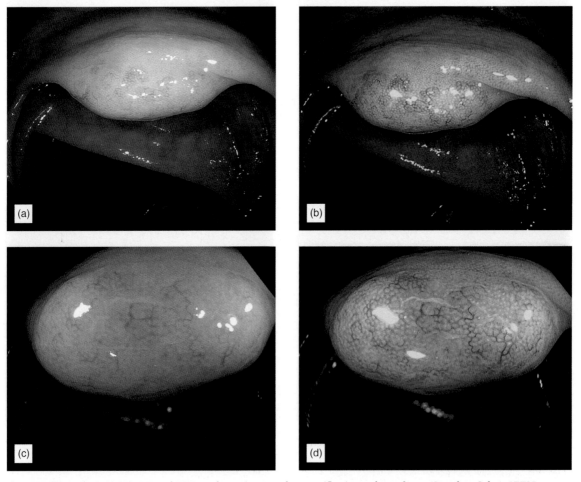

Figure 17.167 (a–d) H190 SSA, WL and NBI near focus views regular magnification and near focus. (Jonathan Cohen, NYU Langone School of Medicine.)

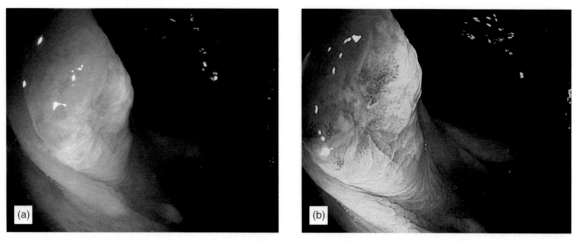

Figure 17.168 (a, b) SSA, WL and NBI with nodular appearance and mucoid appearance to surface H190. (Jonathan Cohen, NYU Langone School of Medicine.)

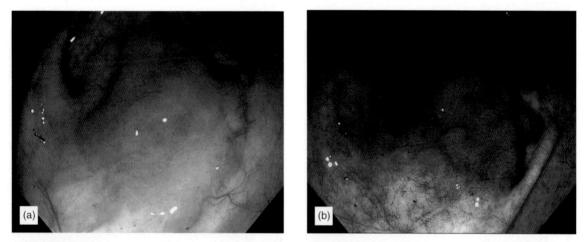

Figure 17.169 (a, b) A 20-mm flat SSA in the cecum, WL and NBI H190 views. Clear mucous cap, nodular surface, and retention of stool remnant film on lesion are clues to detection. (University of Amsterdam.)

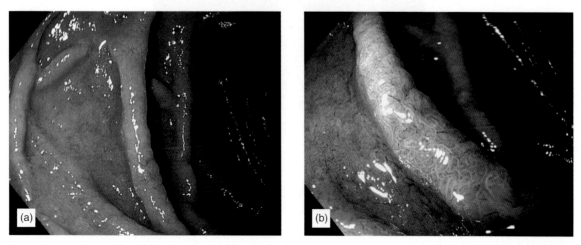

Figure 17.170 (a, b) SSA along fold, WL and NBI H190 near-focus views. Findings on normal magnification WL are subtle and easily missed without careful inspection and consideration of the surface texture of each fold. (Michael Wallace, Mayo Clinic Jacksonville.)

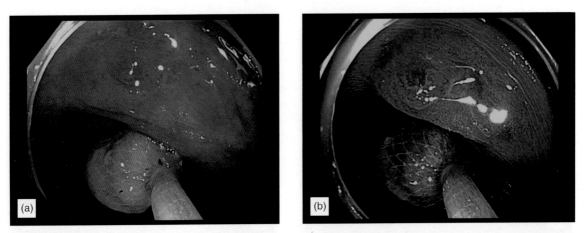

Figure 17.171 (a, b) A 2-cm rectal SSA with low-grade and focal high-grade dysplasia here being retrieved with net H190 WL and NBI views. (University of Amsterdam.)

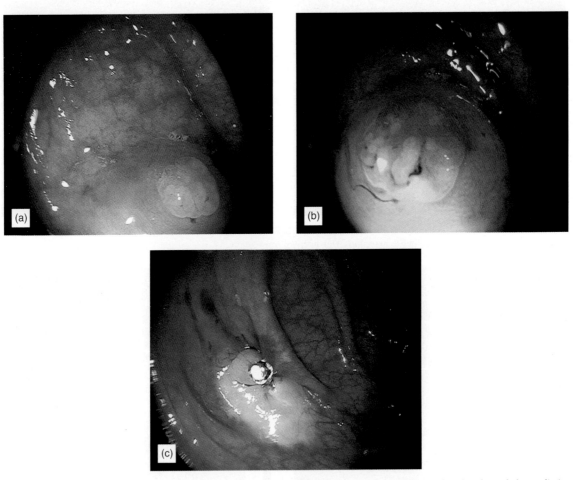

Figure 17.172 Nodular SSA post saline lift in (a) WL H190 and (b) NBI near-focus views. (c) EMR site closed with single hemoclip in setting of planned early resumption of required anticoagulation. (Jonathan Cohen, NYU Langone School of Medicine.)

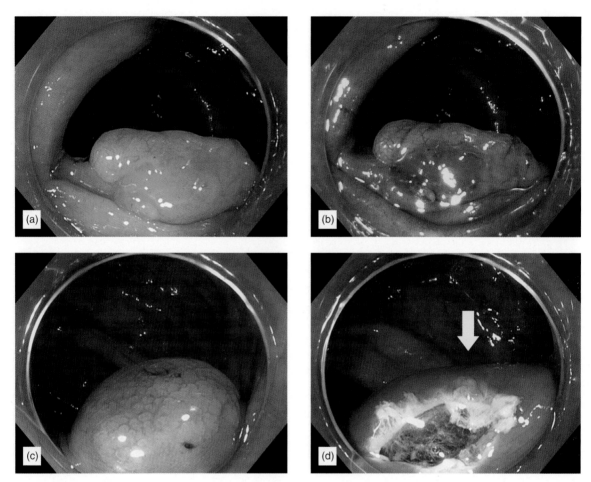

Figure 17.173 (a–d) SSA and margin assessment post resection on WL and NBI H190 views. Submucosal lift accentuates lesion and post-EMR margin resection reveals residual tissue. (Michael Wallace, Mayo Clinic Jacksonville.)

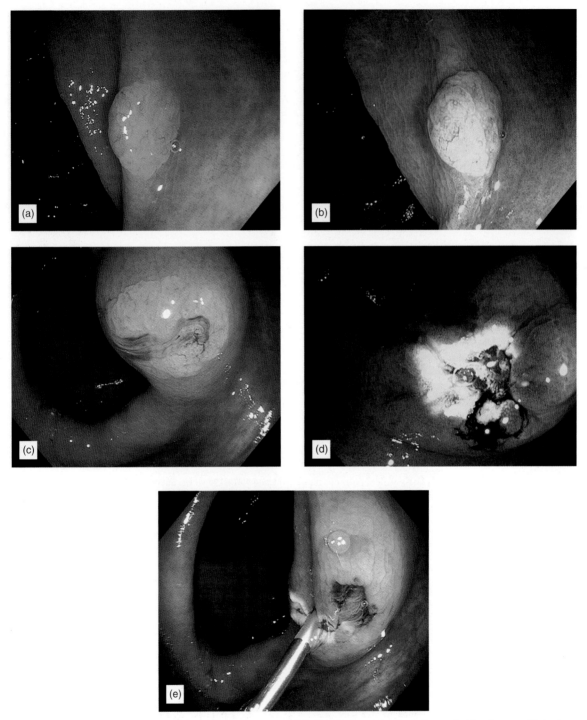

Figure 17.174 (a–e) SSA with fine isolated erratic vessels on WL and NBI H190 views. Margins delineated with submucosal injection. (Jonathan Cohen, NYU Langone School of Medicine.)

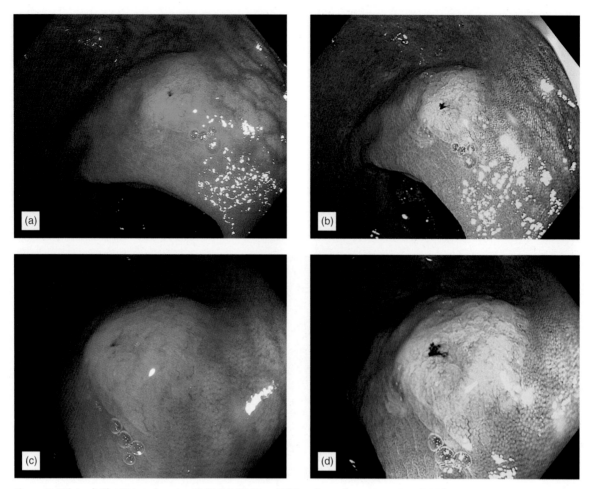

Figure 17.175 (a–d) Flat SSA undergoing EMR, WL H190 and NBI and near-focus views. (continued)

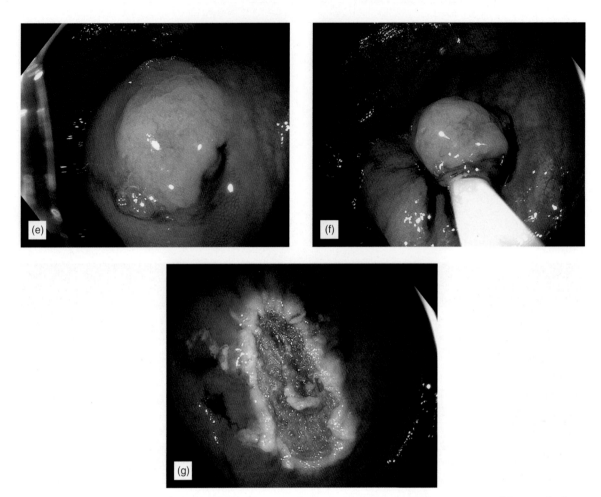

Figure 17.175 (Continued) (e–g) Resection en block of this serrated polyp in WL with post resection assessment of the resection base and margin. (Jonathan Cohen, NYU Langone School of Medicine.)

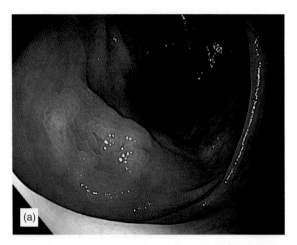 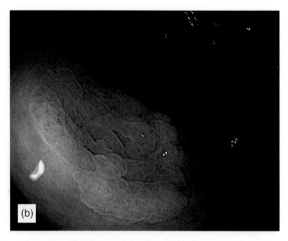

Figure 17.176 (a, b) Right-sided SSA, WL and NBI H190 views. Typical flat and nodular surface pattern requires excellent preparation and careful examination to detect. (Tonya Kaltenbach, Veterans Affairs Palo Alto Health Care System.)

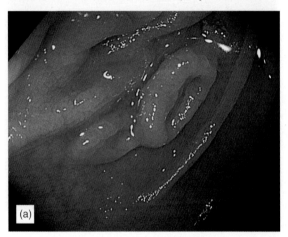 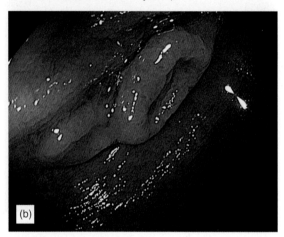

Figure 17.177 (a, b) This SSA looks on first inspection to be an inverted diverticulum H190 WL view. However, close NBI inspection of the rim shows nodular surface, sporadic erratic vessels, and mucous cap suggestive of SSA. (Tonya Kaltenbach, Veterans Affairs Palo Alto Health Care System.)

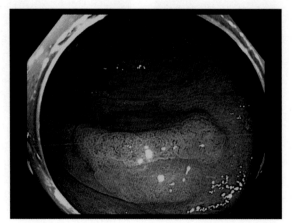

Figure 17.178 NBI normal magnification view through 3-mm cap of ascending colon showing 2.5-cm SSA with low-grade dysplasia. (University of Amsterdam.).

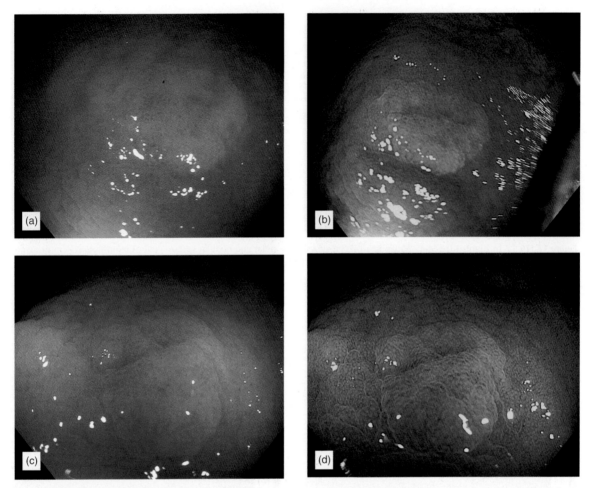

Figure 17.179 (a) Barely visible flat SSA on WL H190 view. (b) NBI view. (c, d) Near-focus WL and NBI views. (Jonathan Cohen, NYU Langone School of Medicine.)

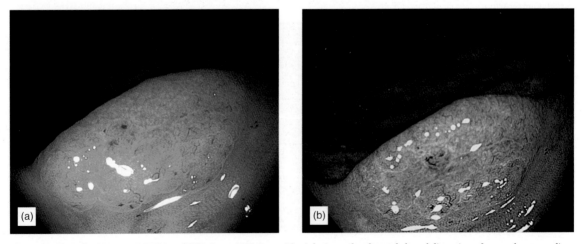

Figure 17.180 (a, b) SSA on WL H190 and NBI views. NBI view with pink rim on border and clear delineation of normal surrounding pit pattern highlights the borders of this lesion prior to EMR. (Tonya Kaltenbach, Veterans Affairs Palo Alto Health Care System.)

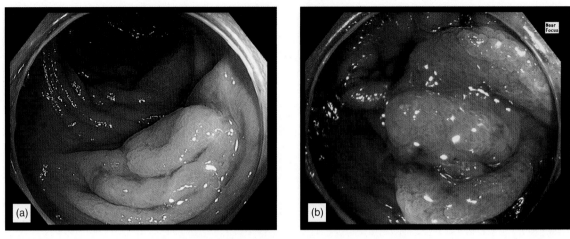

Figure 17.181 (a, b) Large SSA over 2 folds seen on WL H190 and NBI near focus view. (Jonathan Cohen, NYU Langone School of Medicine.)

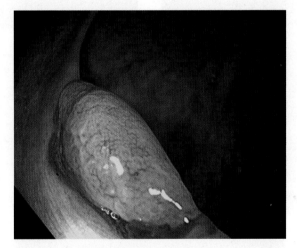

Figure 17.182 NBI use in margin detection may begin with recognition of pink film of residual stool material around the border of a sessile polyp, as shown here around this SSA H190 low magnification view. (Jonathan Cohen, NYU Langone School of Medicine.)

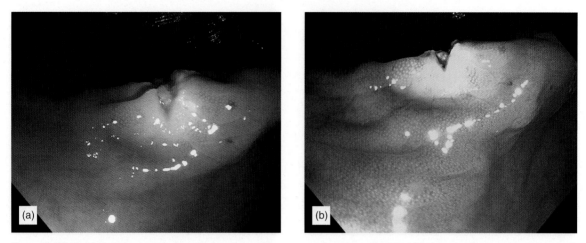

Figure 17.183 (a, b) Examination of edge of polypectomy site post resection. WL and NBI H190 views confirm presence of normal pits reflecting complete resection. (Jonathan Cohen, NYU Langone School of Medicine.)

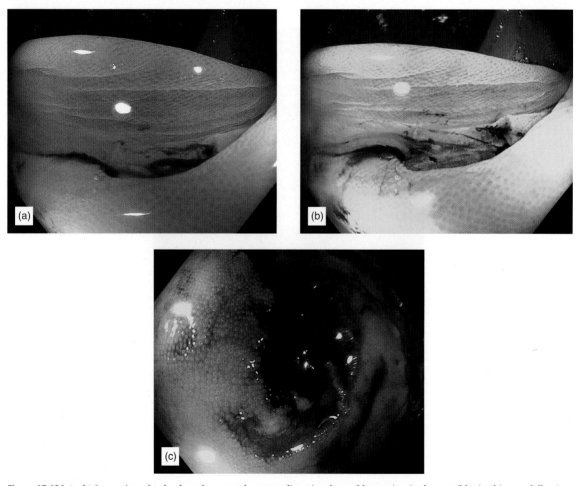

Figure 17.184 (a, b) Inspection of polyp base for normal surrounding pits after cold resection is also possible, in this case following a cold avulsion of a diminutive polyp in one piece WL and NBI H190 views. (c) This NBI near focus image following a cold snare polypectomy clearly demonstrates both the pits en face on the left and in horizontal cross section to the right of the resection margin. (Jonathan Cohen, NYU Langone School of Medicine.)

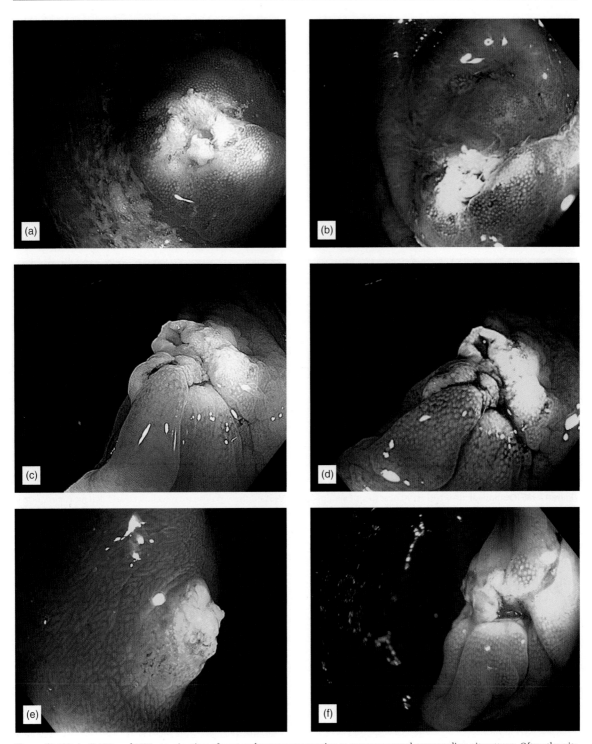

Figure 17.185 (a–j) WL and NBI examination of post-polypectomy margins to ensure normal surrounding pit pattern. Often the pits can be seen under WL but as shown the NBI near focus provides the clearer confirmation of normal pits H190 views. (continued)

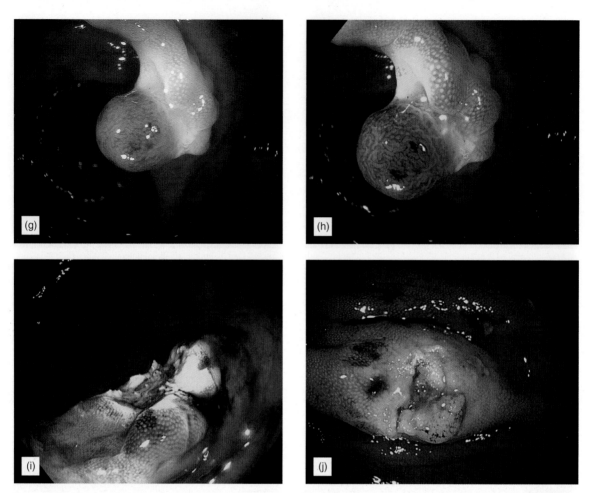

Figure 17.185 (Continued) (g–j) NBI H190 near focus examination of the periphery post snare resection clearly defenestrates normal colon pit pattern. (Jonathan Cohen, NYU Langone School of Medicine.)

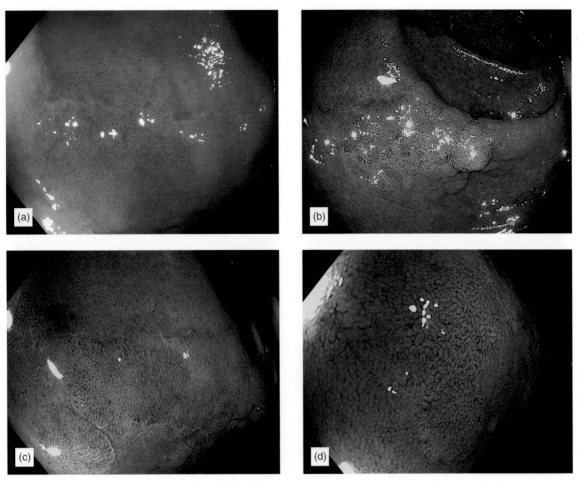

Figure 17.186 (a–d) WL and NBI H190 low magnification and near focus views of LST of the proximal ascending colon. (continued)

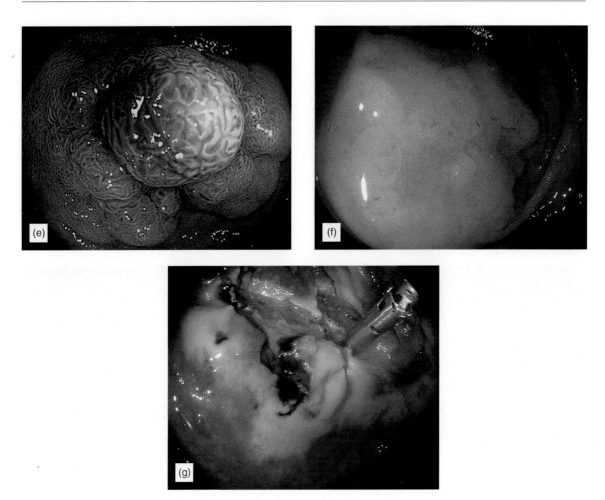

Figure 17.186 (Continued) (e–g) (e) Raised central area in this 3 cm LST raised concern for cancer, but NBI pattern did not. Tubular adenoma and tubulovillous adenoma confirmed on histology (f) WL image post submucosal injection of flat portion of the polyp. (g) post resection. (Dennis Jensen, David Geffen School of Medicine at UCLA.)

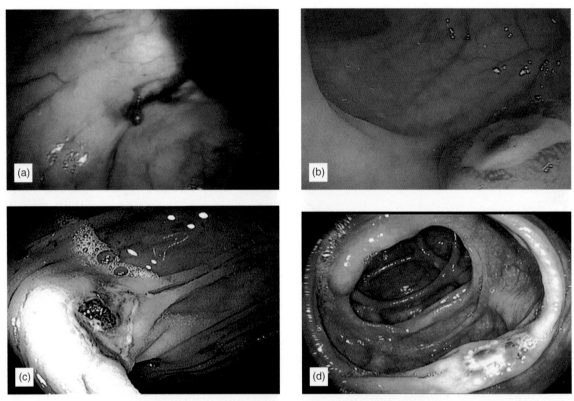

Figure 17.187 (a–d) WL images of endoscopic stigmata for delayed post-polypectomy ulcer bleeding. (a) Active arterial bleeding from under a clot, on urgent colonoscopy several days after outpatient polypectomy in ascending colon. (b) A flat spot on postpolypectomy induced ulcer (PPIU.) (c) An adherent clot on a PPIU. (d) A nonbleeding visible vessel. (Dennis Jensen, David Geffen School of Medicine at UCLA.)

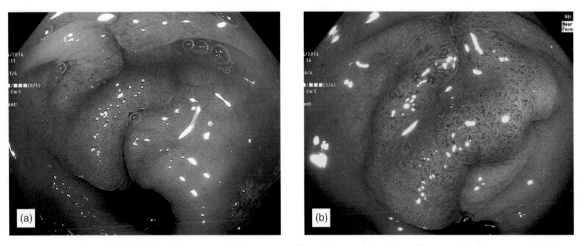

Figure 17.188 Delayed effects of prior biopsy on adenoma. (a) This polyp was biopsied 10 days previously. Neovascularization is noted at the biopsy site. (b) NBI H190 with near focus enhances the vascular appearance and clearly defines the edges of the adenoma. (Jerome Waye, Mount Sinai School of Medicine.)

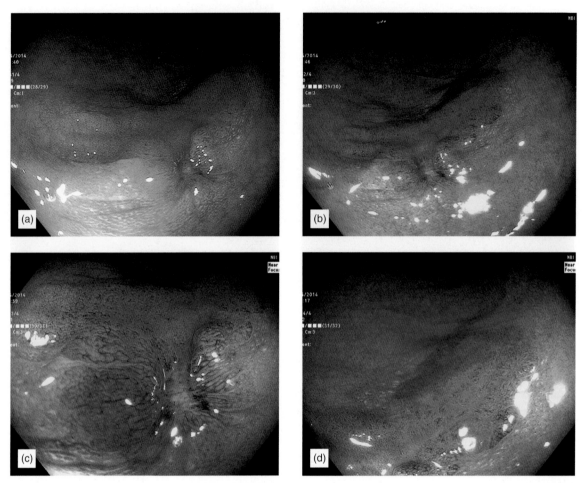

Figure 17.189 Residual adenoma following apparent total polypectomy. (a) A polypectomy 10 days previously declared this polyp to have been completely removed. A scar is present at the incised margin. Neovascularization is present H190 WL low magnification. (b) NBI demonstrates the neovascular reparative process but demonstrates a diffuse flat area of adenoma above the scar site (Paris 0-IIb, LST.) (c) NBI and near focus reveal no residual adenoma below the polypectomy scar but the neovascularization is clearly seen as is the extensive adenoma above the scar. (d) The extent of residual tumor proximal to the polypectomy scar is well demonstrated. (Jerome Waye, Mount Sinai School of Medicine.)

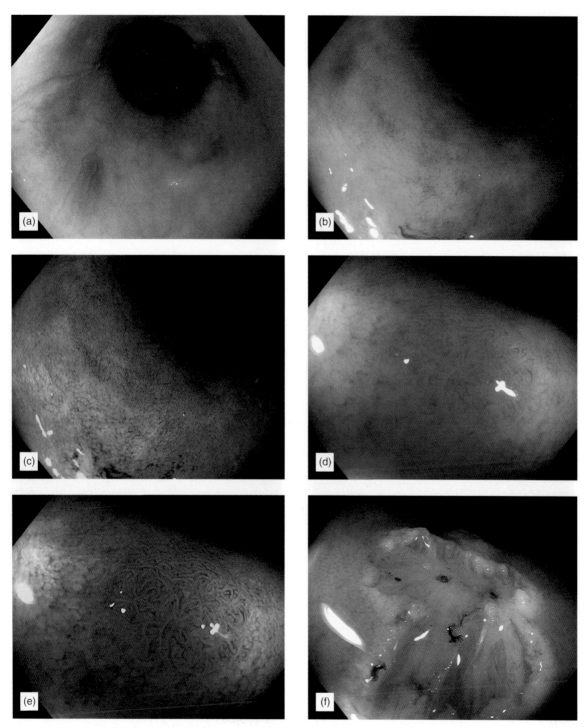

Figure 17.190 (a–f) On H190 WL, subtle recurrent flat adenoma detected between ink marks from prior piecemeal resection of rectal LST. Even with NBI and close examination, lesion is not apparent until near-focus view reveals adenoma. (Jonathan Cohen, NYU Langone School of Medicine.)

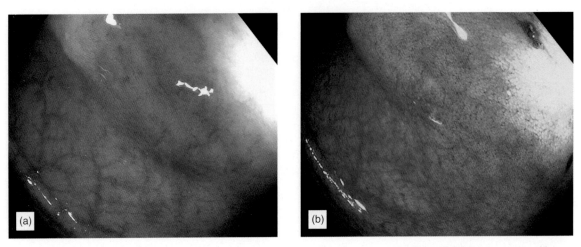

Figure 17.191 (a) Inspection of ink tattoo at site of prior polypectomy on WL H190 view. (b) NBI view: ink tattoo is not readily visible. (Jonathan Cohen, NYU Langone School of Medicine.)

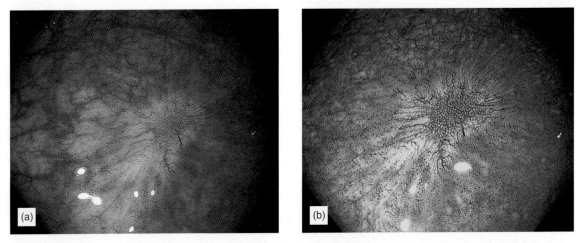

Figure 17.192 (a, b) Post-polypectomy scar on WL and NBI H190 views. (Jonathan Cohen, NYU Langone School of Medicine.)

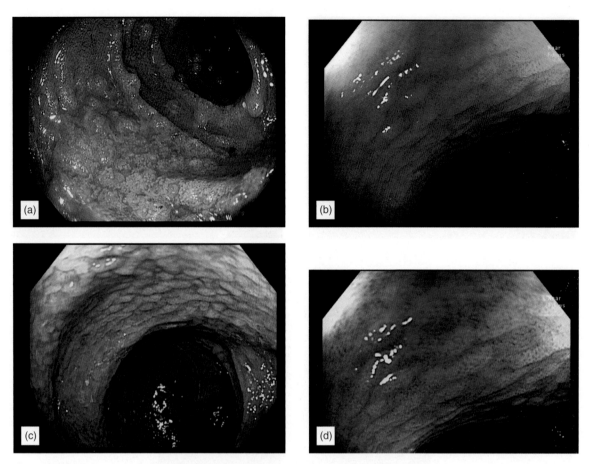

Figure 17.193 (a) Prominent ileal lymphoid tissue in an HIV-positive patient with negative viral load presenting with suspected infectious colitis with prolonged diarrhea. (b–d) Diffuse nodular colon mucosa without ulceration or visible inflammation: H190 WL, NBI, and NBI near-focus views. (Jonathan Cohen, NYU Langone School of Medicine.)

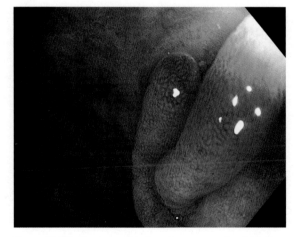

Figure 17.194 Classic psudopolyps in an area of mild inflammation in chronic ulcerative colitis, NBI H180 non-magnification view (Jonathan Cohen, NYU Langone School of Medicine.)

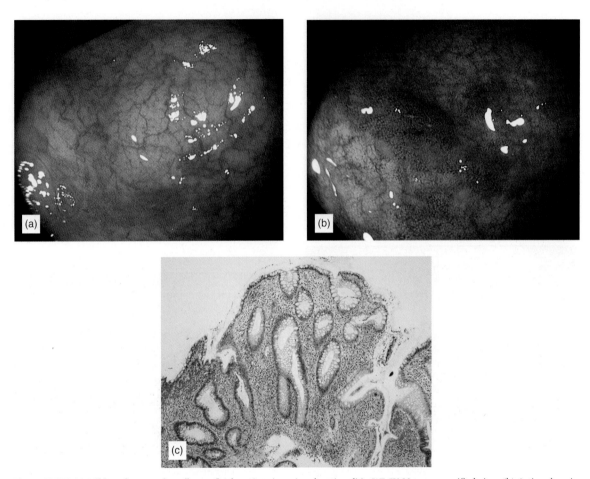

Figure 17.195 (a) Mild erythema and small superficial erosions in active chronic colitis, WL H180 non-magnified view. (b) Active chronic colitis, NBI low-magnification view. (c) Active chronic ulcerative colitis. The mucosal architecture is distorted, with branched glands and abnormal gland spacing, and a mixed acute and chronic inflammatory infiltrate expands the mucosa. (Jonathan Cohen, NYU Langone School of Medicine.)

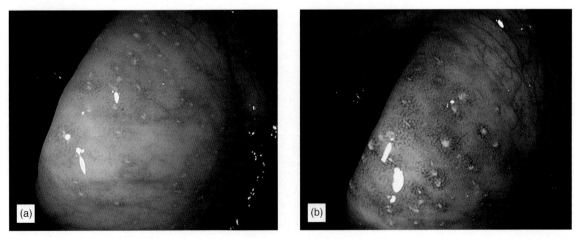

Figure 17.196 (a) WL H180 view of punctate erosions in the cecum of a patient with ulcerative colitis. (b) NBI low-magnification view of punctate cecal erosions in this patient with mildly active ulcerative colitis (Jonathan Cohen, NYU Langone School of Medicine.)

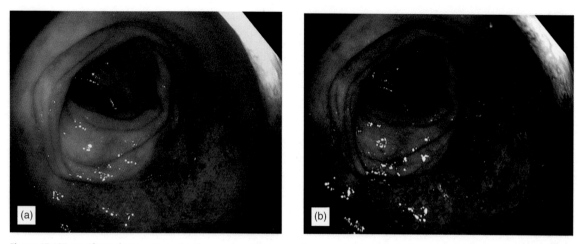

Figure 17.197 (a) Sharp demarcation of inflammation from normal mucosa at the splenic flexure in this patient with left-sided ulcerative colitis WL H180 view. (b) An NBI light view of sharp demarcation between inflamed and normal mucosa at the splenic flexure. (James DiSario, University of Utah Health Sciences Center.)

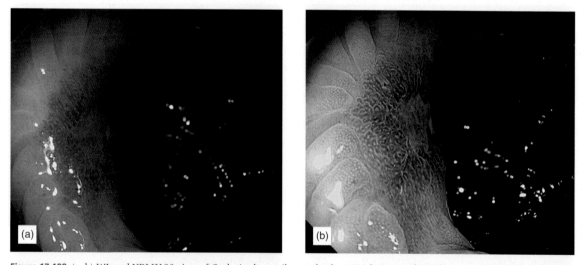

Figure 17.198 (a, b) WL and NBI H190 view of Crohn's ulcer at ileocecal valve. (Krish Ragunath, Wolfson Digestive Disease Centre).

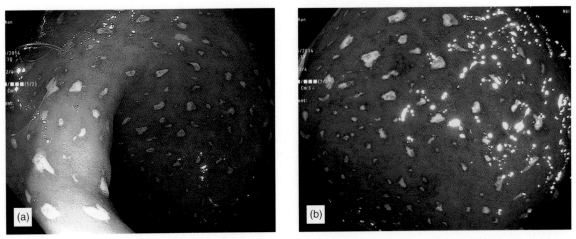

Figure 17.199 Healing ulcerative colitis after a severe flare of activity. (a) Ulcerations in chronic ulcerative colitis are always surrounded by markedly inflamed mucosa. This patient had a recent flare of activity that had been treated with a biological agent and rectal steroid enemas. The multiple ulcerations in this rectal image have no surrounding edema or erythema due to healing of the mucosa before the ulcerations heal WL H190 view. (b) NBI demonstrates engorged vascularity immediately surrounding each ulceration seen as dark areas surrounding each ulcer. This is evidence of the healing phase of the mucosa. (Jerome Waye, Mount Sinai School of Medicine.)

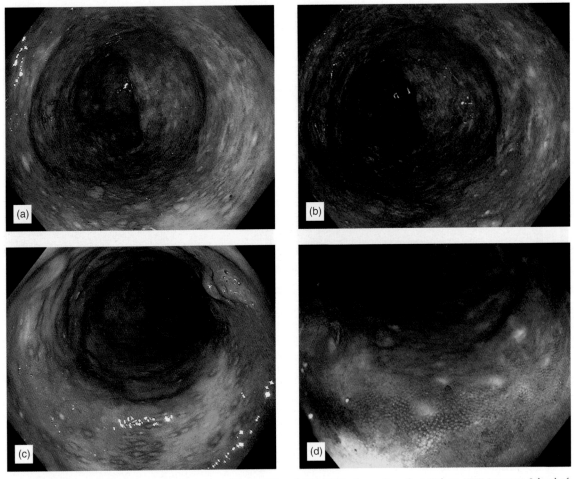

Figure 17.200 (a–d) Moderately active ulcerative colitis on WL and NBI H190 views. (Jonathan Cohen, NYU Langone School of Medicine.)

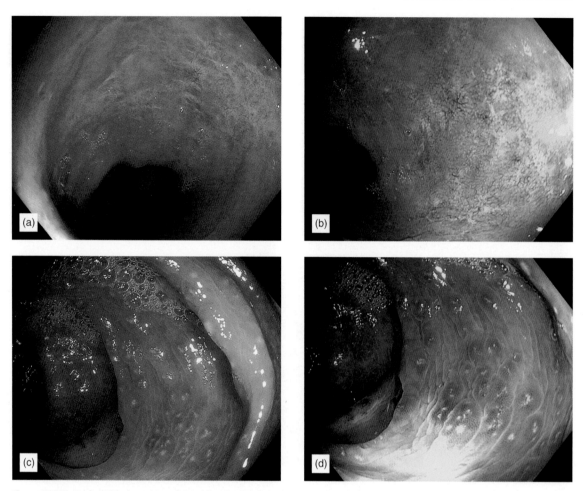

Figure 17.201 (a–d) Mild ulcerative colitis with superficial erosions on WL and NBI H190 views. (Jonathan Cohen, NYU Langone School of Medicine.)

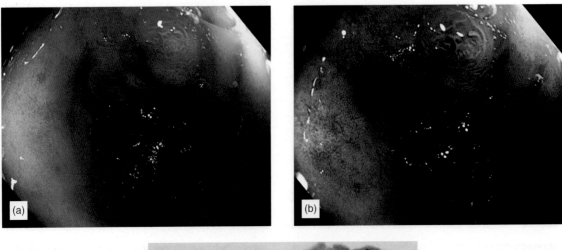

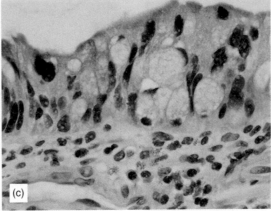

Figure 17.202 (a) Polypoid area in sigmoid colon of patient with ulcerative colitis in remission WL H180 view. (b) High-magnification NBI image of polypoid lesion with irregular vascular pattern and villous-appearing sulci in a patient with chronic ulcerative colitis in remission. (c) High-grade dysplasia in ulcerative colitis. There is loss of polarity in the surface epithelial cells, some of which contain atypical, enlarged hyperchromatic nuclei. (Jonathan Cohen, NYU Langone School of Medicine.)

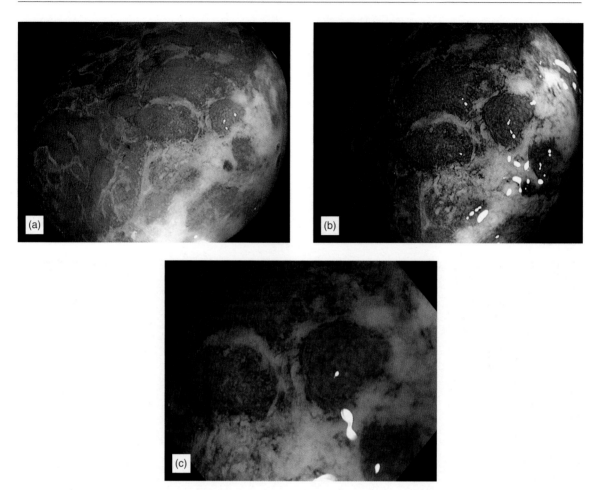

Figure 17.203 (a) Active rectal superficial ulceration with focal polypoid area WL H190 view. (b) Low-magnification NBI view of the focal polypoid area in this patient with active rectal ulceration. (c) High-magnification NBI view of the raised bump in this patient that, in contrast to the raised dysplastic lesion in (a) and (b), shows a regular mucosal pit pattern and normal vessels. (Jonathan Cohen, NYU Langone School of Medicine.)

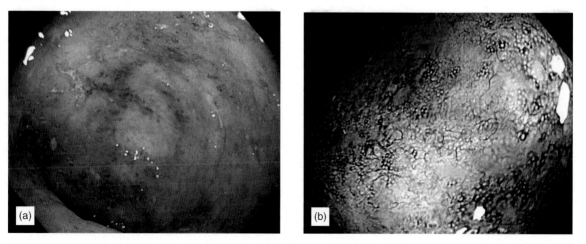

Figure 17.204 (a) Active ulcerative colitis, WL H180 low-magnification view. (b) NBI view of the same area more clearly shows the vascular pattern associated with active inflammation. (Jean-François Rey, Institut Arnault Tzanck.)

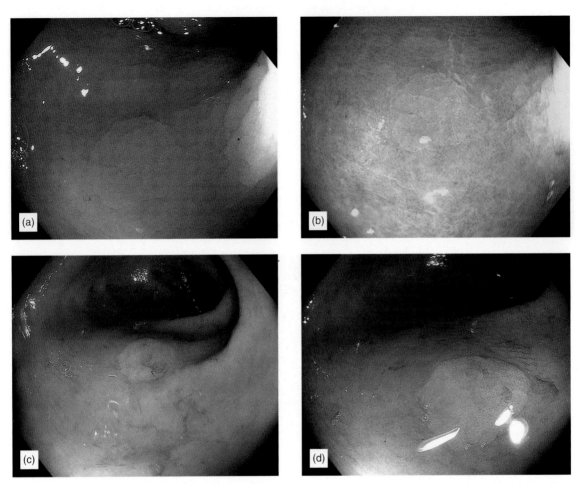

Figure 17.205 Methylene blue chromoendoscopy H190 WL (a) and NBI near focus (b) performed for surveillance in ulcerative colitis revealed this flat right-sided serrated polyp in an area of inactive colitis. (c, d) similar flat polyp revealed with chromoendoscopy WL in low magnification and near focus.

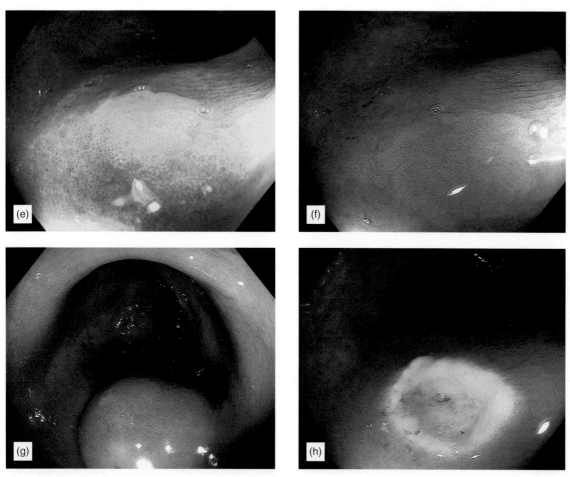

Figure 17.205 (Continued) (e–h) Second polyp detected using NBI H190 near focus and WL with chromoendoscopy, and saline assisted mucosal resection. H 190 views (Jonathan Cohen, NYU Langone School of Medicine.)

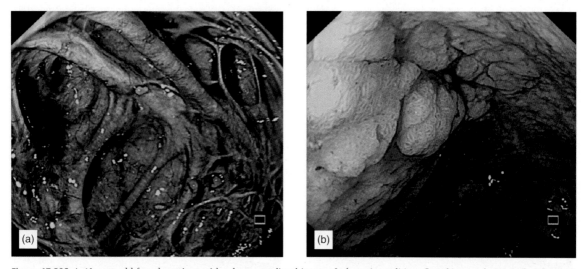

Figure 17.206 A 61-year-old female patient with a long-standing history of ulcerative colitis, a first-degree relative with colorectal cancer at a young age, and a personal history of a flat tubular low-grade dysplastic lesion 2 years prior to this examination. The previous colonoscopy did not show any dysplastic lesions, but scarring (a) and pseudopolyps (b) were seen throughout the colon performed with chromoendoscopy H190 views. (University of Amsterdam.)

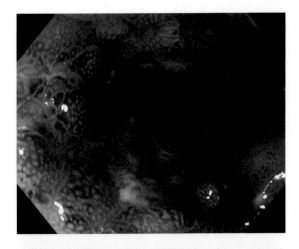

Figure 17.207 High-grade intraepithelial neoplasia (HGIN) in ulcerative colitis: 38-year-old female with 19-year history of ulcerative colitis. Depressed area with villous pattern seen in this NBI H180 view. (University Medical Center Hamburg Eppendorf.)

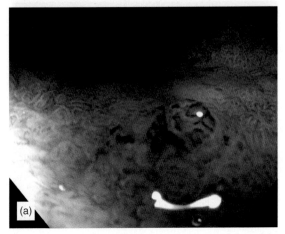

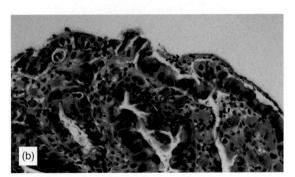

Figure 17.208 (a) HGIN and low-grade intraepithelial neoplasia (LGIN) in long-term ulcerative colitis; image taken from the nearest distance. Elevated area with gyrus-like pattern was HGIN; the surrounding villous area was LGIN NBI H180 view. (b) Gyriform area in the rectum, HGIN. Surrounding villous tissue (not shown) demonstrated LGIN from the same lesion. Neoplastic glands show highly enlarged rounded nuclei with prominent nucleoli. (University Medical Center Hamburg Eppendorf.)

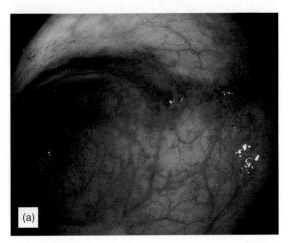

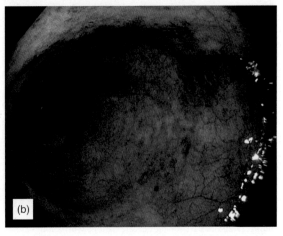

Figure 17.209 (a) WL view of mild colitis due to Crohn's disease with a patchy erythematous appearance. (b) NBI H180 light view of mild Crohn's colitis, with the patchy erythematous area seen as dark discoloration. (James DiSario, University of Utah Health Sciences Center.)

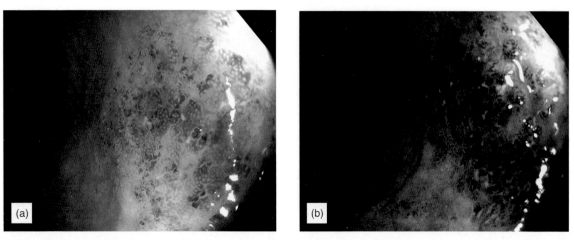

Figure 17.210 (a) WL H180 view of moderate Crohn's colitis with erythema and crypt distortion. (b) NBI light view of moderate Crohn's colitis with the inflamed areas seen in dark green. (James DiSario, University of Utah Health Sciences Center.)

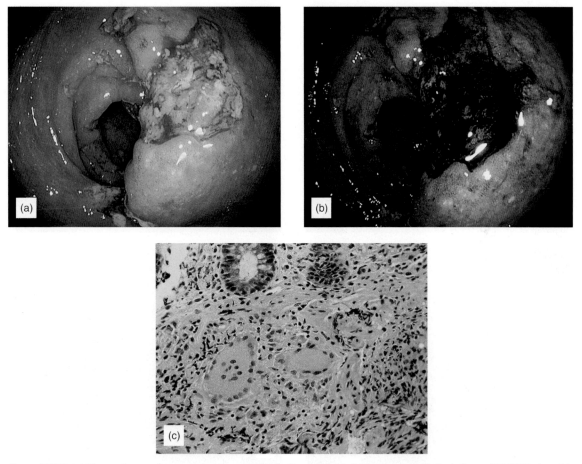

Figure 17.211 (a) Ulcerated cecum in a patient with confirmed celiac disease and ASCA-positive Crohn's disease WL H180 view. (b) NBI view of ulcerated cecum in a patient with confirmed celiac disease and ASCA-positive Crohn's disease. (c) Granulomatous colitis in Crohn's disease. A non-necrotizing granuloma containing multinucleate giant cells is present at the base of the mucosa. (Jonathan Cohen, NYU Langone School of Medicine.)

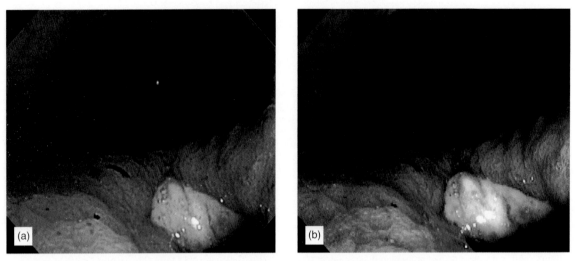

Figure 17.212 (a) Colonic ulcer in Crohn's disease WL H190 view. (b) NBI image. (Mount Sinai School of Medicine.)

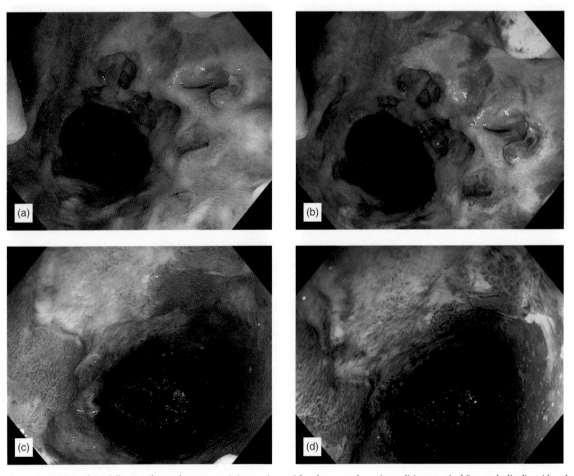

Figure 17.213 Pouchitis following ileoanal anastomosis in a patient with refractory ulcerative colitis on topical 5-acetylsalicylic acid and biological therapy with severe scarring of the distal anal mucosa (a, b) and multiple ulcerations in the more proximal end of the pouch (c–f) with relatively normal distal pouch mucosa H190 views (g.) (Jonathan Cohen, NYU Langone School of Medicine.)

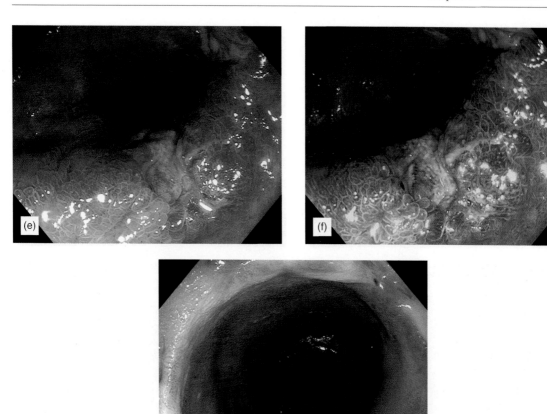

Figure 17.213 (Continued)

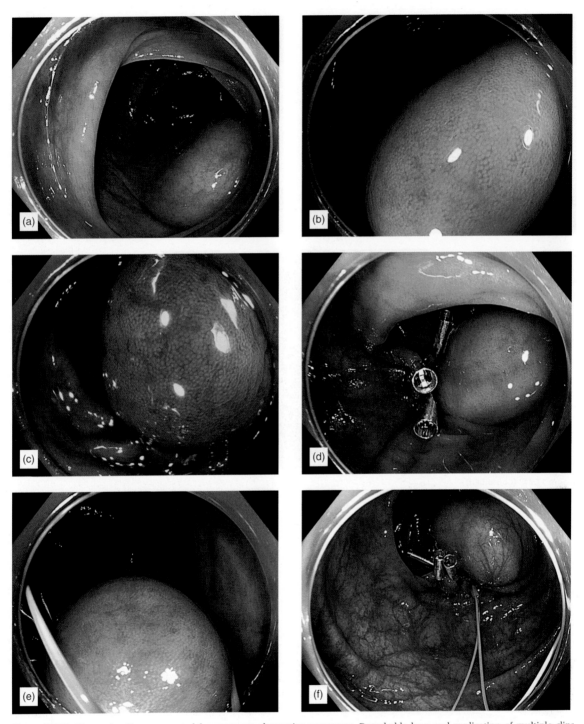

Figure 17.214 Giant colon lipoma resected for recurrent obstructive symptoms. Detachable loop and application of multiple clips across base used to prevent bleeding. (a, b, c) WL and NBI H190 views of lipoma with clear delineation of normal mucosal surface. (d) Clips applied across base. (e) Detachable loop applied over top of lesion. (f, g) Close-up of secure loop and clips at base.

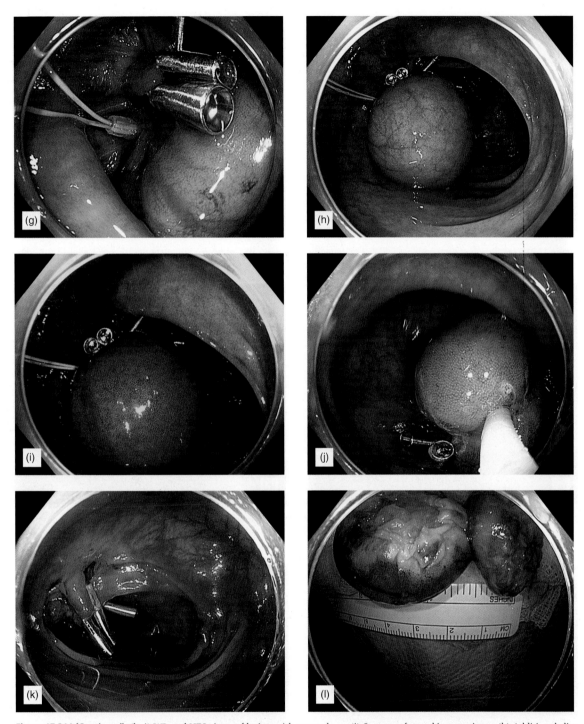

Figure 17.214 (Continued) (h, i) WL and NBI views of lesion with secure base. (j) Snare performed in two pieces. (k) Additional clips placed perpendicular to the base to prevent delayed bleeding. (l) Specimen post resection. (Jonathan Cohen, NYU Langone School of Medicine.)

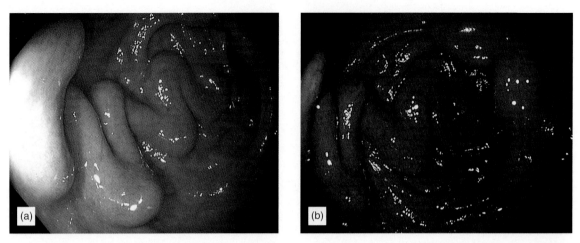

Figure 17.215 (a) Tortuous rectal varix under WL low-magnification H180 HRE view. (b) Low-magnification NBI view of tortuous rectal varix. (Jonathan Cohen, NYU Langone School of Medicine.)

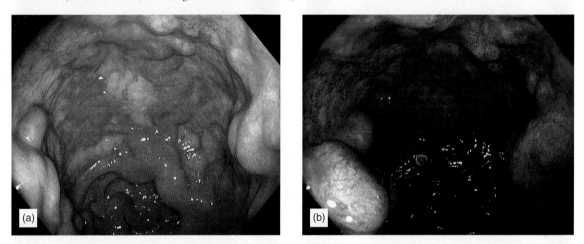

Figure 17.216 Multiple nonbleeding rectal varices seen on (a) WL low-magnification H180 HRE. (b) NBI low-magnification view. (Jonathan Cohen, NYU Langone School of Medicine.)

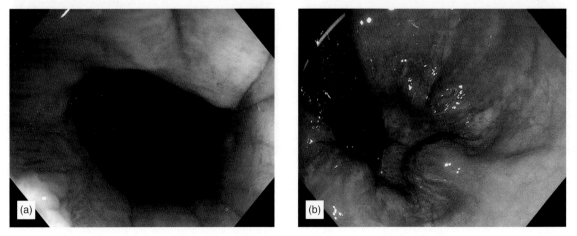

Figure 17.217 (a, b) H190 WL retroflexion views of internal hemorrhoids not seen on anterograde view. (Jonathan Cohen, NYU Langone School of Medicine.)

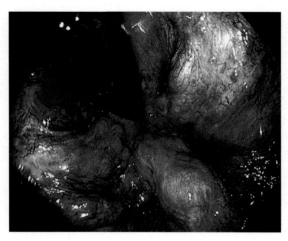

Figure 17.218 NBI H180 image of internal hemorrhoids as seen in retroflexion. (Jonathan Cohen, NYU Langone School of Medicine.)

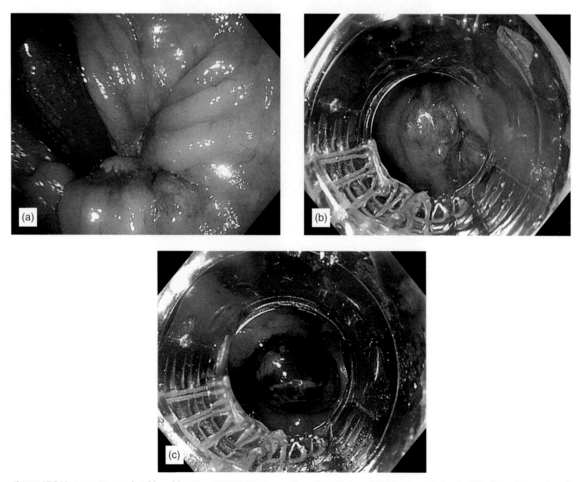

Figure 17.219 (a–e) Hemorrhoid band ligation, WL H190 views. (Jonathan Cohen, NYU Langone School of Medicine.) (continued)

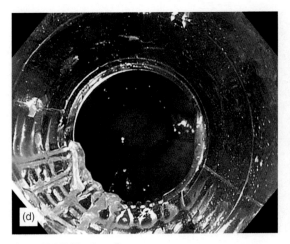

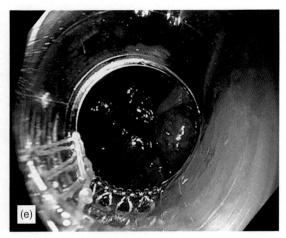

Figure 17.219 (Continued)

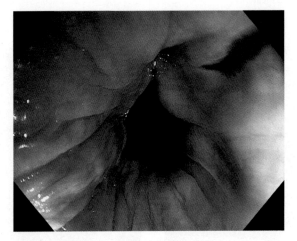

Figure 17.220 HRE WL H190 view of anal fissure. (Jonathan Cohen, NYU Langone School of Medicine.)

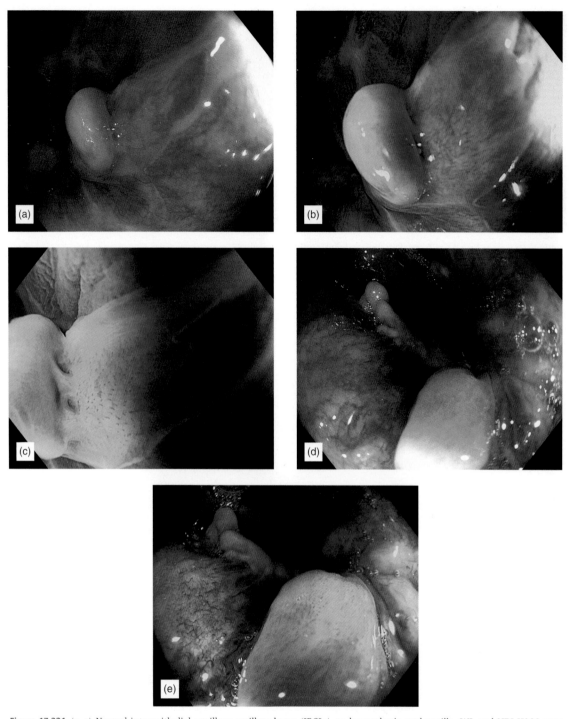

Figure 17.221 (a–e) Normal intraepithelial papillary capillary loops (IPCLs) on hyperplastic anal papilla, WL and NBI H190 near-focus views. (Jonathan Cohen, NYU Langone School of Medicine.)

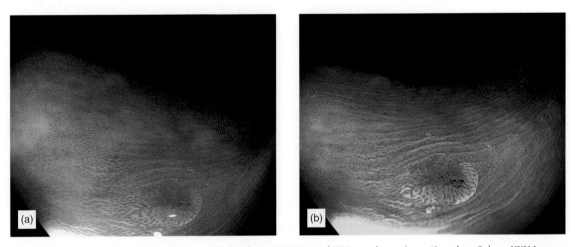

Figure 17.222 (a, b) Rectal papilloma with central dimple in WL H190 and NBI near focus views. (Jonathan Cohen, NYU Langone School of Medicine.)

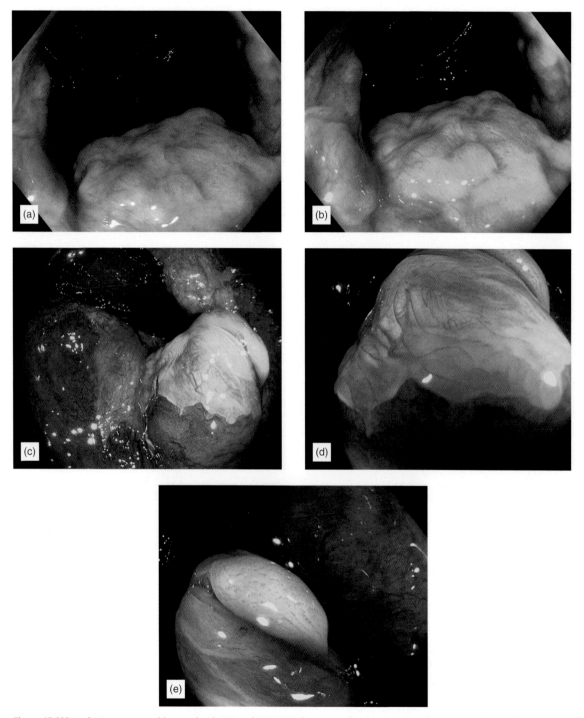

Figure 17.223 (a, b) Large external hemorrhoid, WL and NBI H190 low-magnification anterograde views. (c, d) Retroflexion examination of the squamous vessels enhanced with NBI in normal and near focus. (e) Normal type 1 squamous IPCLs on near-focus NBI view. (Jonathan Cohen, NYU Langone School of Medicine.)

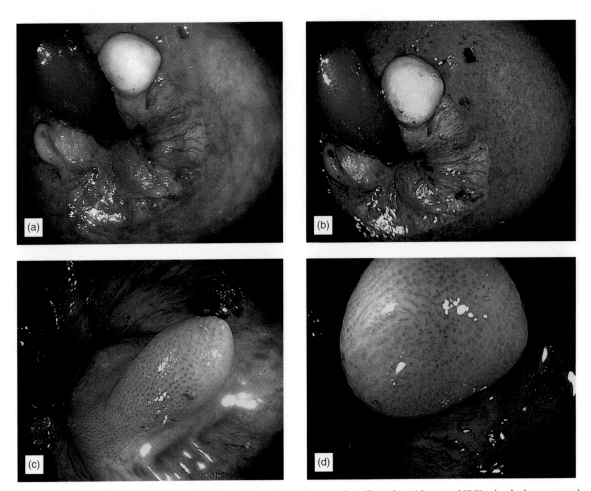

Figure 17.224 Retroflexion WL H190 and NBI views of large hyperplastic anal papilla (a, b), with normal IPCLs clearly demonstrated on near-focus NBI views (c, d). (Jonathan Cohen, NYU Langone School of Medicine.)

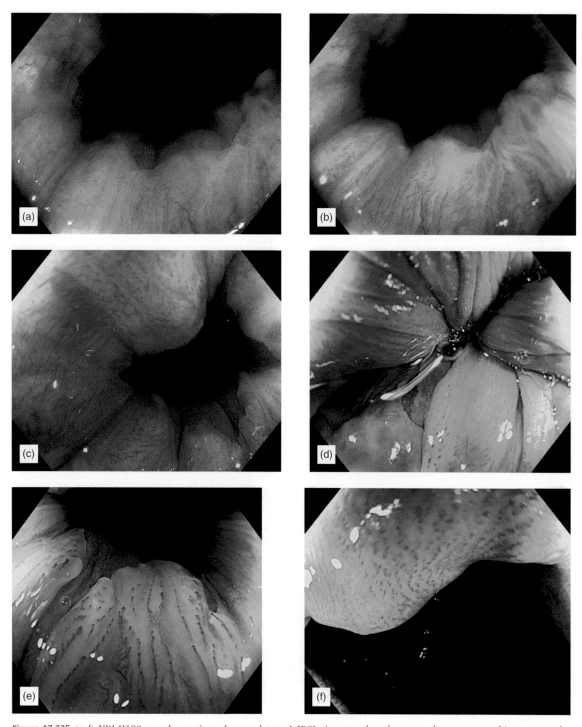

Figure 17.225 (a–f) NBI H190 near-focus view of normal type 1 IPCLs in normal anal mucosa that appear as thin punctate dots perpendicular to the plane of the mucosa and in a regular array. (Jonathan Cohen, NYU Langone School of Medicine.)

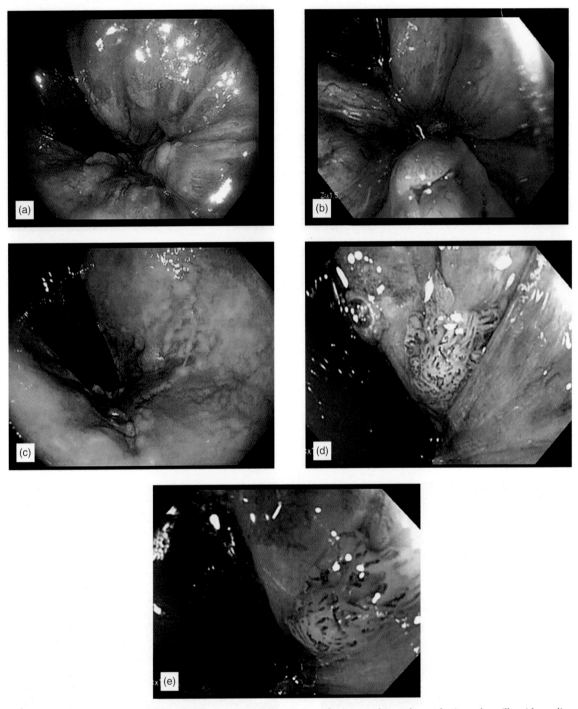

Figure 17.226 (a, b) H180 WL and NBI retroflexion views on screening colonoscopy show a hyperplastic anal papilla with no discernable IPCLs. (c, d) Screening colonoscopy on 52-year-old woman with no risk factors for anal cancer with similar raised area on retroflex view of the dentate line on WL but NBI (d) reveals thick irregular IPCLs confirmed on 1.5′ digital zoom view (e). Pathology of snare resection showed anal intraepithelial neoplasia (AIN) 3, high-grade dysplasia. (Jonathan Cohen, NYU Langone School of Medicine.)

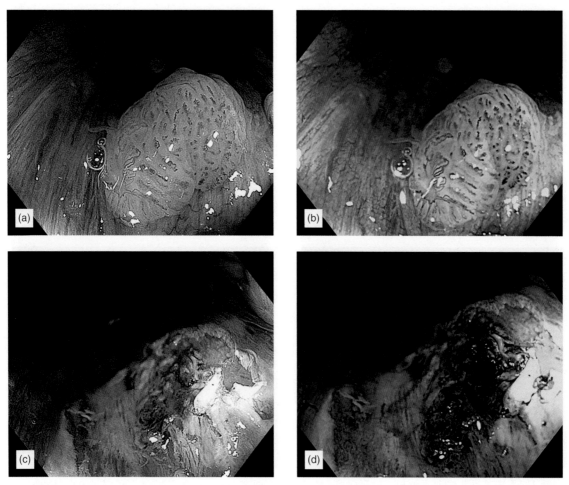

Figure 17.227 Focal raised nodular anal lesion with abnormal IPCL's seen well on both WL and NBI H190 near focus views (a, b). (c, d) shows the cauterized base following snare resection of the lesion in WL and NBI. (Jonathan Cohen, NYU Langone School of Medicine.)

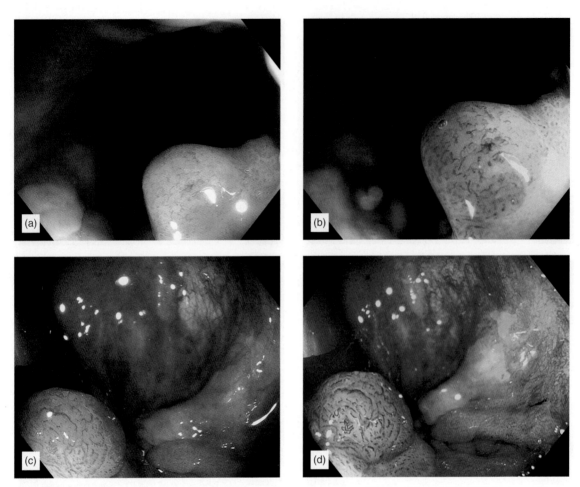

Figure 17.228 Anal high-grade dysplasia identified due to abnormal squamous IPCLs on WL and NBI H190 low magnification anterograde views (a, b) and retrograde views low and high magnification (c–f).

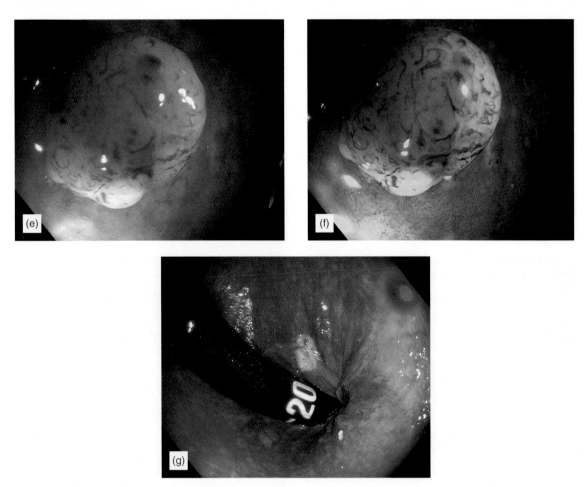

Figure 17.228 (Continued) (e–g) WL and NBI H190 near focus views of the dysplastic anal lesion and retroflexion view in WL post snare resection. (Jonathan Cohen, NYU Langone School of Medicine.)

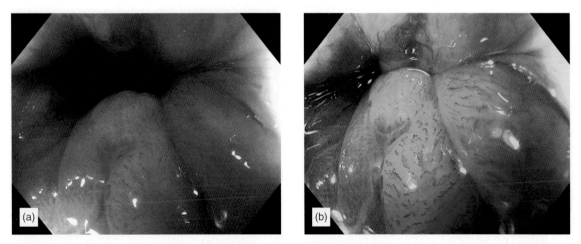

Figure 17.229 (a, b) Flat anal high-grade dysplasia AIN 3 characterized by atypical IPCLs best seen on NBI H190 near focus view. (Jonathan Cohen, NYU Langone School of Medicine.)

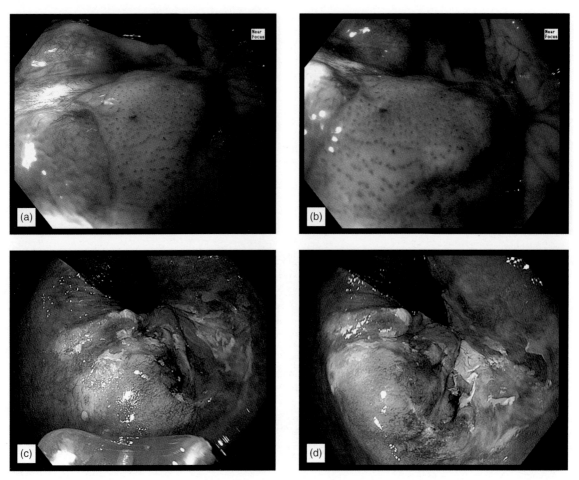

Figure 17.230 A patient with recurrent anal high grade dysplasia seen on NBI H190 near focus as flat localized irregular IPCLs (a, b) underwent RFA with Halo 90 (c, d). (Jonathan Cohen, NYU Langone School of Medicine.)

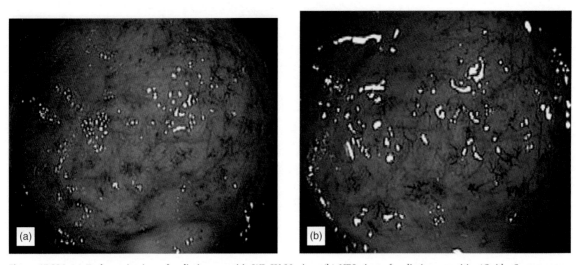

Figure 17.231 (a) Endoscopic view of radiation proctitis WL H180 view. (b) NBI view of radiation proctitis. (Guido Costamagna, Catholic University of the Sacred Heart.)

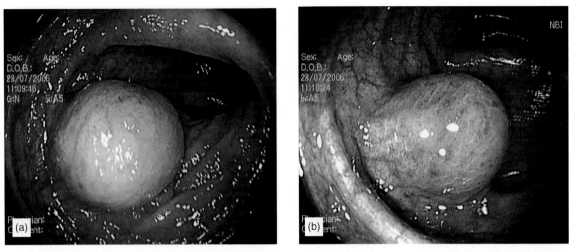

Figure 17.232 (a) WL HRE H180 view of colon lipoma. (b) NBI image of colon lipoma. (Guilherme Macedo, Hospital Sao Marcos.)

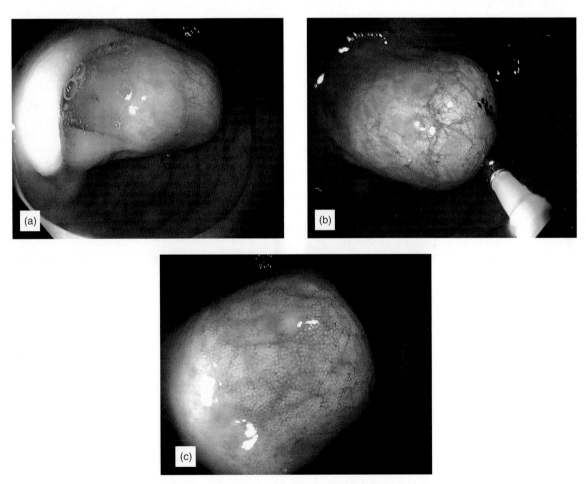

Figure 17.233 (a) This large smooth apparent submucosal nodule is seen next to the appendiceal orifice in WL H180 HRE. (b) NBI view of this lesion which was felt to be firm and without pillowing upon probing with closed biopsy forceps. (c) Magnification 1.5´ NBI view of this suspected submucosal nodule confirms normal colon mucosal pit pattern. (Jonathan Cohen, NYU Langone School of Medicine.)

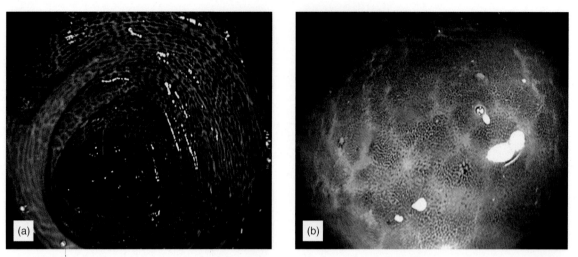

Figure 17.234 (a) NBI non-magnified view of melanosis coli WL H180 view. (b) Melanosis coli, magnified NBI view. (Guilherme Macedo, Hospital Sao Marcos.)

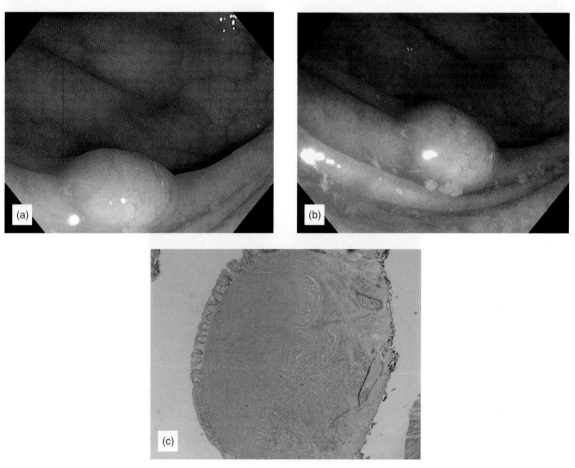

Figure 17.235 (a) WL H180 view of a 3-mm submucosal mass in sigmoid. (b) A 3-mm submucosal carcinoid in sigmoid. NBI confirms normal overyling mucosa. (c) Pathology shows low-grade carcinoid. (Mount Sinai School of Medicine.)

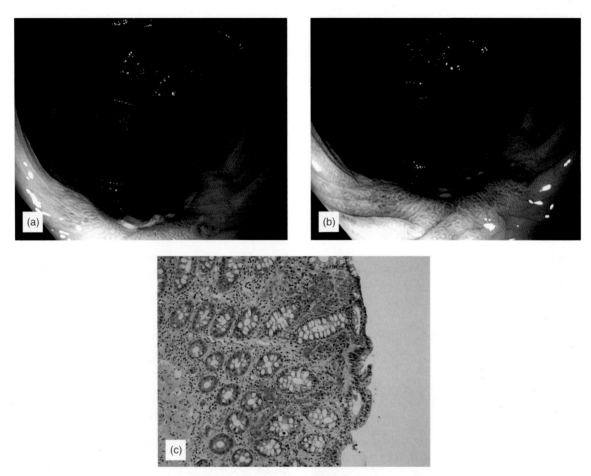

Figure 17.236 (a) Ischemic ulcer of the cecum, WL H190 HRE view. Note the linear ulcer with a white base. (b) Viewed with NBI light. (c) Colonic mucosa with eosinophilia of the lamina propria, mild crypt atrophy, and focal mucosal hemorrhage, 20′ magnification. (James DiSario, University of Utah Health Sciences Center.)

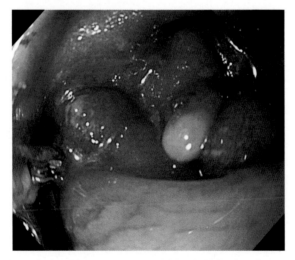

Figure 17.237 Patient with multiple medical problems presenting with left-sided left colon obstruction referred for temporary enteral stent decompression and found to have narrowed inflamed sigmoid with multiple large inflammatory polyps and diverticulosis, without mass or ulceration WL H180 view. (Jonathan Cohen, NYU Langone School of Medicine.)

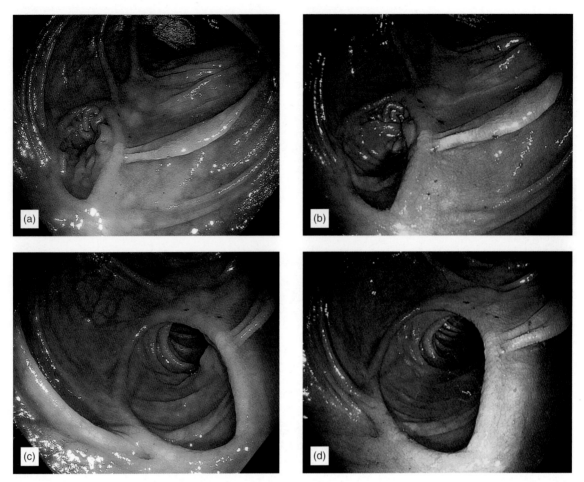

Figure 17.238 (a–d) Normal ileocolonic anastomosis, WL and NBI H190 views. (Jonathan Cohen, NYU Langone School of Medicine.)

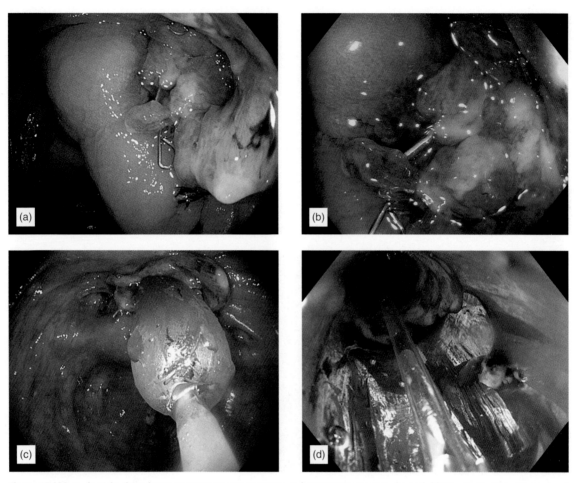

Figure 17.239 (a–d) Tight ileocolonic anastomotic stricture WL and NBI H190 views (a, b) and dilation in Crohn's disease (c, d). (Jonathan Cohen, NYU Langone School of Medicine.)

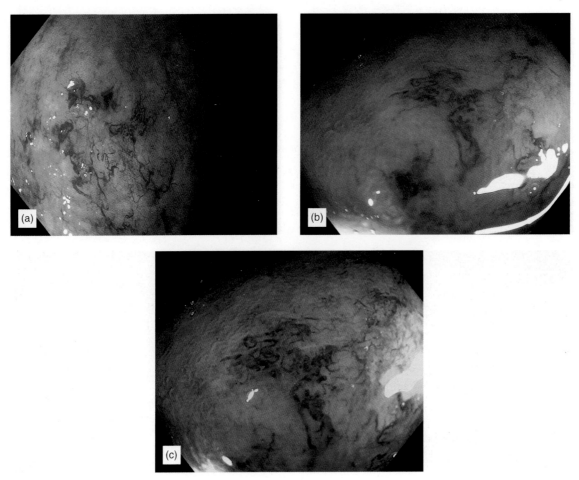

Figure 17.240 (a–c) Isolated, large, nonbleeding, rectal post-radiation telangiectasias on H190 WL and NBI near focus views. (Jonathan Cohen, NYU Langone School of Medicine.)

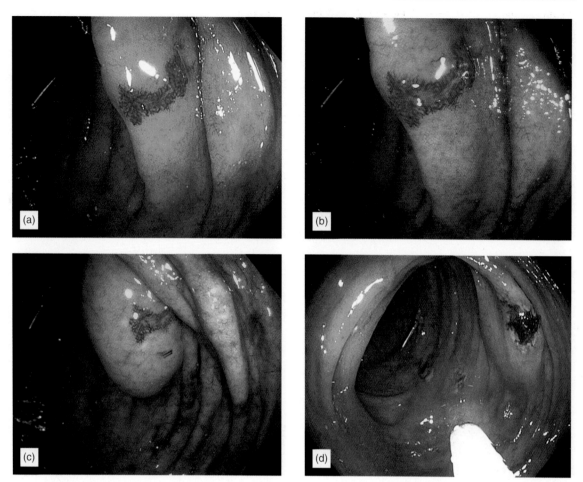

Figure 17.241 (a–d) Isolated large right colon angioectasia, WL and NBI H190 views, showing submucosal lift and treated lesion. (Jonathan Cohen, NYU Langone School of Medicine.)

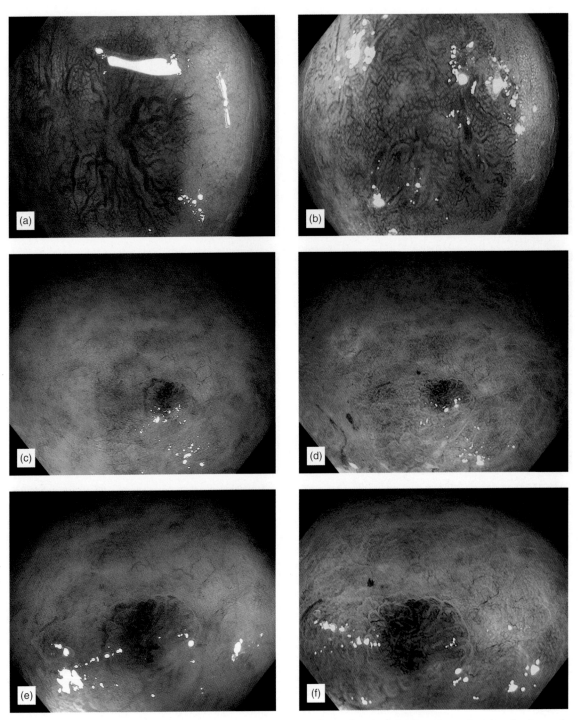

Figure 17.242 (a, b) Giant right colon AVM in WL and NBI H190 near focus view. (c–f) Small angioectasia right colon in regular magnification and near focus WL and NBI. (Jonathan Cohen, NYU Langone School of Medicine.)

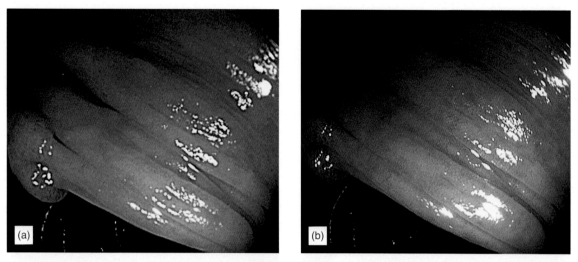

Figure 17.243 Prior India ink tatoo (a) with polyp partially hidden behind a fold WL H190 view. (b) Less visible on NBI non-magnified view. Polyp partially behind fold. (Mount Sinai School of Medicine.)

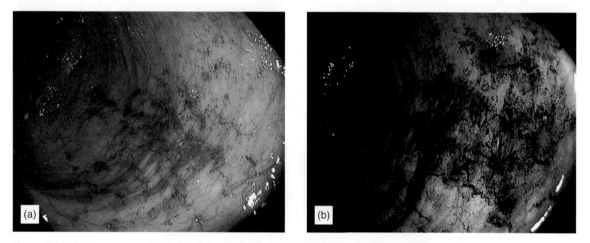

Figure 17.244 (a) Numerous angioectasias of proximal colon with mild oozing, WL H180 view. (b) NBI low-magnification view of proximal colon angioectasias (Jonathan Cohen, NYU Langone School of Medicine.)

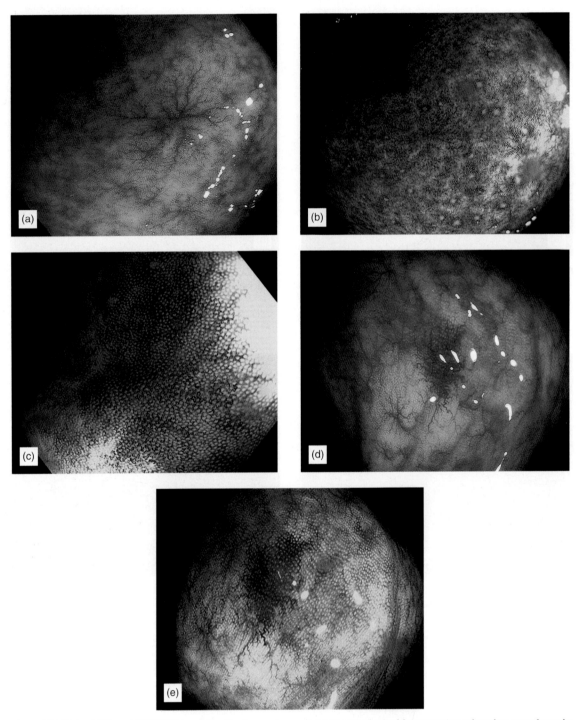

Figure 17.245 (a–e) WL and NBI H190 low magnification and near focus images of portal hypertensive colopathy; apart from the increased vascular pattern with focal appearance similar to angioectasias, the NBI views show numerous flat round pale spots corresponding to normal lymphoid follicles. (Jonathan Cohen, NYU Langone School of Medicine.)

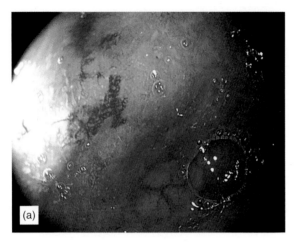 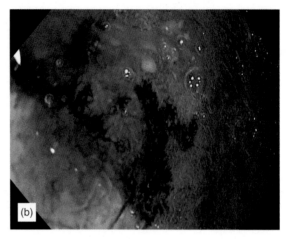

Figure 17.246 (a) Non-magnified WL H180 HRE view of a cecal angioectasia. (b) Magnified 1.5´ NBI image of cecal angioectasia. (Jonathan Cohen, NYU Langone School of Medicine.)

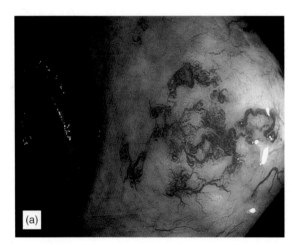 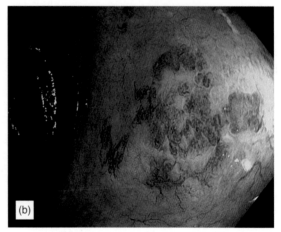

Figure 17.247 Similar large cecal angioectasia in (a) WL HRE and (b) NBI with H190 colonoscope. (Jonathan Cohen, NYU Langone School of Medicine.)

ABBREVIATIONS

AIN	anal intraepithelial neoplasia		IPCL	intraepithelial papillary capillary loop
APC	adenomatous polyposis coli		LGIN	low-grade intraepithelial neoplasia
ASCA	anti-*Saccharomyces cerevisiae* antibodies		LST	lateral spreading tumor
BLI	blue laser imaging		NBI	narrowband imaging
EMR	endoscopic mucosal resection		PPIU	post-polypectomy induced ulcer
ESD	endoscopic submucosal dissection		SSA	sessile serrated adenoma
FAP	familial adenomatous polyposis		WL	white light
HGIN	high-grade intraepithelial neoplasia			
HNPCC	hereditary nonpolyposis colorectal cancer			
HRE	high-resolution endoscopy			

Video clips to accompany this book can be found in the online material at www.wiley.com/go/cohen/NBI

Index

Page numbers in *italics* refer to illustrations; those in **bold** refer to tables

Comprehensive Atlas of High-Resolution Endoscopy and Narrowband Imaging, Second Edition. Edited by Jonathan Cohen.
© 2017 John Wiley & Sons, Ltd. Published 2017 by John Wiley & Sons, Ltd.
Companion website: www.wiley.com/go/cohen/NBI